Other books by
Glade B. Curtis, MD, MPH, OB/GYN,
and Judith Schuler, MS

· · · · · · · · · · · · ·

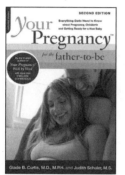

*Your Pregnancy for the
Father-To-Be*
978-0-7382-1275-3

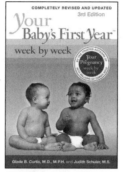

*Your Baby's First Year,
Week by Week*
978-0-7382-1372-9

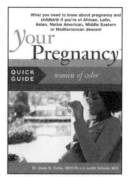

*Your Pregnancy Quick
Guide: Women of Color*
978-0-7382-1060-5

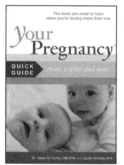

*Your Pregnancy Quick
Guide: Twins, Triplets,
and More*
978-0-7382-1008-7

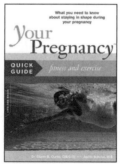

*Your Pregnancy Quick
Guide: Fitness and Exercise*
978-0-7382-0952-4

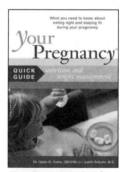

*Your Pregnancy Quick
Guide: Nutrition and
Weight Management*
978-0-7382-0954-8

What Doctors Are Saying About
Your Pregnancy Week by Week

. . . .

"*Your Pregnancy Week by Week* is the primary book I recommend to patients during pregnancy. I know I can trust it. It's organized, up to date, and provides women with terrific information."

—Elizabeth D. Warner, M.D., OB/GYN,
Rochester Gynecologic and Obstetric Associates

"*Your Pregnancy Week by Week* is an extraordinarily well-written and accessible book. Dr. Glade Curtis's years of practice make him familiar with what really concerns patients and with what they most want to know. *Your Pregnancy Week by Week* covers not only the specific issues every pregnant woman experiences, but deals with the whole wide array of potential concerns that can arise in pregnancy. All this, together with the elegant side-bars and skillful drawings, make *Your Pregnancy Week by Week* not only the most comprehensive of the pregnancy books available for the lay public but also the most readable."

—Henry M. Lerner, M.D., OB/GYN, Newton-Wellesley Hospital,
Clinical Instructor in Obstetrics and Gynecology at
Harvard Medical School

"Regular contact with an obstetrician is an important part of a healthy pregnancy. And that's why I can so strongly recommend *Your Pregnancy Week by Week* to patients who want to have a doctor's advice in addition to my own. It's written by a doctor, it's full of trustworthy and up-to-date information, and its 'bedside manner' is excellent."

—Henry Hess, M.D., Associate Clinical Professor of
Obstetrics and Gynecology, University of Rochester
School of Medicine

What Women Are Saying About
Your Pregnancy Week by Week
. . . .

"Most books only give you a month-by-month breakdown of what's going on with baby and mom. I like how this one gives you week-by-week information. I look forward to reading it each week." —Rachel M., Ohio

"*Your Pregnancy Week by Week* has been a good friend. Reading each week and knowing what changes my baby was going through was important to me."
—Anita A., California

"I have other pregnancy books, but when I started reading *Your Pregnancy Week by Week*, I put the others down. This book is excellent. I highly recommend it to all mothers-to-be." —Crystal L., Virginia

"The week-by-week style is wonderful. It lets you know what is happening as it happens."
—Heather H., Louisiana

"I liked how it went week by week because that is how my doctor thinks too."
—Rebecca C., Virginia

"The detailed week-by-week information about changes in me and my baby's changing body was excellent. It gave me something to read weekly, not just monthly."
—Deana S., Massachusetts

"*Your Pregnancy Week by Week* was my second Bible. I used it so much I have almost memorized it! I recommend it to everyone!" —Chrissy M., Illinois

"*Your Pregnancy Week by Week* was very comforting. It put my mind at ease."
—Jennifer W., Kentucky

"This book is full of helpful ideas that both new and experienced mothers-to-be can put to immediate use." —Zenaida M., Florida

"This book is the 'A, B, C book to pregnancy'." —Doris H., Indiana

"Reading this book is like talking to your mom about how it was being pregnant."
—Amanda S., Kentucky

"All the information on a weekly basis is wonderful. I highly recommend this book to every woman expecting." —Theresa C., California

"This book should be read by every mother-to-be. It gives you information week by week instead of month by month, and it helped me so much." —Kristi C., Georgia

Your Pregnancy™
Week by Week

ALSO BY

Glade B. Curtis, M.D., M.P.H., OB/GYN, and Judith Schuler, M.S.

Your Pregnancy™
Week by Week

8TH EDITION

· · · ·

Glade B. Curtis, M.D., M.P.H., OB/GYN
and Judith Schuler, M.S.

Da Capo
LIFE
LONG

A MEMBER OF THE PERSEUS BOOKS GROUP

Your Pregnancy™ is a registered trademark of Da Capo Press
Medical illustrations by Jennifer Fairman, CMI, FAMI
Exercise Illustrations by Neal Rohrer

Set in 10.5 point Minion Pro by the Perseus Books Group

Cataloging-in-Publication data for this book is available from the Library of Congress.

First Da Capo Press edition 2016
ISBN: 978-0-7382-1892-2 (hardcover)
ISBN: 978-0-7382-1893-9 (paperback)
ISBN: 978-0-7382-1894-6 (e-book)

Published by Da Capo Press
A Member of the Perseus Books Group
www.dacapopress.com

Note: The information in this book is true and complete to the best of our knowledge. This book is intended only as an informative guide for those wishing to know more about health issues. In no way is this book intended to replace, countermand or conflict with the advice given to you by your own physician. The ultimate decision concerning care should be made between you and your doctor. We strongly recommend you follow his or her advice. Information in this book is general and is offered with no guarantees on the part of the authors or Da Capo Press. The authors and publisher disclaim all liability in connection with the use of this book.

Da Capo Press books are available at special discounts for bulk purchases in the U.S. by corporations, institutions, and other organizations. For more information, please contact the Special Markets Department at the Perseus Books Group, 2300 Chestnut Street, Suite 200, Philadelphia, PA, 19103, or call (800) 810-4145, ext. 5000, or e-mail special.markets@perseusbooks.com.

10 9 8 7 6 5 4 3 2 1

About the Authors

Glade B. Curtis, M.D., M.P.H., F.A.C.O.G., is board certified by the American Board of Obstetrics and Gynecology and a Fellow of the American Congress of Obstetricians and Gynecologists. He has over 25 years of experience and has participated in more than 5000 deliveries.

Dr. Curtis is a graduate of the University of Utah with a Bachelor of Science and a Master's Degree in Public Health (M.P.H.). He attended the University of Rochester School of Medicine and Dentistry in New York. He interned and was a resident and chief resident in Obstetrics and Gynecology at the University of Rochester Strong Memorial Hospital, Rochester, New York.

Judith Schuler, M.S., has worked with Dr. Curtis for over 25 years as his co-author. They have collaborated together on 18 books dealing with pregnancy, women's health and children's health.

Ms. Schuler earned a Master of Science degree in Family Studies from the University of Arizona in Tucson. Before becoming an editor for HPBooks, where she and Dr. Curtis first began working together, Ms. Schuler taught at the university level in California and Arizona.

Their Goal as Authors

One of Dr. Curtis's goals as a doctor has been to provide patients with information about gynecological and obstetrical conditions they may have, problems they may encounter and procedures they may undergo. In pursuit of that goal, he and Ms. Schuler have co-authored several additional books for pregnant women and their partners, including *Your Pregnancy for the Father-to-Be*; *Your Pregnancy Questions & Answers*; *Your Pregnancy after 35*; *Your Pregnancy—Every Woman's Guide*; *Your Pregnancy Journal*; *Bouncing Back after Your Pregnancy*; *Your Baby's First Year Week by Week* and the *Your Pregnancy Quick Guide*, including *Understanding and Enhancing Your Baby's Development*; *Fitness and Exercise*; *Feeding Your Baby*; *Labor and Delivery*; *Twins, Triplets and More*; *Nutrition and Weight Management*; *Postpartum Wellness*; *Tests and Procedures*, and *Women of Color*.

Acknowledgments

Glade B. Curtis. In this, the 8th edition of *Your Pregnancy Week by Week*, I continue to draw upon the many questions from discussions with my patients and their partners as well as my professional colleagues. I have gained new insights and a greater understanding of the joy and anticipation of impending parenthood. I have rejoiced in my patients' happiness and thank all of them for allowing me to be part of this miraculous process.

Credit must also be given to my understanding and generous wife, Debbie, and our family, who support me in a profession that requires much of them. Beyond that commitment, they have supported and encouraged me to pursue the challenge of this project. Thanks to David Stevens, D.D.S., for his dental expertise. And my parents have always offered their unconditional love and support.

Judith Schuler. I wish to thank my friends, family members and people I have met all over the world who have shared with me their questions and concerns about their journey through pregnancy. They have helped me immensely in our efforts to provide for all our readers the pregnancy information they seek.

To my son, Ian, thank you for your interest, friendship and love. And thanks to Bob Rucinski for helping me in so many ways—for your professionalism, your expertise and your encouragement.

Contents

Preparing for Pregnancy

Nothing compares with the miracle of pregnancy. Physically and mentally preparing for this experience can improve your chances of having a healthy pregnancy and giving birth to a healthy baby.

Your lifestyle affects you and your baby, so choose to live healthfully. The first 3 to 8 weeks of pregnancy are the most critical; you may not even know you're pregnant during this important time. By the time you realize it, you may be 4 to 8 weeks pregnant. Many important things can happen in the first few weeks of pregnancy.

Pregnancy is a condition, not an illness; you're not sick. However, you will experience major changes. Being in good health before pregnancy can help you deal with physical and emotional changes during pregnancy, and labor and delivery.

Your General Health

In the past, the emphasis was to be healthy *during* pregnancy. Today, most experts suggest looking at pregnancy as lasting 12 months or more, instead of just 9 months; this includes a 3-month preparation period.

Some medical experts suggest all women of childbearing age should live their lives as if they were trying to get pregnant. Why? Because 50% of all pregnancies are unplanned. That means half of all mothers-to-be may not have been taking the best care of themselves, which could impact baby. Live every day as if this is the day you get pregnant, and you'll help make certain any child you give birth to has a good start in life.

Prepare for Pregnancy

There are a lot of things you can do to get ready for pregnancy, such as reaching your ideal weight before you get pregnant. Overweight women often have more pregnancy complications. Underweight women may have a harder time getting pregnant.

Eat lots of fruits and vegetables, and choose foods low in saturated fat. Begin exercising regularly, and stick with it. Exercise 30 minutes a day, at least 5 days a week. Exercising before and during

1

Tip for Prepregnancy

. . . .

Even though you aren't pregnant, treat your body as if you were. When you do get pregnant, you'll be on the right track for eating, exercising and avoiding harmful substances.

pregnancy can help you feel good for the entire 9 months.

See your healthcare provider to talk about any medicine you take regularly. If you have medical problems, get them under control. Schedule medical tests before you stop contraception. Be sure you're up to date on vaccinations. Have your immunity to rubella and chicken pox checked. If you need vaccinations, find out how long you have to wait after you have them before you try to get pregnant.

Find out your HIV status. Know your blood type and the blood type of your baby's father. Together with your partner, write down your family medical histories.

Ask your healthcare provider to check your iron level, and get a thyroid test. Check your cholesterol level; high cholesterol may contribute to high blood pressure during pregnancy.

Take time off the pill—at least 3 months. Keep a record of your fertility cycle by using charts. Or check your fertility cycle with ovulation-predictor devices. See the discussion in Appendix A.

Stop taking your daily multivitamin, and start taking prenatal vitamins. More is not better in pregnancy. Take folic acid—400mcg/day is recommended—to help prevent some types of birth defects. Taking folic acid before pregnancy gives you protection during the first 28 days of pregnancy, which is very important.

Stop taking aspirin and ibuprofen. Instead, use acetaminophen (Tylenol)—this may help reduce chances of miscarriage—but use sparingly. Be careful about taking some herbs, such as St. John's wort, saw palmetto and echinacea; they may interfere with conception.

Have a dental checkup, and have any treatments you need. Get gum disease under control; if you have it during pregnancy, it may increase your risk of problems.

Stop smoking. Avoid second-hand and third-hand smoke. Stop drinking alcohol. Stay away from hazardous chemicals at work and at home. Reduce stress in your life.

Some of the above actions may be hard to begin during pregnancy. If you know you're healthy, you won't have to worry about the risks they may pose while you're pregnant.

. . . .

The father-to-be can have an impact on his partner's ability to get pregnant and to have a healthy pregnancy. To learn more, read the information in the fertility discussion, Appendix A.

. . . .

See Your Healthcare Provider before Pregnancy

See your healthcare provider before you get pregnant. Have a checkup and discuss pregnancy plans. You'll know when you do get pregnant, you're in good health.

Your general medical history will be covered. You may be asked many things about your health and lifestyle. Your answers provide clues as to what needs to be done once you do get pregnant to keep you healthy.

Your healthcare provider will ask you about your gynecologic history. Answer all questions as clearly and honestly as you can to help him or her understand how pregnancy may affect you. Areas often covered include date of your last menstrual period, how long your cycle lasts, the age at which menstruation began, questions about Pap smears and any STDs you may have had. A pregnancy history will also be taken.

If you've had any surgeries in the past, you'll be asked about it. Previous Cesarean delivery or other surgeries may affect your pregnancy, so be sure to share this information.

Your healthcare provider will also want to know about your family's medical history, especially on your side of the family. Talk to your mother, aunts and sisters about pregnancy complications they may have had. It's good to know if anyone in the family had twins, triplets or more. If birth defects occurred, get as much information as possible about them. If there's a history of inherited problems in your family or your partner's family, tell your healthcare provider.

Be prepared to talk about any medicine you take and any tests you may be having. Cover all medical problems you're being treated for. Include all over-the-counter medicines, herbs, supplements and vitamins you may use. It's easier to answer questions about these things before you get pregnant rather than after you are pregnant.

Don't be surprised if you're asked about your lifestyle and any substances you take or use. These include cigarettes, alcohol, illicit drugs, legal drugs you may be using, your exercise program, your job and chemical substances you may be exposed to at work or at home. Domestic violence may also be addressed because it can often appear for the first time or it can escalate during pregnancy.

Be honest in your answers; your healthcare provider is trying to evaluate your situation. Concealing facts because you're embarrassed or scared doesn't help you or the baby you hope to conceive.

. . . .

If you're stressed out, it may be harder to get pregnant. Studies show chances of getting pregnant improve when stress is lowered, so try to reduce the amount of stress in your life.

. . . .

If You Have Problems

The odds of getting pregnant in any menstrual cycle are about 20 to 25%; nearly 60% of all couples conceive within 6 months. If you have trouble getting pregnant, talk to your healthcare provider. If you're over 35, your healthcare provider may be able to advise you about lifestyle changes and other factors that could increase pregnancy chances.

If your menstrual cycle is longer than 36 days or shorter than 23 days, ovulation may be an issue. Your healthcare provider can advise you of various ways to determine whether you are ovulating and when you ovulate. Also see the discussion in Appendix A.

. . . .

You will find many boxes in each weekly discussion that will provide you with information you will not find in the text. Our boxes do not repeat information contained in a discussion. Each box is unique, so read them for specific information.

. . . .

Tests for You

Have a physical exam before you get pregnant. A Pap smear and a breast exam should be included in this physical. Lab tests may include tests for rubella, blood type and Rh-factor. If you're 40 or older, a mammogram is also a good idea.

If you think you may have been exposed to HIV or hepatitis, ask about testing. If you have a family history of other medical problems, such as diabetes, ask about tests to rule them out. If you have a chronic medical problem, such as anemia, your healthcare provider may suggest other tests.

Ask for a pregnancy test before having an X-ray, CT scan or MRI; this includes dental X-rays. Use reliable contraception before these tests to make sure you're not pregnant. Schedule a test right after the end of your period. If you need a series of tests, continue birth control.

Possible Prepregnancy Tests

Your healthcare provider may do a lot of tests at a prepregnancy visit to identify any problems that could affect your pregnancy so you can deal with them now instead of later. You may have had some of these tests in the past, and they may not need to be repeated. Tests may include a physical exam, pelvic exam and a Pap smear, breast exam (mammogram if you are at least 40), rubella (German measles) and varicella (chicken pox) tests, blood type and Rh-factor. Other tests may be done if you have risk factors, including HIV/AIDS, a hepatitis screen, vaccination and immunization screens, and screening for sexually transmitted diseases. Screening tests for genetic disorders based on racial and ethnic background and/or family history may also be done.

Tests for Women of Color and Jewish Women

If you are a woman of color (Black/African American, Latina/Hispanic, Native American/Alaska Native, Asian/Pacific Islander or Mediterranean) or are of Jewish descent, you may be advised to have some tests to help determine whether you could pass a particular disease or condition to your baby. For example, if you are of Mediterranean descent, you may be told a screening test for beta-thalassemia is a good idea. Asian/Pacific Islanders might be screened for alpha-thalassemia. If you're Black/African American, your healthcare provider may suggest screening for sickle-cell disease.

Although a woman of Jewish descent may not be a woman of color, there are diseases that might affect her. The American Congress of Obstetricians and

Gynecologists recommends Tay-Sachs-carrier screening be offered before pregnancy to women who are at high risk. This includes those of Ashkenazi Jewish, French-Canadian or Cajun descent, and those with a family history of Tay-Sachs disease.

If you have any questions about these conditions, discuss them with your healthcare provider. He or she can give you information and guidance.

Discontinuing Contraception

It's important to continue some form of contraception until you're ready to get pregnant. If you're in the middle of treatment for a medical problem or if you're having tests, finish the treatment or tests before trying to conceive. (If you're not using some form of birth control, you're basically trying to get pregnant.)

After stopping your regular contraceptive, use some other birth-control method until your periods become normal. You can choose from condoms, spermicides, the sponge or a diaphragm.

If you use birth-control pills, patches or rings, most healthcare providers recommend you have two or three normal periods after you stop using them before trying to get pregnant. If you get pregnant immediately, it may be hard to determine when you conceived. This can make it harder to figure out your due date. It may not seem important now, but it'll be very important during pregnancy and before you deliver.

If you have an IUD (intrauterine device), have it taken out before you try to conceive. The best time to remove an IUD is during a menstrual period.

If you use an implantable contraception device, have at least two or three normal menstrual cycles after it's removed before trying to get pregnant. It may take a few months for your periods to return to normal. If you get pregnant immediately, it may be difficult to determine when you got pregnant and what your due date is.

Depo-Provera should be discontinued for at least 3 to 6 months before trying to conceive. Wait until you have had at least two or three normal periods.

- -

You may have heard a couple shouldn't have sex too often when they're trying to conceive. One study found having sex several times in one week may actually increase a man's sperm production by as much as 30%.

- -

Your Health before Pregnancy

Discuss any chronic medical problems you have with your healthcare provider. You may need extra care before and during pregnancy. Some common chronic medical problems are discussed below.

If you have *anemia*, you don't have enough hemoglobin in your blood to carry oxygen to your body's cells. Symptoms include weakness, fatigue, shortness of breath and pale skin. It's possible to develop anemia during pregnancy because the baby makes great demands on your body for iron. If you have low iron levels, pregnancy can tip the balance and make you anemic.

If you have a family history of anemia (such as sickle-cell disease or thalassemia), discuss it with your healthcare provider before you get pregnant. If you take hydroxyurea, discuss whether you should continue using it.

Most *asthma* medications are safe to take during pregnancy, but talk to your healthcare provider about your medication. Try to get asthma under good control before trying to get pregnant.

Bladder infections, such as urinary-tract infections (UTIs), may occur more often during pregnancy. If a urinary-tract infection is not treated, it can cause a kidney infection. Kidney stones may also cause problems during pregnancy.

If you have an occasional bladder infection, don't be alarmed. Your healthcare provider will decide whether further testing is necessary before you become pregnant. If you've had kidney or bladder surgery, major kidney problems or if your kidney function is less than normal, tell your healthcare provider. It may be necessary to evaluate your kidney function with tests before you become pregnant.

Celiac disease affects the small intestine and interferes with nutrient absorption; it occurs when you eat gluten. If you have celiac disease, discuss any intestinal problems you have. It's best to have the disease under control for 1 to 2 years before pregnancy to help heal your digestive tract. Good nutrient absorption helps ensure the good health of you and your baby. If you can manage your celiac disease and take in enough of the nutrients your body needs before pregnancy, you decrease your risks of problems.

It may be harder for you to become pregnant if you have *diabetes*. If your diabetes is not under control when you get pregnant, the risk increases of having a child with a birth defect. Most healthcare providers recommend having diabetes under control for at least 2 to 3 months before pregnancy begins. Get your blood sugar under control, manage blood pressure, reach a healthy weight and take care of any other problems you may have. When diabetes is not under control, you increase the chance of problems, many of which occur during the first trimester (the first 13 weeks of pregnancy).

If you're diabetic, you may have more prenatal visits and more testing during pregnancy. Your healthcare provider may have to work very closely with the healthcare provider who treats your diabetes. Pregnancy may increase your need for insulin. Being pregnant increases your body's resistance to insulin; some oral antidiabetes medications can cause problems for your baby. You may have to check your blood sugar several times a day.

Before you become pregnant, talk to your healthcare provider about therapies for treating *epilepsy*. Some anticonvulsant medicine shouldn't be used during pregnancy. If you take several medications in combination, you may be advised to take only one.

Seizures can be dangerous to a mother and baby. It's important for you to take your medication regularly and as prescribed by your healthcare provider. Do not decrease or discontinue any medication on your own!

Consult your physician about any *heart condition* before you become pregnant. Some heart problems may be serious during pregnancy and may require antibiotics at the time of delivery. Other heart problems may seriously affect your health. Your healthcare provider will advise you.

High blood pressure, or *hypertension*, can cause problems for a pregnant woman and her growing baby. If you have high blood pressure before pregnancy, you'll need to work with your healthcare provider(s) to lower your blood pressure. If necessary, start exercising now and lose any extra weight. Take blood-pressure medication as prescribed.

Some high-blood-pressure medications are safe to take during pregnancy; others are not. Do not stop or decrease any medication on your own! If you're planning pregnancy, ask your healthcare provider about your medication.

Lupus treatment may involve taking steroids. There is an increased risk of problems in women with lupus, which requires extra care during pregnancy. If you take methotrexate, discontinue it before you try to get pregnant. Don't just stop taking it. Talk to your healthcare provider so you can plan alternative treatment.

If you have *rheumatoid arthritis,* discuss the medicine you take to treat your disease. Some medication can be dangerous to a pregnant woman. If you take methotrexate, talk to your healthcare provider.

About 15 to 20% of all pregnant women suffer from *migraine headaches.* If you take medication for migraines, check with your healthcare provider now so you'll know whether the one you take is safe to use during pregnancy.

Thyroid problems can appear as either too much or too little thyroid hormone. Pregnancy can change medication requirements, so you should be tested before pregnancy to determine the correct amount of medication for you. You will also need to be checked during pregnancy.

If you've had back surgery, discuss pregnancy plans with your surgeon. If you had surgery on your lower back, you may be advised to wait 3 to 6 months before trying to become pregnant. If you had fusion surgery, the wait is often 6 months to a year. Waiting lets your back heal before taking on the stress of pregnancy. You may have fewer problems or complications. Be sure to check with your surgeon before you plan to become pregnant.

. . . .

If you have psoriasis, it's very important to discuss treatment options with your healthcare provider before you get pregnant. Some medications you may take can cause birth defects; others may be considered if your psoriasis is severe.

. . . .

Current Medications

It's important for you and your healthcare providers to consider the possibility

Be Careful with Medications

· · · · · · · · · · ·

Before pregnancy, play it safe with medicines. Keep in mind the following.
- If you use birth control, don't stop unless you want to get pregnant.
- Take prescriptions exactly as they are prescribed.
- Tell your healthcare provider if you think you might be pregnant or if you are not using birth control when a medication is prescribed.
- Don't self-treat or use medicine you were given for other problems.
- Never use someone else's medication.
- If you're unsure about taking something, call your healthcare provider before you use it!

of pregnancy each time you are given a prescription or advised to take a medicine. When you're pregnant, many things change with regard to medication usage.

Medicine that is safe when you aren't pregnant may have harmful effects during pregnancy. Most organ development in the baby occurs in the first 13 weeks of pregnancy. This is an important time to avoid exposing baby to unnecessary or harmful substances. You'll feel better and do better during pregnancy if you have medication use under control before you try to get pregnant.

Some medicine is intended for short-term use, such as antibiotics for infections. Others are for chronic or long-lasting problems, such as high blood pressure or diabetes. Some medications are safe and may help make your pregnancy successful. Other medications may not be safe to take during pregnancy.

Vaccinations

At your prepregnancy visit, check to see whether you're up to date on vaccinations.

If you need any, use reliable contraception because it's better to receive vaccinations for various diseases before you get pregnant than during pregnancy. Some vaccinations cannot be given to pregnant women; others can. A good rule of thumb is to complete vaccinations at least 3 months before trying to get pregnant.

An exception to this rule is the flu vaccine; you can get it at any time during pregnancy. However, don't get the nasal mist type of flu vaccine—it's not advised for pregnant women. If you're advised to take the flu vaccine because of your job or for some other reason, go ahead. It will help protect you and baby.

Genetic Counseling

If you're planning your first pregnancy, you're probably not considering genetic counseling. However, there may be circumstances in which genetic counseling could help you and your partner make informed decisions about having children.

Genetics is the study of how traits and characteristics are passed from parent to child through chromosomes and genes.

Genetic counseling is an information session between you and your partner and a genetic counselor or group of counselors.

The occurrence of birth defects is actually very low—they occur in less than 0.5% of all births. The primary goal in genetic counseling is prevention and/or early diagnosis of these problems. Certain groups have a higher incidence of problems, and certain medications, chemicals and pesticides can put a couple at risk.

Genetic disorders may be caused in various ways. If you have an *inherited disorder*, it comes from your parents. A *chromosomal disorder* can happen even when parents don't have any risk factors. *Multifactorial disorders* can occur from more than one source; the cause is generally unknown.

Genetic counseling aims to help you and your partner understand what might happen in your particular situation. A counselor won't make decisions for you; he or she will give you information on tests you might take and what results may mean. Don't hide information you feel is embarrassing or hard to talk about. It's important to tell a counselor what he or she needs to know.

Most couples who need genetic counseling do not find out they needed it until after they have a child born with a birth defect. You might consider genetic counseling if any of the following apply to you.

- You will be at least 35 years old at the time of delivery.
- You have delivered a child with a birth defect or have a family history of inherited deafness.
- You or your partner have a birth defect.
- You or your partner have a family history of Down syndrome, mental retardation, cystic fibrosis, spina bifida, muscular dystrophy, bleeding disorders, skeletal or bone problems, dwarfism, epilepsy, congenital heart defects or blindness.
- You and your partner are related (consanguinity).
- You have had recurrent miscarriages (usually three or more).
- You and your partner are descended from Ashkenazi Jews.
- You or your partner are Black/African American.
- Your partner is at least 40 years old.

Research indicates it may be the *father's age* more than the mother's age that is the most important factor in a baby being born with a genetic disorder. The risk of a child developing autism or schizophrenia increases significantly as the father's age increases. These errors are not believed to be inherited; rather, they occur in the sperm or at the time of fertilization. Because sperm are constantly being produced, as compared to eggs a woman is born with, it has been found sperm from older men carry more genetic errors. More research is needed to understand the risks fully.

Some information may be difficult to gather, especially if you or your partner are adopted. You may know little about your family's medical history. Discuss this with your healthcare provider before you get pregnant. If you learn about the chances of problems before pregnancy, you won't have to make difficult decisions after you get pregnant.

Genetic Testing

Your genetic counselor may discuss various tests with you. More than 1000 disorders can be detected using genetic tests, but most are rare. The conditions regularly tested for include cystic fibrosis, Down syndrome, neural-tube defects, thalassemia, Tay-Sachs and sickle-cell disease.

There are three types of tests—carrier tests, screening tests and diagnostic tests. *Carrier tests* involve testing both partners to determine if either or both is a carrier of a particular genetic defect. *Screening tests* may be done during pregnancy to determine whether there is an increased risk of a problem; it does not identify the problem. *Diagnostic tests* often determine whether a problem is present.

Pregnancy after 35

More women are choosing to marry after they have established a career, and more couples are choosing to start their families at a later age. Today, healthcare providers are seeing more older first-time mothers; many have safe, healthy pregnancies. You may also want to read our book, *Your Pregnancy after 35*, which focuses primarily on pregnancy in older women.

An older woman considering pregnancy often has two major concerns: she wants to know how the pregnancy will affect her and how her age will affect her pregnancy. A pregnant woman older than 35 may face increased risks.

You may find it easier to be pregnant when you're 20 than it is when you're 40. You may have a job or other children making demands on your time. You may find it harder to rest, exercise and eat right. But these concerns shouldn't dissuade you from having children when you're older.

We know older women are at higher risk of giving birth to a child with Down syndrome. Various tests may be offered to an older woman during pregnancy to determine whether a baby will have Down syndrome. It's the most common chromosomal defect detected by amniocentesis.

The risk of delivering a baby with Down syndrome increases as you get older. But there's a positive way to look at these statistics. If you're 45, you have a 97% chance of *not* having a baby with Down syndrome. If you're 49, you have a 92% chance of delivering a child without Down syndrome. If you're concerned about the risk of Down syndrome because of your age or family history, discuss it with your healthcare provider.

Research shows a father's age is important. Chromosomal abnormalities that cause birth defects occur more often in older women and in men over 40. Some researchers recommend men father children before age 40, but there's still some controversy about this.

If you're older, you can maximize your chances of having a successful pregnancy by being as healthy as possible before you become pregnant. Paying

Green-Tea Warning
. . . .

Don't drink green tea while you're trying to get pregnant—not even a glass or two! It may increase your chances of having a baby with a neural-tube defect. The problem is the antioxidant in green tea decreases the effectiveness of folic acid. Enough folic acid during the first few weeks of pregnancy may help lower the risk. Wait until after baby's birth to drink green tea again.

attention to general recommendations for your diet and health care is also important in preparing for pregnancy.

Your Weight before Pregnancy

Most people feel better when they eat a well-balanced diet. Planning and following a healthy eating plan before pregnancy helps provide your growing baby good nutrition during the first few weeks or months of pregnancy.

Usually a woman takes good care of herself once she knows she's pregnant. By planning ahead, you can be sure baby has a healthy environment for the entire 9 months of pregnancy, not for just the 6 or 7 months after you find out you're pregnant.

Weight Management

Some researchers believe your weight may affect your chances of getting pregnant. Being underweight or overweight can alter sex hormones, your menstrual cycle, ovulation and may even affect the lining of your uterus. Any of these can make it harder for you to get pregnant.

If you're underweight, your body may not produce enough hormones for you to ovulate every month. You may also have problems getting the best nutrition for your baby.

If you're overweight, you may have a harder time getting pregnant. Overweight is defined as having a body-mass index (BMI) between 26 and 30. Obesity is defined as having a BMI over 30. See the discussion in Week 14.

Examine your eating habits. Determine what you need to work on to make your food intake healthy for you and baby. It may be very helpful to lose weight before trying to get pregnant, which may help reduce pregnancy complications and birth defects.

Consult your healthcare provider if you're thinking about starting a special diet to lose or to gain weight before you try to get pregnant. Dieting may cause a drop in vitamins and minerals that both you and your developing baby need.

If You've Had Weight-Loss Surgery

Some women have weight-loss surgery to help them lose weight. Bariatric surgery is defined as "surgery related to the prevention and control of obesity and related diseases." Women who have had bariatric surgery have been shown to have less-complicated pregnancies

Can You Help Avoid Morning Sickness in Pregnancy?

· · · · · · · · · · ·

If you eat high amounts of saturated fat—the kind found in cheese and red meat—in the year before you get pregnant, you may have severe morning sickness during pregnancy. If you're planning to get pregnant, cut down on these foods. Taking a multivitamin regularly before you get pregnant may also lower your risk.

than obese women who don't have surgery.

With *gastric-bypass surgery*, a surgeon closes off part of the stomach, which reduces its size. Making it smaller seems to trigger hormones that control metabolism and feelings of hunger. *Gastric banding* involves placing a silicone band around the upper part of the stomach. This creates a small sac that restricts how much food you can eat. The band remains forever, unless it is removed by surgery. A plastic tube connects the band to an apparatus under the skin so the doctor can tighten or loosen the band as needed.

If you had gastric-bypass surgery to lose weight, you may be at increased risk of getting pregnant after the procedure. This happens because you lose weight, which may lead to more-regular ovulation. This could result in pregnancy.

If you plan to become pregnant soon, having gastric-banding surgery may be your best choice. Unlike gastric-bypass surgery, gastric banding is fully reversible. It's possible to have your stomach-outlet size opened so you can meet the increased nutritional needs of pregnancy.

Put off pregnancy for 12 to 18 months following surgery because this is the time you will be losing weight very rapidly. You may not have sufficient nutrients available for you and your growing baby.

Your Lifestyle

Be Careful with Vitamins, Minerals and Herbs

Don't self-medicate with large amounts or unusual combinations of vitamins, minerals or herbs. Certain vitamins, such as vitamin A, can cause birth defects if used in excessive amounts. Some experts believe some herbs can temporarily reduce fertility in men and women, so you and your partner should avoid St. John's wort, echinacea and gingko biloba.

Stop all extra supplements at least 3 months before pregnancy. Eat a well-balanced diet and take a multivitamin or prenatal vitamin. Most healthcare providers are happy to prescribe prenatal vitamins if you're planning a pregnancy.

Folic acid is a B vitamin (B_9) that can contribute to a healthy pregnancy. Taking folic acid for at least 1 year before pregnancy may help reduce your risk of certain birth defects and pregnancy problems. If you take 0.4mg (400 micrograms) of folic acid each day before pregnancy, it may help protect your baby against birth defects of the spine and

Dad Tip
. . . .

If your partner is making lifestyle changes to prepare for pregnancy, such as giving up smoking or not drinking alcohol, support her in her efforts. Quit these habits if you share them.

brain, called *neural-tube defects*. Once pregnancy is confirmed, it may be too late to prevent these problems.

In the United States, many food products are fortified with folic acid. Eat a well-balanced, varied diet to help you reach your goal. Many foods that contain folate (the natural form of folic acid found in food) include asparagus, avocados, bananas, black beans, broccoli, citrus fruits and juices, egg yolks, green beans, leafy green vegetables, lentils, liver, peas, plantains, spinach, strawberries, tuna, wheat germ, yogurt and fortified breads and cereals.

Begin Good Eating Habits

A woman often carries her prepregnancy eating habits into pregnancy. Many women eat on the run and pay little attention to what they eat most of the day. Before pregnancy, you may be able to get away with this; however, because of increased demands on you and the needs of your baby, it won't work when you do become pregnant. Eat a balanced diet. Going to extremes with vitamins or fad diets may be harmful.

If you have various problems, such as polycystic ovarian syndrome, some foods may improve your chances of conceiving. Foods to consider adding to your diet include broccoli, spinach, cabbage, nuts, fruit, kelp, nori, beans and fish.

Before getting pregnant, talk to your healthcare provider if you have special dietary needs. This includes being a vegetarian, how much exercise you do, whether you skip meals, your diet plan (are you trying to lose or gain weight?) and any special needs you might have. If you eat a special diet because of medical problems, discuss it with your healthcare provider.

While you're trying to get pregnant, don't eat more than 12 ounces of fish a week. Avoid fish not recommended during pregnancy. See the discussion in Week 26.

Exercise

Exercise is good for you. Benefits may include weight control, a feeling of well-being and increased stamina or endurance, which will become important later in pregnancy.

Begin exercising regularly before you get pregnant. Make adjustments in your life so you can include regular exercise. It will help you now and make it easier to stay in shape during pregnancy. Find exercise you like and will continue to do on a regular basis, in any kind of weather. Focus on improving strength in your lower back and abs to help during your pregnancy.

Don't exercise to an extreme; it may cause problems. Avoid intense training.

Are You in the Military?

· · · · · · · · · · ·

Are you currently serving in the U.S. Armed Forces or planning to enter one of the services soon? Studies show women who get pregnant while on active duty may face many challenges, including some risks to the baby.

The pressure to meet military body-weight standards can affect your health. You may have low iron stores and lower-than-normal folic-acid levels. Some jobs may be hazardous, such as standing for a long time, heavy lifting or exposure to certain chemicals.

If you plan to get pregnant during your service commitment, work hard to reach your ideal weight a few months before you conceive, then maintain that weight. Take in enough folic acid and iron by eating well-balanced meals. You may also want to take a prenatal vitamin. If you're concerned about hazards related to your work, discuss it with a superior. Find out whether you're pregnant before getting any vaccinations or inoculations.

It's important to take care of yourself and your baby. Also see the discussion in Week 14.

Don't increase your exercise program. Skip playing competitive sports that involve pushing yourself to the max.

If you have concerns about exercise before or during pregnancy, talk to your healthcare provider. Exercise you can do easily before pregnancy may be more difficult for you during pregnancy. The American Congress of Obstetricians and Gynecologists (ACOG) has proposed guidelines for exercise before and during pregnancy. Ask your healthcare provider for a copy.

Substance Use

We know a lot about the effects of drugs and alcohol on pregnancy. We believe the safest approach to drug or alcohol use during pregnancy is no use at all.

Tell your healthcare provider about substance abuse, and deal with problems now. Your baby goes through some of its most important developmental stages in the first 13 weeks of your pregnancy. Stop using any substance you don't need at least 3 months before trying to conceive!

There is help for those who use drugs—if you need to, seek help before you get pregnant. Preparing for pregnancy may be a good reason for you and your partner to change your lifestyle.

Smoking can damage your eggs and ovaries. If you stop smoking for at least 1 year before trying to get pregnant, you increase your chances of conceiving. You also reduce your odds of having a miscarriage.

Smoking cigarettes and exposure to cigarette smoke deplete folic acid from your body. Mothers who smoke during pregnancy may have low-birthweight babies or babies with other problems. Ask for help to stop smoking before you become pregnant.

Most experts agree there is no safe amount of alcohol to drink during pregnancy. Alcohol crosses the placenta and

Protecting Yourself from STDs
• • • • • • • • • • •

Protect yourself against STDs. Use a condom, and limit the number of sexual partners you have. Have sexual contact only with those people you're sure don't sleep around. Get tested if you have a chance of having an infection, even if you don't have symptoms, and ask for treatment if you think you need it.

affects baby. Heavy drinking during pregnancy can cause fetal alcohol syndrome (FAS) or fetal alcohol exposure (FAE); both are discussed in Weeks 1 & 2. *Stop drinking now!*

If you use cocaine during the first 12 weeks of pregnancy, you increase your risk of problems. Women who use cocaine throughout pregnancy also have a higher rate of problems. Stop using cocaine before you stop using birth control. Damage to a baby can occur as early as 3 days after conception!

Marijuana can cross the placenta, enter a baby's system and have long-lasting effects. If your partner smokes marijuana, encourage him to stop. One study showed the risk of SIDS was twice the average for children if their father smoked marijuana.

Work and Pregnancy
You may need to consider your job when you plan a pregnancy. Some jobs might be considered harmful during pregnancy. Some substances you might be exposed to at work, such as chemicals, inhalants, radiation or solvents, could pose a problem. Consider things you're exposed to at work as part of your lifestyle. Chemical exposure can impact a pregnancy. Risks are highest for women with increased on-the-job exposure.

Continue reliable contraception until you know the environment at work is safe.

Women who stand for long periods have smaller babies. A job that involves standing a great deal may not be a good choice during pregnancy. Talk to your healthcare provider about your work situation.

Check the types of benefits or insurance coverage you have and your company's maternity-leave program. Most programs allow some time off work. Prenatal care and baby's birth could cost you several thousand dollars if you don't plan ahead.

• •
If you're self-employed, you won't be qualified to receive state disability payments. You may want to think about a private disability policy to cover you for any problems before birth and for time off after baby arrives. The glitch here is that the policy must be in place before you get pregnant.
• •

Sexually Transmitted Diseases
Infections or diseases passed from one person to another by sexual contact are called *sexually transmitted diseases (STDs)*. These infections may affect your ability to get pregnant and can harm a growing baby. The type of contraception you use may have an effect on the

Should a Man Prepare for Pregnancy?

· · · · · · · · · · ·

Is a father-to-be's health important in getting pregnant? Research over the years has proved a man's health before pregnancy is just as important as a woman's! We know about 40% of all infertility problems are caused by a father-to-be. And because it takes 74 days for sperm to mature, anything a man ingests or is exposed to during that time can impact sperm, which can affect pregnancy.

A man's eating habits, exercise routine and vitamin/supplement intake is very important in preparing for pregnancy. So are lifestyle issues, such as the use of tobacco and/or marijuana products, alcohol intake and use of some over-the-counter and prescription medications.

So when should a man start preparing for pregnancy? He should start at least 3 months before conception—that's the same amount of time as a woman needs to prepare. A dad-to-be should be as healthy as possible before pregnancy, and he should continue these habits until pregnancy is achieved. By doing so, he will help give baby the best start in life.

likelihood of getting an STD. Condoms and spermicides can lower the risk. You're more likely to get a sexually transmitted disease if you have more than one sexual partner.

Some STD infections can cause pelvic inflammatory disease (PID). An infection can result in scarring and blockage of the tubes. This can make it difficult or impossible to get pregnant or make you more susceptible to an ectopic pregnancy. Surgery may be necessary to repair damaged tubes.

The Centers for Disease Control (CDC) recently released an advisory to all women of childbearing age. Experts at the CDC recommend a woman of childbearing age who is sexually active and not using birth control abstain from drinking alcohol. Because 50% of all pregnancies are unplanned, following this advisory could help protect the 2 million babies conceived every year by women who are not planning a pregnancy. If a woman who doesn't use birth control lives every day as if this is the day she could get pregnant, she could go a long way in giving her baby a healthy start in life!

Weeks 1 & 2

Pregnancy Begins

This is an exciting time for you—having a baby growing inside you is an incredible experience! Our goal is to help you understand and enjoy your pregnancy. In this book, you will learn what is going on in your body and how your baby is growing and changing.

Material in this book is divided into weeks because this is the way healthcare providers look at pregnancy. It makes sense to look at changes in you and baby the same way. This also lets you and your partner follow your changes and baby's growth more closely. Weekly illustrations help you see how you and baby change and grow. Weekly topics cover areas of special concern as well as how big your baby is, how big you are and how your actions affect your baby.

The information in this book is not meant to replace any discussion with your healthcare provider—discuss any and all concerns with him or her. Use this material as a starting place in your dialogue. It may help you put your concerns or interests into words.

the following symptoms and you believe you might be pregnant, contact your healthcare provider:

- missed menstrual period
- nausea, with or without vomiting
- food aversions or food cravings
- fatigue
- frequent urination
- breast changes and breast tenderness
- new sensitivity or feelings in your pelvic area
- metallic taste in your mouth

What will you notice first? It's different for every woman. When your period doesn't begin, you may think of pregnancy.

. . . .

Although this book is designed to take you through your pregnancy by examining one week at a time, you may seek specific information. Because the book cannot include everything you need before you know you're looking for it, check the Index for a particular topic. We may not cover the subject until a later week.

. . . .

Signs and Symptoms of Pregnancy

Many changes in your body can indicate pregnancy. If you have one or more of

When Is Your Baby Due?

The beginning of a pregnancy is actually figured from the *beginning* of your last menstrual period. For your

Tip for Weeks 1 & 2
· · · · · · · · · · ·

Over-the-counter pregnancy tests are reliable and can be positive (indicate pregnancy) as early as 10 days after conception. Even pregnancy tests from a dollar store have proved accurate.

healthcare provider's calculations, you are pregnant 2 weeks before you actually conceive! Pregnancy lasts about 280 days, or 40 weeks, from the beginning of the last menstrual period. This can be confusing, so let's look at it more closely.

Your due date is important in pregnancy because it helps determine when to perform certain tests or procedures. It also helps estimate the baby's growth and may indicate when you're overdue—this will be really important to you as delivery time approaches.

Your due date is only an estimate, not an exact date. Only 1 out of 20 women actually delivers on her due date. You may see your due date come and go and still not have your baby. Think of your due date as a goal—a time to look forward to and to prepare for.

Most women don't know the exact date of conception, but they usually know the beginning of their last period. This is the point from which a pregnancy is dated. Figuring a due date can be tricky because periods and menstrual histories can be uncertain.

Calculate your due date by counting 280 days from the first day of bleeding of your last period. Dating a pregnancy this way gives the gestational age (menstrual age), which is the way most healthcare providers keep track of time during pregnancy. It's different from ovulatory age (fertilization age), which is 2 weeks shorter and dates from the actual date of conception.

Some medical experts suggest instead of a "due date," women be given a "due week"—a 7-day window of time during which delivery may occur. This time period would fall between the 39th and 40th weeks. Because only 5% of women deliver on their actual due date, a 7-day period could help ease a mom-to-be's anxiety about when baby will be born.

You may hear references to your stage of pregnancy by *trimester.* Trimesters divide pregnancy into three periods, each about 13 weeks long, to help group together developmental stages.

You may even hear about *lunar months,* referring to a complete cycle of the moon, which is 28 days. Because pregnancy is 280 days from the beginning of your period to your due date, pregnancy lasts 10 lunar months.

Using a 40-week timetable, you actually become pregnant during the third week. Details of your pregnancy are discussed week by week beginning with Week 3. Your due date is the end of the 40th week. Each weekly discussion includes the actual age of your growing baby. For example, in Week 8, you'll see the following:

Definitions of Time
• • • • • • • • • •

Gestational age (menstrual age)—Begins the first day of your last period, which is actually about 2 weeks *before* you conceive. This is the age most healthcare providers use to discuss your pregnancy. The average length of pregnancy is 40 weeks.

Ovulatory age (fertilization age)—Begins the day you conceive. The average length of pregnancy is 38 weeks or 266 days.

Trimester—Each trimester lasts about 13 weeks. There are three trimesters in a pregnancy.

Lunar months—A pregnancy lasts an average of 10 lunar months (28 days each).

Week 8 [gestational age]
Age of Fetus—6 Weeks [fertilization age]

This tells you how old your developing baby is at any point in your pregnancy.

No matter how you count the time of your pregnancy, it's going to last as long as it's going to last. But a miracle is happening—a living human being is growing and developing inside you! Enjoy this wonderful time in your life.

Your Menstrual Cycle

Menstruation is the normal periodic discharge of blood, mucus and cellular debris from the uterus. Two important cycles occur during the menstrual cycle—the *ovarian cycle* and the *endometrial cycle*. The ovarian cycle provides an egg for fertilization, and the endometrial cycle provides a suitable site for implantation of the fertilized egg inside your uterus.

There are about 2 million eggs in a newborn girl at birth. This decreases to about 400,000 in girls just before puberty. The maximum number of eggs is actually present before birth. When a female fetus is about 5 months old (4 months before birth), she has about 6.8 million eggs!

About 25% of women have lower-abdominal pain or discomfort on or about the day of ovulation, called *mittelschmerz*. It may be caused by irritation from fluid or blood from the follicle when it ruptures. The presence or absence of this symptom is not considered proof ovulation did or did not occur.

Your Health Can Affect Your Pregnancy

Your health is one of the most important factors in your pregnancy and is important to the development and well-being of your baby. Healthy nutrition, proper exercise, sufficient rest and taking care of yourself all affect your pregnancy. Throughout this book, we provide information about medicine you may take, tests you may need, substances you might use and many other topics that may concern you. This information helps you be aware of how your actions affect your health and the health of your developing baby.

Dad Tip
· · · · · · · · · · ·

You may find you'll need to make some changes in your life during your partner's pregnancy. You may have to change how often you participate in various activities or when you do them. You may not be able to travel as much for work or pleasure. But remember—pregnancy only lasts 9 months. Supporting your pregnant partner can make both of your lives better.

Your Healthcare Provider

You have many choices when it comes to choosing your doctor or other healthcare provider for your pregnancy. An *obstetrician* is a doctor who specializes in the care of pregnant women, including delivering babies. Obstetricians are medical doctors or doctors of osteopathic medicine who have graduated from an accredited medical or osteopathic school and have fulfilled the requirements for a medical license. Both have completed further training after medical school (residency).

Perinatologists are obstetricians who specialize in high-risk pregnancies. Few women require a perinatologist (only 1 out of 10). If you're worried about past health problems, ask your healthcare provider whether you need to see a specialist.

An added credential is *board certification*. Not all doctors who deliver babies are board certified; it's not a requirement. Board certification means your doctor has put in extra time preparing for and taking exams to qualify him or her to care for pregnant women and to deliver their babies. If your doctor has passed his or her boards, you will see the initials F.A.C.O.G. after the doctor's name. This means he or she is a Fellow of the American Congress of Obstetricians and Gynecologists. Your local medical society can also give you this information.

Some women choose a *family practitioner* for their care. In some cases, an obstetrician may not be available, and a family practitioner may serve as internist, pediatrician and obstetrician/gynecologist. Many family practitioners are experienced at delivering babies. If problems arise, you may be referred to an obstetrician. This may also be the case if a Cesarean delivery is needed.

Pregnant women sometimes choose a *certified nurse-midwife*, an *advance-practice nurse* (NP) or a *physician assistant* (PA) for their prenatal care. These healthcare professionals have additional training and certification in a medical specialty. See the discussion of each and the type of care they provide that begins on page 26.

It's important to be able to communicate with your healthcare provider. You need to be able to ask any questions you or your partner may have. You should be able to express your concerns and talk about what's important to you. Don't be afraid to ask any question; your healthcare provider has probably already heard it.

Your healthcare provider has experience involving many pregnancies and is drawing on this for your well-being. He or she has to consider what is best for you and your baby while trying to honor any "special" requests you may have. A request may be unwise or risky for you, but it's important to ask about it ahead of time. If a request is possible, you can plan for it together, barring unforeseen developments.

How do you find someone who "fits the bill"? If you already have a healthcare provider you're happy with, you may be all set. If you don't, call your local medical society. Ask for references to professionals who are taking new patients for pregnancy. Or ask friends and family members who have recently had a baby to suggest someone. Another healthcare provider, such as a pediatrician or internist, may also provide a reference.

When you pick a healthcare provider, you usually also pick a hospital. Things to consider include how close the facility is to you, policies regarding your partner and his participation, and whether your insurance covers the healthcare provider and the hospital.

You will find many boxes in each weekly discussion; they provide you with information you will not find in the text. Our boxes do not repeat information contained in a discussion. Each box is unique, so read them for specific information.

How Your Actions Affect Your Baby's Development

It's never too early to start thinking about how your activities and actions can affect your growing baby. Many substances you normally use may have negative effects on your baby, including drugs, tobacco, alcohol and caffeine. Below are discussions of cigarette smoking and alcohol use. Either of these activities can harm a developing baby. Other substances are discussed throughout the book.

A symptom is something you feel or can see. A sign is something other people observe. A headache is a symptom; a red rash is a sign.

Cigarette Smoking

Smoking cigarettes narrows blood vessels, reducing the amount of oxygen and nutrients your baby receives. Smoking also causes blood to clot. These two effects are the reason smoking cigarettes is especially harmful during pregnancy.

Over 10% of all pregnant women smoke; some experts put the number at 20%. A pregnant woman who smokes 20 cigarettes a day (one pack) inhales tobacco smoke more than 11,000 times during an average pregnancy! Cigarette smoke crosses the placenta to the baby; when you smoke, so does your baby!

Smokers may have more complications during pregnancy than nonsmokers. Infants born to mothers who smoke weigh less by nearly half a pound.

Some people believe it's OK to use smokeless tobacco products during pregnancy. It's not! Use of any smokeless tobacco product contributes to nicotine in the bloodstream, which is one of the main causes of problems.

Tobacco smoke contains over 250 harmful substances that may damage a

Stop-Smoking Aids
· · · · · · · · · · ·

You may be wondering whether you can use the patch, gum or stop-smoking pill during pregnancy to help you stop smoking. This is something to discuss with your healthcare provider.

Nicotrol, available as an inhaler, nasal spray, patch or gum, is sold under the brand names Nicoderm and Nicorette; it's also sold generically. Nicotrol preparations contain nicotine and are *not* recommended for use during pregnancy.

Zyban (bupropion hydrochloride) is a nonnicotine aid to help a person stop smoking. It's also sold as the antidepressant Wellbutrin or Wellbutrin SR. It's *not* recommended for pregnant women.

Chantix (varenicline tartrate) is another prescription medication available to help someone stop smoking. It doesn't contain nicotine, but it's *not* recommended for pregnant women. Studies show it may reduce a fetus's bone mass and cause low birthweight.

Nicotine-replacement therapy may be suggested if a woman can't stop smoking on her own. Studies show the benefits of these products may outweigh the risks, but some experts disagree. They don't believe nicotine addiction can be stopped by nicotine, which is contained in sprays, inhalers, patches and gum. Discuss the situation with your healthcare provider if you have questions.

developing baby. The incidence of SIDS (sudden-infant-death syndrome) after birth may be higher, and babies may be more excitable as infants. The nicotine you take in during pregnancy could lead to nicotine withdrawal in baby after birth. One study showed smoking cigarettes increases a woman's risk for stillbirth (fetal death after 20 weeks of pregnancy). This risk also increases if a woman is exposed to second-hand smoke.

Children of smokers are more likely to suffer acute ear infections and respiratory problems. Studies show if you smoke during pregnancy, your child may be a smoker as an adult. And if baby's dad smoked before conception and smokes during pregnancy, the child also has a higher risk of developing problems.

Even if you don't smoke, you may be at risk. Some studies show a nonsmoker and her unborn baby exposed to second-hand smoke (cigarette smoke in the air) are exposed to nicotine and other harmful substances. In addition, third-hand smoke can be harmful; it occurs when tobacco toxins stick to fabric, hair, skin and other surfaces, even after smoke has disappeared. It can be as harmful as second-hand smoke. A clue to the presence of third-hand smoke is smell—if you can smell it, it's still there.

What can you do? The answer sounds simple but isn't—*quit smoking*. In more realistic terms, if you smoke, cut down or stop smoking before or during pregnancy. Withdrawal symptoms from smoking are normal, but they're a sign your body is healing. Cravings may be strongest during withdrawal, but after a few weeks, symptoms will decrease. Maybe your pregnancy can serve as good reason for everyone in the family to stop smoking!

Electronic Cigarettes. *Electronic cigarettes*, also called *e-cigarettes*, are now being sold in the United States. These "cigarettes" look similar to real cigarettes, but they are very different. Electronic cigarettes use a battery to heat a small cylinder filled with liquid nicotine, a man-made substitute or a nicotine-free substance. The cylinder also contains propylene glycol (PEG), which is used to make theatrical smoke. The heated material is released as a vapor the user inhales; vapor that looks like smoke is exhaled.

Although sellers claim electronic cigarettes are safe, there is no proof they won't cause harm. They do not have FDA approval here in the United States, and their sales and importation have been banned in Canada.

Are electronic cigarettes a safe alternative for pregnant women to use? We cannot advocate their use during pregnancy because we have no information on how the ingredients in these cigarettes can affect a developing fetus. The warnings about cigarette smoking and tobacco use during pregnancy can probably also be applied to these new devices.

Don't take any chances with your developing baby's health and growth by using these products.

Alcohol Use

Drinking alcohol during pregnancy carries many risks. In fact, some experts believe alcohol may be one of the worst substances a developing baby can be exposed to. Babies born to mothers who drink while they're pregnant may suffer the effects of their mother's drinking for the rest of their lives.

. . . .
It's probably OK to eat a food that contains alcohol if it has been baked or simmered for at least 1 hour.
. . . .

Drinking during pregnancy has been linked to behavior problems in a child, various birth defects, facial disfigurement and interruption in brain development and development of baby's nervous system. Taking drugs with alcohol increases the risk of damage to baby. As a safeguard, be very careful about over-the-counter cough and cold remedies; many contain alcohol—some as much as 25%!

Some pregnant women want to know if they can drink socially. We don't know of any safe amount of alcohol a woman can drink during pregnancy. So for the health and well-being of your baby, don't drink *any* alcohol.

Use of alcohol in pregnancy can lead to *fetal alcohol syndrome* and *fetal alcohol exposure* in baby. Both are discussed below. They are considered part of *fetal alcohol spectrum disorder (FASD)*, which covers the range of effects that can occur.

Fetal alcohol syndrome (FAS) is characterized by smaller growth before and after birth; heart, limb and facial problems may also be present. An FAS child may have behavior, speech and motor-function problems. Fifteen to 20% of them die soon after birth. Most studies indicate a woman would have to drink four to five drinks a day for FAS to occur.

Mild defects are the result of *fetal alcohol exposure (FAE)*. This condition can result from intake of very little alcohol. The condition has led many researchers to conclude there is no safe level of alcohol consumption during pregnancy. For this reason, all alcoholic beverages in the United States carry warning labels that advise women to avoid drinking alcohol during pregnancy.

. . . .

The American Academy of Pediatrics (AAP) has weighed in on the use of alcohol during pregnancy. Pediatricians believe the use of alcohol by a pregnant woman should be avoided. There is no benefit to mom or baby if alcohol is consumed during a pregnancy.

. . . .

Nonalcoholic Beer and Wine. We've had women ask us if drinking nonalcoholic beer and wine is OK during pregnancy. They believe because it is labeled "nonalcoholic," it doesn't contain any alcohol. They are wrong.

Nonalcoholic beer and wine start out as alcoholic beverages. After they are produced, nearly all of the alcohol is removed. Note we said "nearly all" of the alcohol. Some alcohol does remain; in fact, to be labeled *nonalcoholic* under federal law, a beverage can contain up to a half of one percent (0.5%) of alcohol in the final product. It can only be labeled *alcohol-free* if it contains no alcohol at all.

. . . .

A beer or wine can only be labeled alcohol-free *if it contains no alcohol whatsoever.*

. . . .

Because we don't know how much alcohol it takes to cause problems, why take a chance with your baby's future life? If you drink any alcohol during pregnancy and your baby is negatively affected, you bear the burden. You are responsible for everything you eat, drink or take in during your pregnancy. Will that glass of wine or that beer be worth it in the end if your baby has problems? For that reason, we must advise pregnant women to also avoid nonalcoholic beer and wine during their pregnancies.

Your Nutrition

Your nutrition is very important during pregnancy. You will probably need to increase your caloric intake during pregnancy to meet demands. During the first trimester (first 13 weeks), you should eat a total of about 2200 calories a day. During the second and third trimesters, you probably need an additional 300 calories each day.

Extra calories give you energy to support your growing baby and the changes in your body. Your baby uses the calories to create and to store protein, fat and carbohydrates. It needs energy for its body processes to function.

You can meet most nutritional needs by eating a well-balanced, varied diet. The quality of your calories is important. If a food grows in the ground or on a tree (meaning it's fresh), it's probably better for you than if it comes out of a box or can.

Be cautious about adding the extra 300 calories to your nutrition plan—it doesn't mean doubling your portions. A medium-sized apple and a cup of low-fat yogurt add up to 300 calories!

You Should Also Know

There are two types of prenatal tests—*screening* and *diagnostic*. *Screening tests* assess your risk of having a baby with a certain birth defect; these tests can provide basic information to determine if more testing is necessary. *Diagnostic tests* can provide nearly definite results. Unfortunately, some prenatal diagnostic tests carry a very small risk of miscarriage. These various tests are described in some of the following weeks.

Healthcare Professionals Who May Care for You

Certified Nurse-Midwives. Many doctors in the United States have certified nurse-midwives on staff. A certified nurse-midwife (CNM) is a registered nurse (RN) who has received additional training delivering babies and providing prenatal and postpartum care to women.

In a normal, uncomplicated pregnancy, many or most of your prenatal visits may be with a CNM, not the physician. This may include labor and delivery. You may find this is a good thing—often a CNM has more time to spend with you, answering questions and addressing your concerns.

A CNM will consult with a physician about specifics of a particular pregnancy and about the labor and delivery of a woman. Most midwives can help you explore birthing methods, including natural childbirth, and pain-relief methods for labor and delivery, including the use of epidurals.

A word of warning: Not all people who call themselves midwives are certified nurse-midwives. Some are not even registered nurses. Be sure to check the credentials of any nurse-midwife you are considering for your care.

If it's important to you, a midwife may be able to help you make your baby's birth one the entire family can participate in or experience. A certified nurse-midwife can also address issues of family planning and birth-control counseling and other gynecological care, including breast exams, Pap smears and other screenings. CNMs can prescribe medications; each state has specific requirements.

Today, over 7000 certified nurse-midwives practice in all 50 states; they attend nearly 10% of all births, mostly in hospitals. Certified nurse-midwives work in private practice (usually associated with a physician), hospitals, birthing centers and clinics.

To receive certification, a person must first have a bachelor's degree and be a registered nurse. He or she must then complete a master's degree or doctorate program from an accredited institution, which usually takes 1 to 4 years. CNMs can be men or women—about 2% of all certified nurse-midwives are male.

Advance-Practice Nurses. An advance-practice nurse, also called a *nurse practitioner (NP)*, has received postgraduate education in a medical specialty and holds either a master's degree or a doctorate. An NP is licensed through a state nursing board.

Nurse practitioners focus on individualized care. In a normal, uncomplicated pregnancy, many or most of your prenatal visits may be with a nurse practitioner, not the physician. This may include labor and delivery. You may find this is a good thing—often these healthcare providers have more time to spend with you, answering questions and addressing your concerns.

To be a nurse practitioner in obstetrics and gynecology, a person must be nationally certified and educated to care for and to treat women's health issues (WHNP). Nurses may also be certified registered nurse anesthetists (CRNAs) who administer anesthetics for various procedures, including pain relief for labor and delivery.

In the United States, state regulations determine whether NPs work independently of doctors or must work with them. A nurse practitioner may work in various institutions, including private medical practices, clinics, health centers, urgent-care centers and health maintenance organizations (HMOs).

Physician Assistants. A physician assistant or physician associate (PA) is a qualified healthcare professional who may take care of you during pregnancy. He or she is licensed to practice medicine in association with a licensed doctor. In a normal, uncomplicated pregnancy, many or most of your prenatal visits may be with a PA, not the physician. This may include labor and delivery. You may find this is a good thing—often these healthcare providers have more time to spend with you, answering questions and addressing your concerns.

Most PAs work in doctors' offices, clinics, urgent-care facilities and/or hospitals. Physician assistants care for people who have conditions (pregnancy is a condition they see women for), diagnose and treat illnesses, order and interpret tests, counsel on preventive health care, perform some procedures, assist in surgery, write prescriptions and do physical exams. A PA is *not* a medical assistant, who performs administrative or simple clinical tasks.

PA training takes 2 to 3 years after receiving an undergraduate degree. A graduate of a physician-assistant program receives a master's degree. Some programs also offer a clinical doctorate degree (Doctor of Science Physician Assistant, or DScPA). There are also specialty programs or residencies some PAs choose to take to specialize in a certain area. They usually last an additional year.

A PA is licensed by the medical board of each state. After graduating from an accredited program, a PA must pass a qualifying exam-administered Physician Assistant National Certifying Exam (PANCE) before being certified.

Weekly Exercises

Each weekly discussion contains an exercise description and an illustration, if one applies, for safe exercises to do during pregnancy. If you're healthy and have no pregnancy problems, experts agree you can probably exercise moderately for at least 30 minutes five times a week or more. Studies show active pregnant women often have fewer problems during pregnancy, and exercise doesn't increase a baby's risk for problems. If you exercised before pregnancy, continue exercising during pregnancy; you'll get many of the same benefits you did before you became pregnant.

Discuss exercise at your first prenatal appointment. Your healthcare provider may have suggestions for your particular situation. Exercises we include in this book are nonweightbearing and should cause few problems, so you can probably do them until your first prenatal visit. Be sure to discuss aerobic and weightbearing exercise with your healthcare provider at that time.

Exercise to condition, strengthen and tone various muscle groups, many of which you'll want to strengthen for your comfort during pregnancy. In addition, some exercises strengthen muscles you use during labor and delivery. It's never too early to get started!

You may decide to set up a routine of exercises to do, adding and deleting some as you get bigger. Some of the exercises are done standing, some sitting, some kneeling and some lying down. We suggest you leaf through each week and choose the exercises that appeal to you.

We advise every pregnant woman to read and practice the Kegel exercise (Week 14) to help strengthen pelvic-floor muscles. Practicing throughout pregnancy can help in many ways, especially with incontinence during and after pregnancy. Actually, it's an exercise every woman, no matter what her age, should practice every day.

Chart Your Pregnancy Weight Gain

• • • • • • •

If you want to chart your pregnancy weight gain, we've provided a chart below for that purpose. Weeks listed are selected based on when you may have a prenatal appointment. If your appointment doesn't fall on that exact week, cross out the number of the week we have listed and mark in the number of the week you saw your healthcare provider.

Weight before pregnancy begins _____

Week	Weight at Each Prenatal Appointment	Weight Gain
8		
12		
16		
20		
24		
28		
30		
32		
34		
36		
37		
38		
39		
40		

Total pregnancy weight gain_____

Week 3

Age of Fetus—1 Week

How Big Is Your Baby?

The embryo is very small—at this point, it's only a group of cells, but it's growing rapidly. It's the size of the head of a pin and would be visible to the naked eye if it weren't inside you. The group of cells doesn't look like a fetus or baby; it looks like the illustration on page 31. During this first week, the embryo is about 0.006 inch (0.150mm) long.

How Big Are You?

It's too soon to notice any changes. Few women know they have conceived. Remember, you haven't even missed a period yet.

How Your Baby Is Growing and Developing

Fertilization is the joining together of one sperm and an egg. We believe it occurs in the middle part of the Fallopian tube, called the *ampulla*, not inside the uterus. Sperm travel through the uterine cavity and out into the tube to meet the egg.

When the sperm and egg join, the sperm passes through the outer layer of the ovum, then digests its way through another layer of the egg. Although several sperm may penetrate the outer layers of the egg, usually only one sperm enters the egg and fertilizes it. The egg reacts by making changes in the outer layers so no other sperm can enter.

Once the sperm is inside the egg, the chromosomes of the male and female pronuclei combine into one. Extremely small bits of information and characteristics from each partner mix. This chromosomal information gives each of us our unique characteristics. The usual number of chromosomes in a human being is 46. Each parent supplies 23 chromosomes. Your baby is a combination of chromosomal information from you and your partner.

The developing ball of cells is called a *zygote*. The zygote passes through the uterine tube on its way to the uterus; the division of cells continues. These cells are called a *blastomere*. As the blastomere divides, a solid ball of cells is formed, called a *morula*. Gradual accumulation of fluid within the morula results in the formation of a *blastocyst*.

During the next week, the blastocyst travels through the uterine tube to the uterus (3 to 7 days after fertilization in

Boy or Girl?

· · · · · · · · · · ·

Your baby's sex is determined at the time of fertilization by the type of sperm (male or female) that fertilizes the egg. A Y-chromosome sperm produces a boy, and an X-chromosome sperm produces a girl.

the tube). The blastocyst lies free in the uterine cavity as it continues to grow and to develop. About a week after fertilization, it attaches to the uterine cavity (implantation), and cells burrow into the lining of the uterus.

Changes in You

Some women can tell when they ovulate. They may feel mild cramping or pain, or they may have an increased vaginal discharge. Occasionally when the fertilized egg implants in the uterine cavity, a woman may notice a small amount of bleeding.

It's too early for you to notice many changes. That lies ahead! (See the discussion in Weeks 1 & 2 for signs and symptoms of pregnancy.)

How Your Actions Affect Your Baby's Development

Aspirin Use

We advise caution with the use of aspirin during pregnancy because it can increase bleeding. If you take aspirin, your baby may be at higher risks for some problems.

Studies show aspirin and nonsteroidal anti-inflammatory medications (NSAIDs), such as Advil, Motrin and Aleve, may increase the risk of

miscarriage. The risk is highest when taken soon after conception. Aspirin also causes changes in blood clotting. This is important to know if you bleed during pregnancy or if you're at the end of pregnancy and close to delivery.

Read labels on every medicine you take to see whether it contains aspirin; some OTC medications do. It's also important to watch your salicylate intake. Salicylate is contained in Pepto-Bismol, Kaopectate and some skin products.

· ·

There may be situations in which aspirin use is helpful and may be good insurance against some pregnancy problems. Talk to your healthcare provider if you have questions.

· ·

If you need a pain reliever or fever reducer and can't reach your healthcare provider for advice, acetaminophen (Tylenol) is an over-the-counter medicine you can use for a short while.

In some cases, small doses of aspirin may be acceptable during pregnancy. If you are at risk for pre-eclampsia, talk to your healthcare provider about taking low-dose aspirin—*baby* aspirin—every day. Studies show it may reduce the risk by as much as 25%. You are at higher risk for pre-eclampsia if you had it in a previous pregnancy, you're carrying more than one baby or if you had high blood pressure or diabetes when you

———— *Blastomere*

Nine-cell embryo 3 days after fertilization.
The embryo is made up of many blastomeres;
together they form a blastocyst.

got pregnant. However, don't take any aspirin without discussing it with your healthcare provider first!

Marijuana Use during Pregnancy

Marijuana use by you can disrupt baby's brain development and can cause many problems. Smoking marijuana during pregnancy has been tied to an increased risk of stillbirth (fetal death after 20 weeks of pregnancy). One study shows that risk can be three times higher if a woman smokes pot during pregnancy. And the more marijuana a woman smokes, the higher the risk.

With the legalization of marijuana in some places in the United States, the risk of fetal exposure to marijuana may become more common as consumers are able to buy pot legally. And it's not just a mom-to-be smoking marijuana that puts the fetus at risk. Eating foods laced with marijuana and second-hand marijuana smoke may also increase a woman's risk of stillbirth.

Exercise during Pregnancy?

Exercise is important to many pregnant women. Studies show more than 60% of all pregnant women exercise. However, statistics also show only 15% of pregnant women engage in 30 minutes of moderate exercise five or more times a week, and only 25% of all pregnant women get enough exercise. The aim of exercise during pregnancy is to stay fit. And exercise may give your baby a healthier start in life.

You can benefit from exercise. Exercise can relieve back pain, increase stamina and muscle strength, and improve circulation and flexibility. You may also have less nausea and constipation; you may sleep better and feel less tired. Women who are physically fit are better able to perform the hard work of labor and delivery.

Exercising may also reduce your chances of having some pregnancy problems. Healthy women who exercise during the first 20 weeks of pregnancy may reduce their risk of developing preeclampsia by as much as 35%. It may also reduce stress and help lower your blood pressure.

Exercise may help you control your weight during pregnancy, and you may have an easier time losing weight after pregnancy. You might even return to your prepregnancy shape faster.

There are many types of exercise to choose from; each offers its own advantages. If you haven't been involved in regular, strenuous exercise before pregnancy, walking and swimming are probably about as involved as you should get with exercise. If you have questions, talk them over with your healthcare provider at your first prenatal visit.

Aerobic exercise is very popular with women who want to stay in shape. Muscle-building exercises are also a popular way to tone muscles and to increase strength. Many women combine the two. Good exercise choices for pregnant women include brisk walking, stationary bicycling, swimming and aerobic exercise designed specifically for pregnant women.

Exercise during pregnancy is not without some risk, however, so listen to your body. Risks include increased body temperature, decreased blood flow to the uterus and possible injury

Tip for Week 3
. . . .

Before you begin any exercise program, discuss it with your healthcare provider. Together you can develop a program that takes into account your level of conditioning and your exercise habits.

to the mother's abdominal area. There are some precautions to take if you exercise. Don't let your body temperature rise above 102F (38.9C). Keep workouts short, especially during hot weather. If you do free weights, sit down when you can. Wear some type of tummy support. In your third trimester, don't lift more than 15 pounds of weight; instead, increase the number of reps. Stretch and warm up muscles before exercising, and cool down after exercising. These activities may help you avoid injury.

There are other types of exercise you might enjoy; a balance ball may be a good choice. Exercising on a big exercise ball is easy on your back, and it helps strengthen core muscles. Some women use them during labor to help relieve pain!

Pregnancy yoga or Pilates classes may be good choices during your first trimester. Ten minutes of yoga or Pilates increases your blood flow and stretches muscles. Try water aerobics to help relieve back and pelvic pain.

Before beginning any exercise program, consult your healthcare provider. If you get the go-ahead, begin exercising gradually. Start with 15-minute workout sessions, with 5-minute rest periods in between. Check your heart rate every 15 minutes.

Break workouts into smaller increments to fit them into your day. Four 10-minute walks may be easier to accomplish than one 40-minute walk. Wear comfortable clothing during exercise, including clothing that is warm enough or cool enough, and good, comfortable athletic shoes with maximum support. Drink water before, during and after exercising. Dehydration may cause contractions.

. . . .

If you feel tired, don't skip a workout! Instead, decrease how hard you exercise or for how long. Sometimes stretching may be all you're up for. Try to stretch at least a couple of times a week. Stretching may lower stress levels and help calm you.

. . . .

You may feel better if you can remember to contract your abdomen and buttocks to help support your lower back. Never hold your breath while you exercise, and don't get overheated. Be careful getting up and lying down. After 16 weeks of pregnancy, don't lie on your back while exercising. This can decrease blood flow to the uterus and placenta. When you finish exercising, lie on your left side for 15 to 20 minutes.

. . . .

You will find many boxes in each weekly discussion that will provide you with information you will not find in the text. Our boxes do not repeat information contained in a discussion. Each box is unique, so read them for specific information.

. . . .

Stop exercising and consult your healthcare provider if you experience bleeding or loss of fluid from the vagina, shortness of breath, dizziness, severe abdominal pain or any other pain or discomfort while exercising. Exercise only under your healthcare provider's supervision if you experience (or know you have) an irregular heartbeat, high blood pressure, diabetes, thyroid disease, anemia or any other chronic medical problem. Discuss exercise if you have a history of three or more miscarriages, an incompetent cervix, intrauterine-growth restriction (IUGR), premature labor or any abnormal bleeding during pregnancy.

Your Nutrition

Folic-Acid Use

Folic acid, also referred to as *folate, folacin* or *vitamin B9*, is very important during pregnancy. *Folate* is the form of folic acid found in food. Folic acid is the synthetic version of this B vitamin. It's important to take folic acid before trying to get pregnant and during early pregnancy because this is when it is most helpful.

To help prevent neural-tube defects, take 400mcg (0.4mg) of folic acid a day, beginning before pregnancy and continuing through the first 13 weeks. This is suggested for *all* pregnant women. *Neural-tube defects* occur in a baby during early pregnancy, often before you even suspect you might be pregnant. The most common is spina bifida. Once pregnancy is confirmed, it may be too late to prevent neural-tube problems.

A pregnant woman's body excretes four or five times the normal amount of folic acid, and it isn't stored in the body for long, so you need to replace it every day. A prenatal vitamin contains 0.8mg to 1mg of folic acid; this is usually enough for a woman with a normal pregnancy.

Folic-acid deficiency can result in anemia in you. Extra folic acid may be needed with multiple fetuses or if you suffer from Crohn's disease.

We know some medications interfere with folic-acid metabolism. Ask your healthcare provider about any medications you take. Smoking cigarettes removes folic acid from the body. Second-hand smoke can also reduce folic-acid levels. In addition, drinking green tea can keep your body from absorbing folic acid, so avoid it.

In the United States, many grain products, including flour, breakfast

Some Information May Scare You
· · · · · · · · · · ·

In an effort to give you as much information as possible about pregnancy, we include serious discussions throughout the book that some might find "scary." The information is not included to frighten you; it's there to provide facts about particular medical situations that may occur during pregnancy.

If a woman experiences a serious problem, she and her partner will probably want to know as much about it as possible. If a woman has a friend or knows someone who has problems during pregnancy, reading about it might relieve her fears. We also hope our discussions can help you start a dialogue with your doctor if you have questions.

Nearly all pregnancies are uneventful, and serious situations don't arise. However, please know we have tried to cover as many aspects of pregnancy as we possibly can so you'll have all the information at hand that you might need and want. Knowledge is power, so having various facts available can help you feel more in control of your own pregnancy. We hope reading information helps you relax and have a great pregnancy experience.

If you find a serious discussion frightens you, don't read it! Or if the information doesn't apply to your pregnancy, just skip over it. But realize information is there if you want to know more about a particular situation.

cereals and pasta, are fortified with folic acid. The number of babies born with neural-tube defects has decreased by nearly 20% since the fortification program began.

Eating 1 cup of fortified breakfast cereal, with milk, and drinking a glass of orange juice supplies about half of your folic-acid requirement for one day. Folate is found naturally in many foods, such as fruits, legumes, brewer's yeast, soybeans, whole-grain products and dark, leafy vegetables. A well-balanced diet can help you reach your folic-acid-intake goal. Also see the list of foods that are good folate sources in *Preparing for Pregnancy*.

Green-Tea Warning
Avoid green tea during pregnancy. Studies show women who consume as little as one or two cups of green tea a day within 3 months of conception and during the first trimester *double* the risk of having a baby with neural-tube defects. The antioxidant in green tea interferes with the body's use of folic acid.

Green tea may also interfere with blood tests; it can alter blood-sugar levels that could mess up a diabetes test. In addition, it may interfere with blood clotting. So wait until after pregnancy to have your green tea.

You Should Also Know
Bleeding and Spotting during Pregnancy
Bleeding and spotting during pregnancy cause concern. *Bleeding* is vaginal bleeding that is usually as heavy as, or heavier than, a menstrual period. *Spotting* is

Benefits of Pregnancy
· · · · · · · · · · ·

There are many benefits to being pregnant. Allergy and asthma sufferers may feel better because natural steroids produced during pregnancy help reduce symptoms. Pregnancy may help protect against ovarian cancer. The younger a woman is when she starts having babies and the more pregnancies she has, the greater the benefit.

Migraine headaches often disappear during the second and third trimesters. Menstrual cramps are a thing of the past. An added benefit—they may not return after baby is born!

Endometriosis (when endometrial tissue attaches to parts of the ovaries and other sites outside the uterus) causes pelvic pain, heavy bleeding and other problems during menstruation for some women. Pregnancy can stop the growth of endometriosis.

Having a baby may protect you against breast cancer. Researchers believe high levels of protein secreted by the growing baby may be associated with a lower risk for younger moms. The protein may interfere with estrogen's role in causing breast cancer.

vaginal bleeding that is usually lighter than a regular menstrual period.

In the first trimester, bleeding or spotting can make you worry about the possibility of miscarriage. As your uterus grows, the placenta forms and vascular connections are made; bleeding may occur then. During the second trimester, bleeding may happen with sexual intercourse or a vaginal exam. Bleeding during the third trimester can be a sign of placenta previa or the onset of labor.

· ·

Strenuous exercise or intercourse may cause some bleeding. If this occurs, stop your activities and check with your healthcare provider.

· ·

If you experience any type of bleeding during pregnancy, it is not unusual. Some researchers estimate 20% of all pregnant women bleed during the first trimester. Not all women who bleed have a miscarriage.

Call your healthcare provider if you experience any bleeding. If bleeding causes your healthcare provider concern, he or she may order an ultrasound exam. Sometimes ultrasound can show a reason for bleeding, but during early pregnancy, there may be no detectable cause.

Most experts suggest resting, decreasing activity and avoiding intercourse if bleeding occurs.

Exercise for Week 3

· · · · · · ·

Facing a wall, stand a couple of feet away from it, with your hands in front of your shoulders. Place your hands on the wall, and lean forward. Bend your elbows as your body leans into the wall. Keep your heels flat on the floor. Slowly push away from the wall, and stand straight. Do 10 to 20 times. *Develops upper-back, chest and arm strength, and relieves lower-leg tension.*

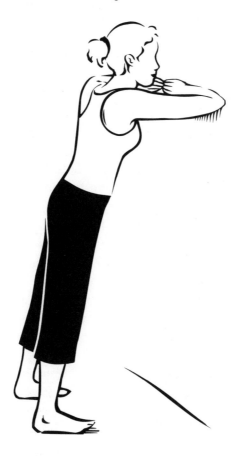

· · · · · · ·

Week 4

Age of Fetus—2 Weeks

If you've just found out you're pregnant, you might want to begin by reading the previous chapters.

How Big Is Your Baby?

Your developing baby's size varies from 0.014 inch to about 0.04 inch (0.36mm to about 1mm) in length. One millimeter is half the size of a letter "o" on this page.

How Big Are You?

At this point, your pregnancy doesn't show. The illustration on page 40 gives you an idea of how small your baby is, so you can see why you don't notice any changes.

How Your Baby Is Growing and Developing

Fetal development is in the very early stages, but great changes are taking place! The blastocyst is embedded more deeply into the lining of your uterus, and the amniotic sac, which will fill with amniotic fluid, is starting to form.

The placenta is also forming; it plays an important role in hormone production and transport of oxygen and nutrients. Networks that contain maternal blood are becoming established.

Development of baby's nervous system (brain and other structures, such as the spinal cord) begins.

Germ layers are forming; they develop into specialized parts of baby's body, such as organs. The three germ layers are the *ectoderm*, *endoderm* and *mesoderm*.

The ectoderm becomes the nervous system (including the brain), the skin and the hair. The endoderm develops into the lining of the gastrointestinal tract, the liver, pancreas and thyroid. The mesoderm becomes the skeleton, connective tissues, blood system, urogenital system and most of the muscles.

. . . .

By the time you miss a period, 80% of baby's organ development has already occurred.

. . . .

Changes in You

You're probably expecting a period around the end of this week. When it doesn't occur, pregnancy may be one of the first things you think of.

The area on the ovary where the egg comes from is called the *corpus luteum*. If you become pregnant, it is called the *corpus luteum of pregnancy.* The corpus luteum forms immediately after ovulation at the site where the egg is released. It looks like a small sac of fluid. It rapidly changes in preparation for producing hormones, such as progesterone, to support a pregnancy before the placenta takes over.

We believe the corpus luteum is important in the early weeks of pregnancy because it produces progesterone. The placenta takes over this function between 8 and 12 weeks of pregnancy. Around the sixth month of pregnancy, the corpus luteum shrinks.

How Your Actions Affect Your Baby's Development

During pregnancy, nearly every parent worries about whether baby will be perfect. Most parents worry unnecessarily. Major birth defects occur in few births. Most birth defects occur during the first trimester (the first 13 weeks of pregnancy).

Structural birth defects occur when some part of the baby's body is not formed correctly or is missing. Heart defects and neural-tube defects are common structural defects. *Genetic defects* are caused by a mistake in a gene. Some are inherited; others occur when the egg and sperm join. Exposure to some chemicals and/or toxic agents account for other birth defects. Additional defects may occur if a pregnant woman is exposed to a particular infection, such as rubella (German measles).

Teratology is the study of abnormal fetal development. A *teratogen* is a substance that can cause birth defects. Some substances may cause major defects if exposure occurs at a specific time in fetal development but are not harmful at other times. By the 13th week, baby has completed major development. After that time, the effect of a substance may be smaller growth or smaller organ size. One example is rubella. It can cause birth defects, such as heart malformations, if the baby is infected during the first trimester. Rubella infection later in pregnancy is less serious.

Women's responses to substances, and the amount they are exposed to, vary greatly. Alcohol is a good example. Large amounts appear to have no effect on some babies, while other babies can be harmed by very low amounts.

Medicine and Drug Use

Information about the effects of a specific medication or drug on a pregnancy comes from cases of exposure before the pregnancy was discovered. These "case reports" help researchers understand possible harmful effects but leave gaps in our knowledge. For this reason, it can be

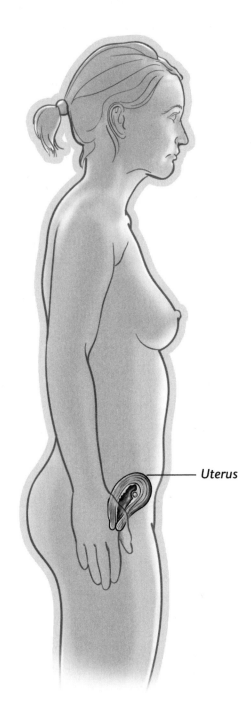

Uterus

Pregnancy at around 4 weeks
(fetal age—2 weeks).

Grandma's Remedy
· · · · · · · · · · ·

If you want to avoid using medication, try a folk remedy. To help relieve constipation, drink an 8-ounce glass of water with 2 teaspoons of apple-cider vinegar. Drink one glass in the morning and another at night.

difficult to make exact statements about a particular substance and its effect. The chart on pages 44 and 45 lists possible effects of drugs and other substances.

If you use drugs, be honest with your healthcare provider. Tell him or her about anything you take or have taken that may affect your baby. The victim of drug use is your baby. A drug problem may have serious consequences that can be best dealt with if your healthcare provider knows about your drug use in advance.

Your Nutrition

You probably won't be able to eat all you want during pregnancy, unless you are one of the lucky women who doesn't have a problem with calories. Even then, you must pay strict attention to the *types* of foods you choose.

To stay healthy during pregnancy, eat nutritious foods. Avoid those with empty calories (lots of sugar and fat). Choose fresh fruits and vegetables. Avoid caffeine when possible. We discuss many of these subjects in later weeks.

You Should Also Know

Weight Gain

Gaining weight during pregnancy is necessary for your health and the health of your growing baby. Getting on the scale and seeing your weight rise may be very hard for you. Recognize now it's OK to gain weight. You don't have to let yourself go, but you need to gain enough weight to meet the needs of your pregnancy. We know the amount of weight you gain directly affects the birthweight of your baby.

Many years ago, women were not allowed to gain much weight—sometimes only 12 to 15 pounds for their entire pregnancy! Today, we know restricting weight gain to this extent is not healthy for you or baby. However, you shouldn't gain too much weight.

Gaining too much weight during pregnancy may increase your risk for developing gestational diabetes. If you gain more weight than your healthcare provider recommends during your pregnancy, baby may be bigger, which can have a negative effect for the rest of his or her life. Research indicates bigger-than-average babies may become overweight as children.

· ·
You may be eating for two during pregnancy, but you don't have to eat twice as much, just twice as smart!
· ·

Experts agree if a woman gains more than 50+ pounds during a full-term pregnancy with one baby, her baby

has an increased chance of weighing 9
pounds or more at birth. In addition, on
average, for each kilogram (2.2 pounds)
of weight these women gain, the baby
gains ¼ ounce.

Many women do not lose their pregnancy weight before they get pregnant
again, so they start the next pregnancy
heavier and gain even more weight.
Not shedding those extra pounds after
pregnancy contributes to a higher risk
of problems for you.

Environmental Pollutants and Pregnancy

An environment that is healthful for you
will be healthy for your growing baby.
Some environmental pollutants may be
harmful to you and baby. It's important
to avoid exposure to them.

We don't know about the safety of
many chemicals. It's best to avoid exposure when possible, but it may not be
possible. If you know you'll be around
various chemicals, wash your hands well
before eating. Not smoking cigarettes
also helps.

Lead Toxicity. The toxicity of lead has
been known for centuries. In the past,
most lead exposure came from the at-
mosphere. Today, exposure comes from
many sources.

Lead is easily transported across the
placenta to the baby. Toxicity can occur as
early as the 12th week of pregnancy, which
could result in lead poisoning in the baby.
If you might be exposed to lead in your
workplace, discuss it with your healthcare
provider.

Some latex paints contain lead. You
may want to avoid using some oil-based
paints and solvents. Solvents are chemicals that dissolve other substances. Read
labels.

Drinking water may contain lead if
your home has brass faucets, lead pipes
or lead solder on copper pipes. Run
water for 30 seconds before you use it to
reduce levels of lead; cold water contains
less lead than hot water.

If you use crystal goblets, they contain lead. Some scented candles have
wicks that contain lead. You could increase your exposure to lead with either.

**Some Other Pollutants to Avoid during
Pregnancy.** Mercury has a long history as
a potential poison to a pregnant woman.
Reports of fish contaminated with mercury have been linked to problems in
babies.

Our environment has been significantly contaminated with PCBs
(polychlorinated biphenyls). PCBs are
mixtures of several chemical compounds.

Most fish, birds and humans now have measurable amounts of PCB in their tissues. This is another reason to limit your intake of fish during pregnancy.

Arsenic may be hiding outdoors in your back yard—furniture, decks and play sets made from pressure-treated lumber may be preserved with chromated copper arsenate. Wash your hands thoroughly after you've been outside, and cover picnic tables with tablecloths when you eat on them. Apply a polyurethane sealant once a year.

Pesticides cover a large number of agents used to control unwanted plants and animals. Human exposure is common because pesticides are used extensively. Those of most concern contain several agents—DDT, chlordane, heptachlor, lindane and others.

Do You Take Paxil?

If you take the antidepressant Paxil, discuss its use with your healthcare provider immediately. You may need to start other treatment options early in pregnancy. But don't stop taking any antidepressant medication without first consulting your healthcare provider.

Paxil belongs to a class of medications called *selective serotonin reuptake inhibitors*, sometimes abbreviated as *SSRIs*. There is concern about the safety of Paxil during pregnancy. Paxil use in the first and third trimesters may put baby at risk.

Pregnancy Brain

Do you have "pregnancy brain"? Is your thinking fuzzy? Do you daydream a lot? Studies show over 75% of all pregnant women experience problems with their memory. If this happens to you, you're not alone. Because you have so much on your mind, it's easy for you to get distracted. Hormones also play a role. Stress can also impact your memory. So what can you do?

Ask for help if you need it. Friends and family members will probably be very willing to help you. They just need to know what you need from them. Get enough rest and sleep. Fatigue can muddle your thinking. Exercise for at least 30 minutes a day, 5 times a week to help clear your head and provide you and baby many benefits. It may also help you sleep better. As obvious as it may sound, make lists and take them with you. Keep a notebook handy to jot down things you need or want to do.

Effects of Various Substances on Fetal Development

Many substances can affect your baby's early development. Below and on the opposite page is a list of various substances and their effects on a developing fetus.

Substance	Possible Effects on Your Baby
Alcohol	fetal abnormalities, fetal alcohol disorders, intrauterine-growth restriction (IUGR)
Amphetamines	placental abruption, IUGR, fetal death
Androgens male	ambiguous genital development (depends on dose given and when given)
Angiotensin-converting enzyme (ACE) inhibitors (enalapril, captopril)	fetal and neonatal death
Anticoagulants	bone and hand abnormalities, IUGR, central-nervous-system and eye abnormalities
Antithyroid drugs (propylthiouracil, iodide, methimazole)	hypothyroidism, fetal goiter
Barbiturates	possible birth defects, withdrawal symptoms, poor eating habits, seizures
Benzodiazepines (including Valium and Librium)	increased chance of congenital malformations
Caffeine	decreased birthweight, smaller head size, breathing problems, sleeplessness, irritability, jitters, poor calcium metabolism, IUGR, mental retardation, microcephaly, various major malformations
Carbamazepine	birth defects, spina bifida
Chemotherapeutic drugs (methotrexate, aminopterin)	increased risk of miscarriage, birth defects and fetal death
Cocaine/crack	miscarriage, stillbirth, congenital defects, severe deformities in a fetus, long-term mental deficiencies, sudden infant death syndrome (SIDS)
Coumadin derivatives (warfarin)	hemorrhage (bleeding), birth defects, an increase in miscarriage and stillbirth
Cyclophosphomide	transient sterility
Diethylstilbestrol (DES)	abnormalities of reproductive organs (females and males), infertility
Ecstasy	long-term learning problems, memory problems
Folic-acid antagonists (methotrexate, aminopterin)	increased risk of miscarriage, birth defects and fetal death

Glues and solvents	birth defects, including shortened stature, low birthweight, small head, joint and limb problems, abnormal facial features, heart defects
Iodine-131 (after 10 weeks)	adverse effects of radiation, growth restriction, birth defects
Isotretinoin (Accutane)	increased miscarriage rate, nervous-system defects, facial defects, cleft palate, fetal death
Ketamine	behavioral problems, learning problems
Lead	increased miscarriage and stillbirth rates
Lithium	congenital heart disease
Marijuana and hashish	attention-deficit disorder (ADD), attention-deficit hyperactivity disorder (ADHD), memory problems, impaired decision-making ability
Methamphetamines	IUGR, difficulty bonding, tremors, extreme fussiness
Misoprostol	skull defects, cranial-nerve palsies, facial malformations, limb defects
Nicotine	miscarriage, stillbirth, neural-tube defects, low birthweight, lower IQ, reading disorders, minimal-brain dysfunction syndrome (hyperactivity)
Opioids (morphine, heroin, Demerol)	congenital abnormalities, premature birth, IUGR, withdrawal symptoms in baby
Organic mercury	cerebral atrophy, mental retardation, spasticity, seizures, blindness
PCBs	possible neurological problems
Phenytoin (Dilantin)	IUGR, microcephaly
Progestins (high dose)	masculinization of female fetus
Streptomycin	hearing loss, cranial-nerve damage
Tetracycline	hypoplasia of tooth enamel, discoloration of permanent teeth
Thalidomide	severe limb defects
Trimethadione	cleft lip, cleft palate, IUGR, miscarriage
Valproic acid	neural-tube defects
Vitamin A and derivatives (isotretinoin, etritinate, retinoids)	increased miscarriage rate, nervous-system defects, facial defects, cleft palate, fetal death
X-ray therapy	microcephaly, mental retardation, leukemia

(Modified from A.C.O.G. Technical Bulletin 236, Teratology, American Congress of Obstetricians and Gynecologists)

Exercise for Week 4

. . . .

Sit on the floor, bring your feet close to your body and cross your ankles. Apply gentle pressure to your knees or the inside of your thighs. See illustration. Hold for a count of 10, relax and repeat. Do this exercise 4 or 5 times. Then place your hands under your knees, and gently press down with your knees while resisting the pressure with your hands. See illustration. Count to 5, then relax. Increase the number of presses until you can do 10 presses twice a day. *Develops pelvic-floor strength and quadricep strength.*

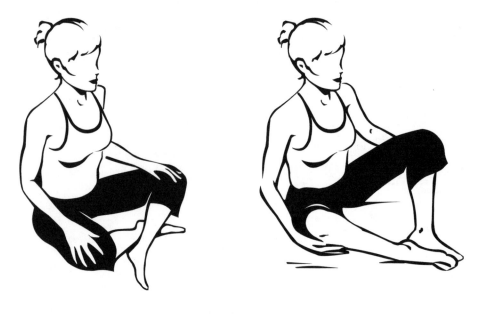

. . . .

Week 5

Age of Fetus—3 Weeks

*If you've just found out you're pregnant, you might want to
begin by reading the previous chapters.*

How Big Is Your Baby?

Your developing baby hasn't grown a lot. By this week, it's about 0.05 inch (1.25mm) long.

How Big Are You?

There are still no big changes in you. Even if you are aware you're pregnant, it will be awhile before others notice your changing figure.

How Your Baby Is Growing and Developing

As early as this week, a plate that will become the heart has developed. Two tubes join to form the heart and begin contracting by day 22 of development. A beating heart is visible as early as 5 to 6 weeks of pregnancy during an ultrasound examination.

Eyes first appear around this time and look like a pair of shallow grooves on each side of the developing brain. These grooves continue to develop and eventually turn into pockets called *optical vesicles*.

The central nervous system (brain and spinal cord) and muscle and bone formation continue. Baby's skeleton is starting to form.

Changes in You

Home pregnancy tests are very sensitive, which makes early diagnosis of pregnancy possible. Tests detect the presence of human chorionic gonadotropin (HCG), a hormone of early pregnancy. A pregnancy test can be positive before you have even missed a period!

Many tests can provide positive results (you're pregnant) 10 days after you conceive. You might want to wait until you miss a period before investing money and emotional energy in any pregnancy test.

The best time to take a home pregnancy test is the first day after your missed period or any time thereafter. If you take the test too early, you may get a result that says you aren't pregnant when you really are! This happens for about 50% of the women who take the test very early.

47

> ## Tip for Week 5
> • • • • • • • • • • •
>
> Pregnancy may affect your sense of smell. You may smell odors more intensely; odors that do not normally affect you may now smell bad. If you're sensitive to the smell of food, try eating a piece of cheddar cheese, some cottage cheese, dry-roasted nuts or cold chicken.

Nausea and Vomiting

An early symptom of pregnancy for some women is nausea, with or without vomiting; it is often called *morning sickness*. About 50% of all pregnant women experience nausea and vomiting, about 25% of pregnant women have nausea only and 25% experience no symptoms. You may get morning sickness if you suffer from motion sickness or migraines before pregnancy.

There is good news about morning sickness—women with nausea and vomiting in pregnancy have a lower incidence of miscarriage. The sicker you are, the less chance you will miscarry.

Morning sickness can occur in the morning or later in the day. It often starts early and improves during the day as you become active. The condition may begin around the 6th week of pregnancy.

Take heart—morning sickness usually improves and disappears around the end of the first trimester (week 13). Hang in there, and keep in mind it is all temporary.

Morning sickness can affect your pregnancy weight gain. For many women with morning sickness, weight gain may not begin until the beginning of the second trimester, when nausea and vomiting often pass.

If morning sickness is wearing you down, call your healthcare provider. Ask about different ways to deal with it. Assurances that this situation is normal and your baby is OK can be comforting.

Did your mother have severe morning sickness when she was pregnant with you or any of your siblings? If so, you may also be more likely to have it.

Hyperemesis Gravidarum. Nausea doesn't usually cause enough trouble to require medical attention. However, a condition called *hyperemesis gravidarum* (severe nausea and vomiting) causes a lot of vomiting, which results in loss of nutrients and fluid. Only 1 to 2% of all pregnant women experience hyperemesis gravidarum. Very high levels of nausea-inducing hormones may be one cause.

You have hyperemesis gravidarum if you're unable to keep down 80 ounces of fluid in 24 hours, if you lose more than 2 pounds a week or 5% of your prepregnancy weight, or if you vomit blood or bile. Contact your healthcare provider immediately!

If symptoms are severe, call your healthcare provider's office as soon as possible. Even though your first prenatal appointment may not be scheduled for a while, there's no reason to suffer. Your healthcare provider will want to know about the problem. You may have to ask to be seen sooner than a normal first prenatal appointment so you can find some relief.

Studies show if you experience hyperemesis gravidarum, your chance of having a daughter increases by more than 75%. Experts believe the cause may be an overabundance of female hormones produced by the baby and mom-to-be in the first trimester.

If you experience severe nausea and vomiting, if you cannot eat or drink anything or if you feel so ill you can't carry on with your daily activities, call your healthcare provider. Call if your urine is dark, you produce little urine, you feel dizzy when you stand up, your heart races or pounds, or you vomit blood or bile.

In severe cases, a woman may need to be treated in the hospital with intravenous fluids and medications. Hypnosis has also been used successfully in treating the problem.

It has been commonly believed symptoms associated with hyperemesis gravidarum disappear after pregnancy. This is the case for most women, but a few women experience symptoms well beyond delivery that can take months to overcome. Symptoms include food aversions, gastroesophageal reflux disease (GERD), digestive problems, nausea, gallbladder issues, fatigue and muscle weakness. Women who received I.V. feedings during pregnancy because they couldn't eat had the highest rate of symptoms.

Recovery can take a few months to as long as 2 years. Some believe it takes 1 to 2 months of recovery for every month you were ill. Women who have nausea and/or vomiting into late pregnancy find it usually takes several months to regain their energy and restore nutritional reserves.

If your hyperemesis gravidarum persists after baby's birth, you may need to see a nutritionist. It is especially important to seek help before you plan another pregnancy. Discuss it with your healthcare provider.

If morning sickness causes you to be absent from your job, the Family and Medical Leave Act (FMLA) states you do not need a healthcare provider's note verifying the problem. Nausea and vomiting during pregnancy is classified as a "chronic condition" and may require you to be out occasionally, but you don't need treatment.

Treating Morning Sickness. There is no completely successful treatment for normal nausea and vomiting. Research has found some women find relief by taking a vitamin B_6 supplement. It's readily available and inexpensive. If vitamin B_6 alone doesn't work, your healthcare provider might want to add an antihistamine.

Diclegis is a prescription medication that is a combination of B_6 and antihistamine. The FDA has approved its use to treat morning sickness. It is useful for women who have not responded to other treatments.

You may also want to ask your healthcare provider about taking PremesisRx, a once-a-day tablet, or Emetrol, an over-the-counter antinausea medication. A different prenatal vitamin might be easier on your stomach. A regular multivitamin—not a prenatal vitamin—or

Some Interesting Facts about Morning Sickness
· · · · · · · · · · ·

- Nausea and vomiting are uncommon in Asia and Africa.
- Morning sickness is more common in women carrying multiples.
- Heartburn and reflux can make morning sickness worse.
- Other conditions can cause nausea and vomiting in early pregnancy, including pancreatitis, gastroenteritis, appendicitis and pyelonephritis, as well as some metabolic disorders.
- If you don't have morning sickness in early pregnancy then experience nausea and vomiting later in pregnancy, it's *not* morning sickness.

a folic-acid supplement during the first trimester may also be better.

· ·

A ReliefBand may help relieve morning sickness. It's worn like a wrist watch on the inside of your wrist. It stimulates nerves with gentle electric signals, believed to interfere with messages between the brain and stomach that cause nausea. It can be used when nausea begins, or you can wear it before you feel ill. It's water resistant and shock resistant, so you can wear it just about any time!

· ·

Acupressure, acupuncture and massage may prove helpful in dealing with nausea and vomiting. Acupressure wristbands, worn for motion sickness and seasickness, and other devices help some women feel better.

This is an extremely important period in the development of your baby. Don't expose baby to herbs, over-the-counter treatments or any other "remedies" for nausea that are not known to be safe during pregnancy.

Some Actions You Can Take. Eat small meals more frequently. Experts agree you should eat what appeals to

you—these foods may be the ones you can keep down more easily right now. If that means sourdough bread and lemon-lime soda, go for it! Some women find protein foods settle more easily in their stomachs; these foods include cheese, eggs, peanut butter and nonfatty meats. A 2-ounce bar of dark chocolate may also help relieve nausea.

Ginger may help reduce vomiting. Make tea from fresh ginger, and drink it to calm your stomach. Taking about 350mg of ginger supplements may also help. Be careful when choosing ginger-root supplements. There's a difference in quality of ginger from different manufacturers. Buy from a reliable company.

If you've heard about Nzu to treat morning sickness, don't use it. It is a traditional remedy from Africa that looks like balls of mud or clay. It's dangerous because it contains high levels of lead and arsenic.

Keep up your fluid intake, even if you can't keep food down. Dehydration is more serious than not eating for a while. If you vomit a lot, you may want to choose fluids that contain electrolytes to help replace those you lose when you vomit. Ask your healthcare provider what fluids he or she recommends.

Other Changes You May Notice

In early pregnancy, you may need to urinate a lot. This can continue during most of your pregnancy. It may really get annoying near delivery as your uterus gets bigger and puts pressure on your bladder.

You may also notice breast changes. Tingling or soreness in the breasts or nipples is common. You may see a darkening of the areola or a lifting of the glands around the nipple. See Week 13 for more information on how breasts are affected by pregnancy.

Another early symptom of pregnancy is tiring easily, which may continue through pregnancy. Take your prenatal vitamins and any other medications prescribed by your healthcare provider. Get enough rest. If you're tired, stay away from sugar and caffeine; either can make the problem worse.

Fatigue in Pregnancy

You may feel exhausted early in pregnancy. It may be hard to get out of bed in the morning, or you may find yourself falling asleep in the middle of the afternoon. Don't worry—this is normal, especially in early pregnancy.

It takes a lot of energy to be pregnant, and your body uses a lot of energy as your baby grows. Your lungs deliver oxygen to you and baby. Your heart works hard to pump the extra (up to 50% extra) blood through your body. All the while, you may have to deal with raging hormones and other demands on your energy levels. It's like you are running a marathon for 9 months!

Take time to deal with your fatigue. Do what you can. Rest during the day if possible. To help fight fatigue, follow the 45-second rule—if it takes 45 seconds or less to take care of something, do it. This may help reduce fatigue and stress.

Many moms-to-be wake up five or more times a night, which can cause fatigue during the day. Baby's movements, leg cramps and shortness of breath may also keep you up later in your pregnancy. A short nap in the middle of the afternoon may pep you up and help make up for lost sleep. It's important to get enough rest, especially late in pregnancy. Research shows women who slept fewer than 6 hours at night were four times more likely to have a Cesarean delivery.

How Your Actions Affect Your Baby's Development

One of the first questions you may ask when you suspect you're pregnant is, "When should I see my healthcare provider?" Good prenatal care is necessary for the health of the baby and mother-to-be. Make an appointment for your first prenatal visit as soon as you're reasonably sure you're pregnant. This could be as early as a few days after a missed period.

Drinking Energy Drinks

Are energy drinks OK for pregnant women to drink? After doing research on these drinks, we have to answer, "No."

If you believe an energy drink is a sports drink, you're wrong. Sports drinks contain electrolytes, which help rehydrate someone who has been perspiring from exercise or because of hot weather. (During pregnancy, it's best to discuss drinking sports drinks with your healthcare provider.)

Energy drinks could more accurately be described as "stimulant beverages." They do not usually contain electrolytes, but they do often contain two or more times the amount of sugar and at least one stimulant, most often caffeine. In some cases, an energy drink has three to five times the amount of caffeine as a cola drink.

Avoid energy drinks during pregnancy because they may raise your blood pressure. You also want to avoid excessive amounts of caffeine, which many of these drinks contain. See the discussion of caffeine in Week 13. Some drinks contain as much as 500mg of caffeine! And to top it off, energy drinks may contribute to tooth decay and cavities because it takes longer for your saliva to neutralize acid in the mouth after drinking an energy drink.

. . . .

If you've been using some type of birth control, tell your healthcare provider. No method is 100% effective. Occasionally a method fails, even oral contraceptives. Don't panic if this happens to you. If you're sure you're pregnant, stop taking the pill and make an appointment as soon as possible.

. . . .

Your Nutrition

As discussed above, you may have to deal with nausea and vomiting during pregnancy. There are quite a few things you can try. Eat small meals frequently to keep your stomach from being over-full. Drink lots of fluid.

Find out what foods, smells or situations nauseate you. Avoid them when possible. Avoid coffee because it stimulates stomach acid. A high-protein or high-carbohydrate snack before bed may help.

Ask your partner to make you some dry toast in the morning before you get up; eat it in bed. Or keep crackers or dry cereal near you to nibble on before you get up in the morning to help absorb stomach acid.

Keep your bedroom cool at night, and air it out often. Cool, fresh air may help you feel better. Get out of bed slowly.

When you feel queasy, eat some soda crackers, cold chicken, pretzels or ginger snaps. Nibble on raw ginger, or pour boiling water over it and sip the "tea." Salty foods help some women with nausea. Lemonade and watermelon may also relieve symptoms. If you take an iron supplement, take it an hour before meals or 2 hours after a meal.

You Should Also Know

Weight Gain during Pregnancy

The amount of weight women gain during pregnancy varies greatly. It may range from weight loss to a total gain of 50 pounds or more, so it is difficult to set one figure as an "ideal" weight gain during pregnancy. But experts agree— gain the recommended weight during pregnancy to have a healthier pregnancy.

How much weight you gain is influenced by your prepregnancy weight.

Pregnancy Weight Gain
. . . .

Weight before pregnancy	Recommended gain during pregnancy (in pounds)
Underweight	28 to 40
Normal weight	25 to 35
Overweight	15 to 25
Obese	11 to 20
Morbidly obese	Your healthcare provider will determine weight gain

Another way to figure how much weight you should gain during pregnancy is to look at your BMI (body mass index). BMI guidelines for weight gain during pregnancy include the following:

BMI of less than 18.5—gain between 28 and 40 pounds
BMI of 18.5 to 25—gain between 25 and 35 pounds
BMI of 26 to 29—gain between 15 and 25 pounds
BMI of 30 to 39—gain between 11 and 20 pounds
BMI of 40 and over—healthcare provider will determine weight gain

Experts agree that what you weigh before pregnancy is the best indicator of how much weight you should gain during pregnancy. In addition, if you're shorter than 5'2" tall, try to gain at the lower end of your weight range.

Statistics show nearly 45% of all pregnant women gain more weight than they should. If you do, your risk of problems goes up. You also put your baby at risk.

Many experts call for a weight-gain figure of 2/3 pound (10 ounces) a week until 20 weeks, then 1 pound a week from 20 to 40 weeks. Other researchers have set up weight-gain guidelines for underweight, normal weight, overweight and obese women. See the box above.

Don't diet while you're pregnant, but do watch what you eat. If you're a normal-weight woman, don't eat more than 2200 to 2500 calories a day during the first trimester of your pregnancy. During the second trimester, increase that amount by about 300 calories a day. In the third trimester, add only an additional 100 calories (beyond the 300 calories you added during the second trimester). By the end of your pregnancy, you should be eating between 2600 and 2900 calories a day.

If you dieted a lot before pregnancy, you may gain more weight than recommended during pregnancy, so pay strict attention to your eating plan. Choose foods for the nutrition they provide. Watch your stress levels, and try not to get too tired. If you're stressed, fatigued or anxious, you may eat more fats, sweets and junk-food snacks. This can lead to gaining too much weight during pregnancy.

If you want to breastfeed, gaining too much weight may contribute to breastfeeding problems. The extra weight may delay your milk from coming in.

If you have any questions, discuss them with your healthcare provider.

. . . .

To help boost energy levels, massage the webbed area between your big toe and the toe next to it. It's an acupressure "sweet" spot that helps increase blood flow to your brain. By doing this, you could increase your energy level by 50%—and it could last up to 2 hours!

. . . .

Ectopic (Tubal) Pregnancy

In a normal pregnancy, fertilization occurs in the Fallopian tube. The fertilized egg travels through the tube to the uterus where it implants on the cavity wall.

An *ectopic pregnancy* occurs in the first 12 weeks of pregnancy when the egg implants outside the uterine cavity, usually in the tube. Ninety-five percent of all ectopic pregnancies occur in the Fallopian tube (hence the term *tubal pregnancy*). The illustration on the opposite page shows some possible locations of an ectopic pregnancy.

We have seen the number of ectopic pregnancies almost triple since 1985. Today about 7 in every 1000 pregnancies is ectopic. Researchers believe STDs (sexually transmitted diseases) are the cause, especially chlamydia and gonorrhea. If you have had an STD, tell your healthcare provider at your first prenatal visit. And tell him or her if you have had a previous ectopic pregnancy; there's a 12% chance it will happen again.

Chances of having an ectopic pregnancy increase with damage to the Fallopian tubes from pelvic inflammatory disease (PID), other infections, infertility, endometriosis and tubal or abdominal surgery. Smoking, exposure to DES (diethylstilbestrol) during your mother's pregnancy and being older may also increase your risk. Use of an IUD also increases the chance of ectopic pregnancy.

Symptoms of ectopic pregnancy include:

• cramps or low-back pain
• tenderness in the lower abdomen
• bleeding or brown spotting
• shoulder pain
• weakness, dizziness or fainting caused by blood loss
• nausea
• low blood pressure

Diagnosing Ectopic Pregnancy. To test for ectopic pregnancy, human chorionic gonadotropin is measured. The test is called a *quantitative HCG*. The level of HCG increases rapidly in a normal pregnancy and doubles in value about every 2 days. If HCG levels do not increase as they should, an ectopic pregnancy is suspected.

Ultrasound testing is helpful. An ectopic pregnancy may be visible in the tube. Blood may be seen in the abdomen.

We are better able to diagnose ectopic pregnancy with laparoscopy. Tiny incisions are made in the area of the bellybutton and in the lower-abdomen area. A doctor looks inside the abdomen at the pelvic organs with a small instrument called a *laparoscope*. An ectopic pregnancy can be seen if one is present.

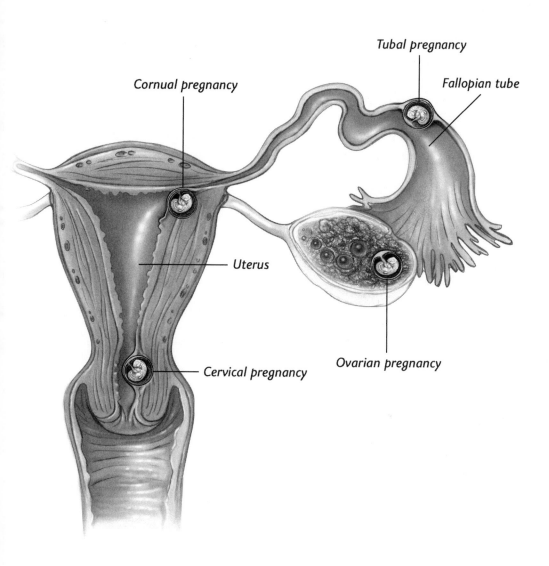

Tubal pregnancy

Cornual pregnancy

Fallopian tube

Uterus

Cervical pregnancy

Ovarian pregnancy

Possible locations of an ectopic pregnancy.

It's best to diagnose a tubal pregnancy before it ruptures and damages the tube. This could make it necessary to remove the entire tube. Early diagnosis also tries to avoid the risk of internal bleeding from a ruptured tube.

Most ectopic pregnancies are detected around 6 to 8 weeks of pregnancy. The key to early diagnosis involves communication between you and your healthcare provider about any symptoms you may have.

Treatment for Ectopic Pregnancy. The goal is to remove the pregnancy while maintaining fertility. Treatment requires anesthesia, laparoscopy or laparotomy (a larger incision and no scope) and recovery from surgery.

A nonsurgical treatment involves the use of methotrexate. It is given by I.V. in the hospital or at an outpatient clinic. Methotrexate ends the pregnancy. HCG levels should decrease after this treatment, and symptoms should improve. If methotrexate is used to treat an ectopic pregnancy, a couple should wait at least 3 months before trying to conceive again.

Exercise for Week 5

· · · · · · ·

Lightly grasp the back of a chair or a counter for balance. Stand with your feet shoulder-width apart. Keep your body weight over your heels and your torso erect. Bend your knees, and lower your torso in a squatting position. Don't round your back. Hold the squatting position for 5 seconds, then straighten to starting position. Start with 5 repetitions and work up to 10. *Strengthens hip, thigh and buttocks muscles.*

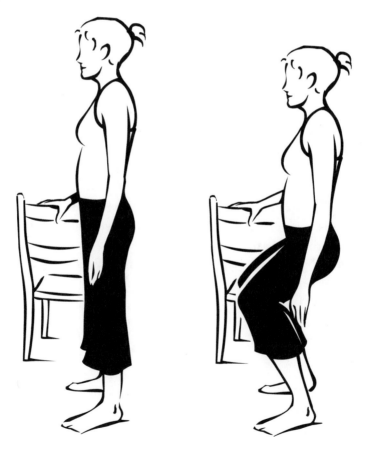

· · · · · · ·

Week 6

Age of Fetus—4 Weeks

If you've just found out you're pregnant, you might want to begin by reading the previous chapters.

How Big Is Your Baby?

Crown-to-rump length is the sitting height or distance from the top of the baby's head to its rump or buttocks. The crown-to-rump length of your baby by this week is 0.08 to 0.16 inch (2 to 4mm).

How Big Are You?

You've been pregnant for 1 month, so you should have noticed a few changes in your body by now. You may have gained a few pounds. Or you may have lost weight. If this is your first pregnancy, your abdomen probably hasn't changed much. You may be gaining weight in your breasts or other places. If you have a pelvic exam, your healthcare provider can usually feel your uterus and note some change in its size.

How Your Baby Is Growing and Developing

During the *embryonic period* (from conception to week 10 of pregnancy, or from conception to week 8 of fetal development), the embryo is most susceptible

to things that can interfere with its development. Most birth defects happen during this critical period.

As the illustration on page 60 shows, baby's body has a head and tail area. Around this time, early brain chambers form. The forebrain, midbrain, hindbrain and spinal cord are established.

The heart tube divides into bulges, which develop into heart chambers, called *ventricles* (left and right) and *atria* (left atrium and right atrium). They form between weeks 6 and 7. Occasionally, with the proper equipment, a heartbeat can be seen on ultrasound by the 6th week. Eyes are also forming, and limb buds appear.

Changes in You

Heartburn

Heartburn discomfort (pyrosis) is one of the most common discomforts of pregnancy. *Heartburn* is defined as a burning sensation in the middle of your chest; it often occurs soon after eating. You may also experience an acid or bitter taste in your mouth and increased pain when you bend over or lie down. During the first trimester, nearly 25% of all pregnant women have heartburn.

Heartburn occurs when your digestive tract relaxes and stomach acid creeps back into the esophagus. It occurs more frequently during pregnancy for two reasons—food moves more slowly through the intestines, and the stomach is squeezed a bit as the uterus gets bigger and moves up into the abdomen.

Symptoms are not severe for most women. Eat small, frequent meals, and avoid some positions, such as bending over or lying flat. Be sure the area from your bellybutton up to your Adam's apple is raised. One sure way to get heartburn is to eat a large meal then lie down flat! (This is true for anyone, not just pregnant women.)

Some antacids offer relief; follow your healthcare provider's advice or package instructions relating to pregnancy. Don't take too much antacid! Avoid sodium bicarbonate because it contains a lot of sodium, which may cause you to retain water.

. . . .
If you have heartburn, cut down on the amount of chocolate you eat because it may make the problem worse.
. . . .

Other actions you take may help with heartburn. Don't overeat, and don't eat late at night. Avoid foods that trigger your heartburn. Be careful with carbonated drinks. Use less fat when cooking.

You can help relieve the problem by trying various things. Wear loose clothing. Stay upright after meals, especially in late pregnancy. Chew gum for 30 minutes after meals and when heartburn strikes. Suck on hard candy. Reduce stress in your life.

For a medicine-free treatment, thoroughly chew 1 or 2 teaspoons of uncooked oat flakes, then swallow. The oatmeal will absorb much of the stomach acid that causes the heartburn. Or mix the juice of ½ lemon and a pinch of salt in 8 ounces of water, and drink it before meals. After meals, 1 teaspoon of honey may help ease discomfort.

Avoid licorice root to treat heartburn; it can raise blood pressure and lower potassium levels. Instead, chew 400 to 800mg of deglycyrrhizinated licorice (DGL) for 20 minutes before meals or before you go to bed. You can use this treatment up to 3 times a day.

When you exercise, don't eat for 2 hours before you begin. Use smooth movement to avoid pushing acids into your esophagus.

GERD. *GERD (gastroesophageal reflux disease)* or *acid-reflux disease* may be mistaken for heartburn during pregnancy. It's very common but often overlooked. The three most common symptoms include heartburn, a sour or bitter taste, and difficulty swallowing. Other symptoms may include persistent cough, hoarseness, upset stomach and chest pain.

Choose foods carefully. Eating too much food that is spicy, highly acidic or high in fat may aggravate acid reflux.

Only your healthcare provider can determine whether you have acid reflux, or GERD, so talk to him or her at a prenatal appointment if it bothers you.

Actual size

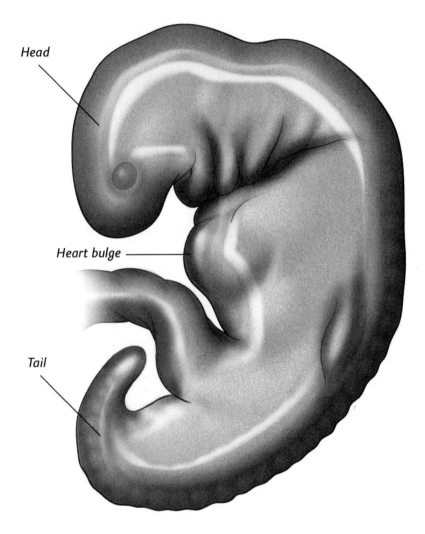

Head

Heart bulge

Tail

Embryo at 6 weeks of pregnancy (fetal age—4 weeks).
It is growing rapidly.

The Difference between Indigestion and Heartburn
. . . .

Some people who suffer from heartburn say they are suffering from indigestion, but indigestion isn't the same thing as heartburn. Although they have similar triggers and treatment may be the same in many instances, they are different. *Indigestion* is a condition; *heartburn* may be a symptom of indigestion.

Indigestion is a vague feeling of discomfort and pain in the upper abdomen and chest. It includes a feeling of fullness and bloating, accompanied by belching and nausea. Occasionally heartburn is a symptom.

Several things can trigger indigestion, including overeating, eating a particular food, drinking alcohol or carbonated beverages, eating too quickly or too much, eating fatty or spicy foods, drinking too much caffeine, smoking or eating too much high-fiber foods. Anxiety and depression can worsen symptoms.

He or she may prescribe a medication that is safe to use during pregnancy. If you now take prescription or over-the-counter medicines to treat your problem, check with your healthcare provider before continuing their use.

Constipation

Your bowel habits will probably change during pregnancy. Most women notice some constipation. Two things add to the problem in pregnancy—increased hormones and blood-volume increase. You may not be drinking enough fluid, which can cause dehydration (and constipation) in you.

Increase your fluid intake. Foods that contain a lot of water include frozen juice treats, watermelon, citrus or a slush made with fresh fruit juice and water. In addition, foods with lots of fiber hold onto water longer, which helps soften your stools.

Exercise may help. It shifts body position, which may stimulate your bowels and increase muscle contractions to help move food through your intestines.

Many healthcare providers suggest a mild laxative if you have problems. Certain foods, such as bran and prunes, can increase the bulk in your diet, which may help relieve constipation.

Don't use laxatives without your healthcare provider's OK. If constipation continues, discuss treatment at a prenatal visit. Try not to strain when you have a bowel movement; straining can lead to hemorrhoids.

How Your Actions Affect Your Baby's Development

Sexually Transmitted Diseases

Infections or diseases passed from one person to another by sexual contact are called *sexually transmitted diseases (STDs)*. These infections can affect your ability to get pregnant. During pregnancy, a sexually transmitted disease can harm your growing baby. Take care of an STD as soon as possible!

About 2 million pregnant women have an STD. That's over 40%! Many don't even know they have one. Ask for a test or treatment if you think you have an STD. Your healthcare provider routinely offers tests for hepatitis B, HIV and syphilis.

Genital Herpes. It's not uncommon for a woman to have genital herpes during pregnancy. If you do, there's a good chance you'll have an outbreak during pregnancy.

Herpes can be dangerous for your baby. If you contract herpes during pregnancy, your baby is at highest risk. If your first outbreak is near delivery, your baby has a higher chance of having problems.

There's no safe treatment for genital herpes during pregnancy. Some women are given valacyclovir during the last month of pregnancy in an attempt to suppress an outbreak. One study found this decreases the chance of an outbreak by nearly 70%. If a woman has a herpes outbreak late in pregnancy, she may have a Cesarean delivery.

Yeast Infections. Monilial (yeast) infections are more common in pregnant women. They have no major effect on pregnancy, but they may cause you discomfort and anxiety.

Yeast infections are sometimes harder to control and may require frequent retreatment or longer treatment during pregnancy. Creams used for treatment are usually safe during pregnancy. Avoid fluconazole (Diflucan); it may not be safe to use during pregnancy. Your partner does not need to be treated.

A newborn infant can get thrush after passing through a birth canal infected with monilial vulvovaginitis. Treatment with nystatin is effective.

Vaginitis. Vaginitis, also called *trichomonal vaginitis* or *trichomoniasis*, is the most common STD among women. It has no major effects on a pregnancy. Treatment includes metronidazole (Flagyl) for you and your partner. Some experts believe metronidazole shouldn't be taken in the first trimester of pregnancy. Most healthcare providers will prescribe metronidazole for a bad infection after the first trimester.

Human Papillomavirus (HPV; Genital Warts). HPV is one of the most common STDs in the United States. In some people, HPV causes venereal (genital) warts, also called *condyloma acuminata*. Genital warts may grow faster during pregnancy because of lowered immunity, pregnancy hormones and increased blood flow to the pelvic area. Warts may enlarge during pregnancy; in rare cases they have blocked the vagina at the time of delivery. If you have many venereal warts, a Cesarean delivery may be necessary.

The Pap smear done at one of your first prenatal visits can assure you that you do not have this problem. If you have genital warts, tell your healthcare provider at your first prenatal appointment. During pregnancy, certain treatments should be avoided.

HPV vaccine is recommended for all males and females between the ages of 9 and 26. It is not recommended during pregnancy. However, it is considered safe during breastfeeding.

Gonorrhea. Gonorrhea presents risks to a woman and her partner, as well as her baby when it passes through the birth canal. The baby may contract *gonorrheal ophthalmia*, a severe eye infection. Eye drops are used in newborns to prevent this problem.

. . . .

Research has determined women with chlamydia or gonorrhea infections before or during pregnancy have a higher risk of complications during pregnancy. Often women diagnosed with gonorrhea have also previously been infected with chlamydia. This is important information, and it may help your healthcare provider anticipate problems in your pregnancy. Be sure to share it with him or her.

. . . .

Syphilis. Detection of a syphilis infection is important for you, your partner and your growing baby. Screening tests for syphilis during pregnancy have reduced the rate of syphilis in babies. If you notice any open sore on your genitals, have your healthcare provider check it. Syphilis can be treated with penicillin and other safe medications.

Chlamydia. Chlamydia is an infection caused by a germ that invades certain types of healthy cells. Chlamydia is passed through sexual activity, including oral sex. Chlamydial infection has been linked to ectopic pregnancy. In one study, 70% of the women who had an ectopic pregnancy also had chlamydia.

Chlamydia is most likely to occur in people who have more than one sexual partner. It may also occur in women who have other sexually transmitted diseases.

Some healthcare providers believe chlamydia occurs more commonly in women who take oral contraceptives. Barrier methods of contraception, such as diaphragms and condoms used with spermicides, may offer some protection from infection.

A mother-to-be can pass the infection to her baby as it comes through the birth canal. It may cause an eye infection in baby, but that's easily treated. A baby may also develop pneumonia.

You may not have symptoms of chlamydia—75% of those infected do not. Symptoms include burning or itching in the genital area, discharge from the vagina, painful or frequent urination, or pain in the pelvic area. Men may also have symptoms.

Chlamydia can be detected by a cell culture. During pregnancy, erythromycin may be the drug of choice, or Zithromax may be prescribed for you and your partner.

After treatment, your healthcare provider may want to do another culture to make sure the infection is gone. The test may be repeated late in pregnancy to be sure you don't have the disease when you go into labor.

. . . .

There is evidence Lyme disease may be transmitted sexually. Studies show the same strain of bacteria in married couples who had unprotected sex. If your partner has had Lyme disease, let your healthcare provider know.

. . . .

Pelvic Inflammatory Disease (PID). Pelvic inflammatory disease (PID) is a severe infection of the upper genital organs involving the uterus, the

Fallopian tubes and even the ovaries. There may be pelvic pain, or there may be no symptoms at all. Infection can result in scarring and blockage of the tubes, making it difficult or impossible to get pregnant or making you more susceptible to an ectopic pregnancy. Surgery may be required to repair damage. Pelvic inflammatory disease (PID) can result from an untreated chlamydia infection. Chlamydia is one of the main causes of PID.

HIV and AIDS. *HIV* (human immunodeficiency virus) is the virus that causes AIDS (acquired immune deficiency syndrome). It's estimated that 6000 babies are born every year to mothers infected with HIV. The CDC now recommends all pregnant women be offered HIV testing. Home testing kits are available; most are very reliable.

After HIV enters a person's bloodstream, the body begins to produce antibodies to fight the disease. A blood test can detect these antibodies. When detected, a person is considered "HIV-positive" and can pass the virus to others. This is not the same as having AIDS.

The virus weakens the immune system and makes it difficult for the body to fight off disease. Gynecological problems can be an early sign of an HIV infection, including ulcers in the vagina, yeast infections that won't go away and severe pelvic inflammatory disease (PID). If you have any of these problems, discuss them with your healthcare provider. Early diagnosis and treatment are crucial.

There may be a period of weeks or months when tests don't reveal the virus. In most cases, antibodies can be detected 6 to 12 weeks after exposure. In some cases, it can take as long as 18 months before antibodies are found.

Once a test is positive, a person may be free of symptoms for some time. Studies indicate taking over-the-counter multivitamins containing vitamins B, C and E every day may delay the progression of HIV and delay the need to start antiretroviral medications.

Two tests are used to determine if someone has HIV—the *ELISA test* and the *Western Blot test*. The ELISA is a screening test. If positive, it should be confirmed by the Western Blot test. Both tests involve testing blood to measure antibodies to the virus.

Before testing, a woman is advised she will be tested for HIV unless she declines—this is called *opt-out testing*. For those at high risk of HIV, experts suggest testing before pregnancy or as early in pregnancy as possible and testing again in the third trimester. Rapid HIV testing during labor is recommended if a woman's HIV status is unknown. This test has the same sensitivity and specificity as the ELISA test, and results are available within 30 minutes.

We know 90% of all cases of HIV in children are related to pregnancy—mother to baby during pregnancy, childbirth or breastfeeding. Research has shown an infected woman can pass the virus to her baby as early as 8 weeks of pregnancy. A mother can also pass HIV to baby during its birth. Breastfeeding is not recommended for women who are HIV-positive.

Research shows the chance of a woman infected with HIV passing the virus to her baby can be nearly eliminated with some medications. However, if an infection is not treated, there's a 25% chance a baby will be born with the virus. If a woman takes AZT during pregnancy and has a Cesarean delivery, she reduces the risk of passing the virus to about 2%! Studies have found no birth defects linked to the use of AZT. Other HIV medications have also been proved safe for use during pregnancy.

If you are HIV-positive, expect more blood tests during pregnancy. These tests help your healthcare provider assess how well you are doing.

The rate of *AIDS* among women has grown to 20% of all reported cases. AIDS can leave a person prone to, and unable to fight, various infections. If you are unsure about your risk, seek counseling about testing for the AIDS virus. Pregnancy may hide some AIDS symptoms, which makes the disease harder to discover.

There is some positive news for women who suffer from AIDS. We know if a woman is in the early course of the illness, she can usually have an uneventful pregnancy, labor and delivery.

Your Nutrition

During your pregnancy, you need to be selective in the foods you choose. Eating the right foods, in the correct amounts, takes planning. Eat foods high in vitamins and minerals, especially iron, calcium, magnesium, folate and zinc. You also need fiber.

Some of the foods you should eat, and the amounts of each, are listed below. Try to eat these foods every day. We discuss food groups in the following weeks. Check weekly discussions for nutrition tips. Foods to help your baby grow and develop include:

- bread, cereal, pasta and rice—at least 6 servings/day
- fruits—3 to 4 servings/day
- vegetables—4 servings/day
- meat and other protein sources—2 to 3 servings/day
- dairy products—3 to 4 servings/day
- fats, sweets and other "empty" calorie foods—2 to 3 servings/day

Understanding Serving Portions
You may believe it will be difficult for you to eat all the portions you need for the health of your growing baby. However, many people don't understand what a "portion" or "serving" really is.

Supersizing and huge portions have skewed our idea of what a normal portion size really is. For example, a blueberry muffin is now about 500 calories. Twenty-five years ago, it was about 200 calories. Look for the following serving sizes when you eat—they're what a "normal" portion size is.

- 1 cup of vegetables—the size of a lightbulb
- 1 serving of juice—a champagne flute
- 1 pancake—the size of a CD
- 1 teaspoon of peanut butter—the end of your thumb
- 3 ounces of fish—an eyeglass case
- 3 ounces of meat—a deck of playing cards
- 1 small potato—a 3x5 index card

Read labels for portion sizes; a common mistake is to read the calorie/nutrient information on a label and not take into account the *number of servings* each package contains. Even a very small package may contain two or more servings, doubling or tripling the calories if you eat the whole thing.

To learn the correct serving size for each of the food groups, check out the USDA's website www.cnpp.usda.gov; it lists actual serving portions. For example, a large bagel may be four to five grain servings! If you don't have access to a computer, ask your healthcare provider for some guidelines or nutrition handouts.

You Should Also Know

Your First Visit to Your Healthcare Provider

Your first prenatal visit may be one of your longest. There's a lot to do. If you saw your healthcare provider before you got pregnant, you may have already discussed some of your concerns.

Feel free to ask questions to get an idea of how your healthcare provider will relate to you and your needs. During pregnancy, there should be an exchange of ideas. Your healthcare provider has experience that can be valuable to you during pregnancy.

At this first visit, you will be asked for a history of your medical health. This includes general medical problems and any problems relating to your gynecological and obstetrical history. You will be asked about your periods and recent birth-control methods. If you've had an abortion or a miscarriage, or if you've been in the hospital for surgery or for some other reason, it's important information. If you have old medical records, bring them with you.

Your healthcare provider needs to know about medicine you take or medication you are allergic to. Your family's medical history may also be important.

Various tests may be done at this first visit or on a subsequent visit. If you have questions, ask them. If you think you may have a "high-risk" pregnancy, discuss it with your healthcare provider.

In most cases, you will be asked to return every 4 weeks for the first 7 months, then every 2 weeks until the last month, then every week. If problems arise, you may be scheduled for more frequent visits.

Ways to Have a Great Pregnancy

Every woman wants to have a happy, healthy pregnancy. Start now to help ensure that yours will be the best it can be!

Dad Tip
· · · · · · · · · · ·

Is your partner suffering from morning sickness? If so, cooking can be a real chore for her. Just looking at food or smelling it can make her feel sick. To help out, bring home your dinner, or cook it yourself. Sometimes it's the only way you'll get any food!

Prioritize and examine what you need to do to help yourself and your growing baby. Do what you need to do, decide what else you can do and let the rest go.

Create memories. It takes some planning, but it's worth it. Relax when you can. Easing the stress in your life is important. Focus on the positive.

Don't be afraid to ask for help. Friends and family will be pleased if you ask them to be involved.

Get information. There are many sources today, such as our books, various magazine articles, television programs, radio interviews and the Internet.

Remember—you're part of a very special miracle that is happening to you and your partner! Enjoy this time of preparation. Concentrate on your couple relationship and on the many changes you will experience in the near future.

Exercise for Week 6

• • • • • • •

Stand with your left side next to the sofa or a sturdy chair. Hold onto the back with your left hand. Standing with your feet shoulder-width apart, step back about 3 feet with your right foot. Bend your leg until your thigh is parallel to the floor. Keep your knee over your toes. Hold for 3 seconds, then as you return to standing position, lift your right leg and squeeze your buttocks muscles for 1 second. Start with 3 repetitions and work up to 6. Repeat for your other leg. *Strengthens hip, thigh and buttocks muscles.*

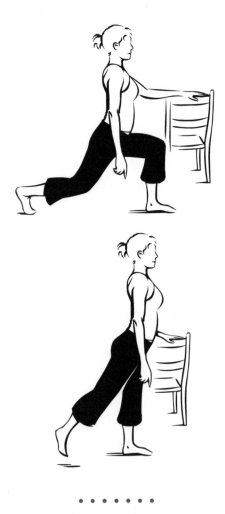

• • • • • • •

Week 7

Age of Fetus—5 Weeks

*If you've just found out you're pregnant, you might want to
begin by reading the previous chapters.*

How Big Is Your Baby?

Your baby goes through an incredible growth spurt around this time. At the beginning of this week, the crown-to-rump length is 0.16 to 0.2 inch (4 to 5mm), about the size of a BB pellet. By the end of the week, your baby has more than doubled in size, to about ½ inch (1.1 to 1.3cm).

How Big Are You?

Although you are probably quite anxious to show the world you're pregnant, there still may be little noticeable change. Changes will come soon.

How Your Baby Is Growing and Developing

Leg buds are beginning to appear as short fins. As you can see on page 70, arm buds have divided into a hand segment and an arm-shoulder segment. The hand and foot have a plate where the fingers and toes will develop.

The heart has divided into right and left chambers. An opening between the chambers called the *foramen ovale* appears. This opening lets blood pass from one chamber to the other, allowing it to bypass the lungs. At birth, the opening closes.

Air passages in the lungs are present. The brain is growing; the forebrain divides into two parts. Eyes and nostrils are developing.

Intestines are forming, and the appendix and pancreas are present. Part of the intestine bulges into the umbilical cord. Later in development, it returns to the abdomen.

Changes in You

Changes occur gradually. You should have gained only a couple of pounds by this time. If you haven't gained weight or if you have lost a couple of pounds, it's OK; it will go the other direction in the weeks to come. You may still have

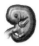

Actual size

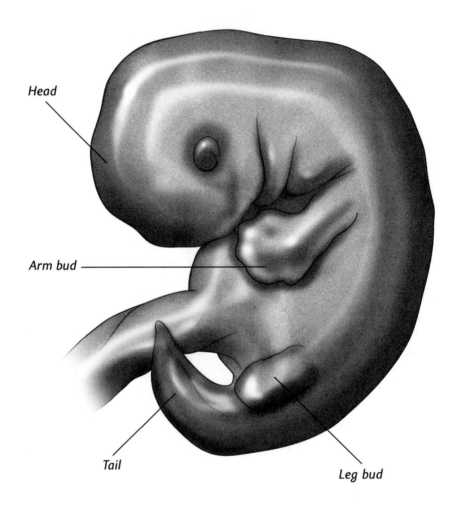

Head

Arm bud

Tail

Leg bud

Your baby's brain is growing and developing.
The heart has divided into right and left chambers.

morning sickness and other symptoms of early pregnancy.

How Your Actions Affect Your Baby's Development

Jewish Genetic Disorders

A group of medical conditions considered genetic disorders occur more commonly among Ashkenazi Jews, who are of eastern European descent. About 95% of the Jewish population in North America is of Ashkenazi heritage. Some of the diseases found in this group also affect Sephardi Jews and non-Jews; however, the conditions are more common among Ashkenazi Jews.

A great deal of research has been done to determine why these disorders occur more frequently in the Ashkenazi Jewish population. Researchers believe two processes are at work—the founder effect and genetic drift.

With the *founder effect*, genes that cause certain problems just happened to occur among the founders of the Ashkenazi Jews. This group emigrated to eastern Europe around 70 A.D. Before they left Palestine, these disorders were probably as common among all other groups in the area. When the Ashkenazi Jews settled together in Europe, they carried these genes.

Because Ashkenazi Jews do not often marry outside their faith or community, the genes were not spread among other communities. This is called *genetic drift*. Presence of the genes was not decreased by introducing genes from outside the community, so many of the problems remained within this group.

Some diseases and conditions occur within other Jewish groups, such as Sephardi Jews. Sephardi Jews are of Spanish or Portuguese descent, and particular disorders occur within this group, probably for the same reasons they occur among Ashkenazi Jews.

Today, various conditions are considered "Jewish genetic disorders." However, we know people of other ethnic backgrounds can inherit some of these diseases. Some diseases and conditions are rare in the general population. These disorders include:

- Bloom syndrome
- factor-XI deficiency
- familial dysautonomia (Riley-Day syndrome)
- Fanconi anemia (Group C)
- Gaucher disease
- glucose-6 phosphate dehydrogenase deficiency (G6PD)
- glycogen storage disease, type III
- mucolipidosis IV
- Niemann-Pick disease (Type A)
- nonclassical adrenal hyperplasia
- nonsyndromic hearing loss
- torsion dystonia

Some very good resources are available to anyone who wants to learn more about Jewish genetic disorders. Two we have contacted for information include:

The Chicago Center
for Genetic Disorders
Ben Gurion Way
One S. Franklin Street, 4th Floor
Chicago, IL 60606
312-357-4718
Email: jewishgeneticsctr@juf.org
www.jewishgeneticscenter.org

Center for Jewish Genetic Diseases
Mount Sinai School of Medicine
Box 1497
One Gustave L. Levy Place
New York, NY 10029
212-659-6774 (Main)
212-241-6947 (Consultation/
    Screening)
www.mssm.edu/jewish_genetics/
Screening tests are available for some of the diseases listed above. One test targets 11 genetic diseases and is designed for couples in which one or both members are of Ashkenazi or Sephardi Jewish descent. Many diseases can be identified before pregnancy or in early pregnancy. Discuss testing with your healthcare provider if you're interested.

Using Over-the-Counter (OTC) Medicines

Nearly 65% of all pregnant women use some sort of medicine during pregnancy, including nonprescription medicine, also called *over-the-counter medication* (OTC). Often, it is used to treat pain and discomfort.

Many people don't think of OTC products as medications and take them willy-nilly, pregnant or not. Some researchers believe over-the-counter medication use actually increases during pregnancy.

Some OTC products may *not* be safe during pregnancy. Use them with as much caution as any other drug! Many products are combinations of medicines. For example, pain medicine can contain aspirin, caffeine and phenacetin. Cough syrups or sleep medications can contain alcohol.

Read package labels and package inserts about safety during pregnancy—nearly all medicines contain this information. Some OTC products can be used safely during pregnancy if you use them wisely. Check the list below:

- analgesics and pain relievers—acetaminophen (Tylenol)
- decongestant—chlorpheniramine (Chlor-Trimeton)
- nasal spray decongestants—oxymetazoline (Afrin, Dristan Long-Lasting)
- cough medicine—dextromethorphan (Robitussin, Vicks Formula 44)
- stomach relief—antacids (Amphojel, Gelusil, Maalox, milk of magnesia)
- throat relief—throat lozenges (Sucrets)
- laxatives—bulk-fiber laxatives (Metamucil, Fiberall)

Never use any medication longer than 3 days without your healthcare provider's OK.

Claritin and Zyrtec are believed to be safe during pregnancy. If you have a yeast infection, ask your healthcare provider about using an over-the-counter treatment, such as Terazol or Monistat.

Avoid sudafed during the first trimester. Primatene Mist is not recommended for use in pregnancy. It may be a good idea to skip Airborne during pregnancy; it hasn't been tested on pregnant women.

If you think your symptoms or discomfort are more severe than they should be, call your healthcare provider.

Tip for Week 7
· · · · · · · · · · ·

Don't take over-the-counter medicines for longer than 48 hours without talking to your healthcare provider. If a problem doesn't get better, your healthcare provider may have another treatment plan for you.

Follow his or her advice, and take good care of yourself.

The Use of Acetaminophen

For years, we have been advising pregnant women acetaminophen (Tylenol) is safe during pregnancy. We're now rethinking that advisory, given the results of recent studies. Experts suggest acetaminophen remains in the body longer in pregnant women because of higher blood volume during pregnancy.

The most dangerous time for a mom-to-be to take acetaminophen appears to be during the second and third trimesters. This is the time a fetus's brain is developing. Studies have shown there may be an increased risk of ADHD (attention-deficit/hyperactivity disorder) in a child if the pregnant woman takes acetaminophen.

Researchers have issued a warning to pregnant women to take as little acetaminophen as possible during pregnancy. If you normally take acetaminophen to treat headaches, fever or aches and pains, it may be best for you to seek natural remedies for these problems when possible. If you do need to take acetaminophen, keep your dose to a minimum, and use it only for a short time.

If the problem doesn't go away, be sure to talk with your healthcare provider about it. He or she will help you explore other treatment options.

It may be easy to overdose on acetaminophen because it is in over 200 products! Taking more than one product to treat a condition or illness could be dangerous because acetaminophen is contained in various products you may take to treat a single problem. Always read labels!

Your Nutrition

Dairy products can be very important during pregnancy. They contain calcium and vitamin D; both are important to you and baby. Calcium helps keep your bones healthy; baby needs it to develop strong bones and teeth. Adequate levels of vitamin D may help decrease your chances of developing pre-eclampsia during pregnancy.

A pregnant woman should take in 1200mg of calcium a day (1½ times the recommended amount for nonpregnant women). Your prenatal vitamin supplies about 300mg, so be sure you eat enough of the right foods to get the other 900mg.

Read food labels to find out how much calcium per serving is in a

Dad Tip
· · · · · · · · · · ·

It's important to know what your partner is talking about when she talks to you about her pregnancy. If she uses terms you don't understand, ask her to explain them. Or take a quick look in our Glossary for a definition, page 433. It helps to become familiar with all the technical pregnancy terms you'll be hearing in the months that lie ahead.

packaged food. Every day, write down the amount of calcium in each food you eat, and keep a running total to be sure you're getting 1200mg. See the box on the opposite page to find out how to figure your daily calcium intake.

Some Good Sources of Calcium. Milk, cheese, yogurt and ice cream are good calcium sources. Other foods that contain calcium include broccoli, bok choy, collards, spinach, salmon, sardines, garbanzo beans (chickpeas), sesame seeds, almonds, cooked dried beans, tofu and trout. Various foods are fortified with calcium, such as some orange juice, breads, cereals and grains. Check your grocery shelves.

Some dairy foods you may choose, and their serving sizes, include the following:

- cottage cheese—¾ cup
- processed cheese (American)—2 ounces
- hard cheese (Parmesan or Romano)—1 ounce
- custard or pudding—1 cup
- milk (whole, 2%, 1%, skim)—8 ounces
- natural cheese (cheddar)—1½ ounces
- yogurt (plain or flavored)—1 cup

If you want to lower calories, choose low-fat dairy products. Calcium content is unaffected in low-fat dairy products. Good choices include skim milk, low-fat yogurt and low-fat cheese.

Increase the amount of calcium you get by adding powdered nonfat milk to recipes, such as mashed potatoes and meat loaf. Make fruit shakes with fresh fruit and milk; add a scoop of ice milk, frozen yogurt or ice cream. Cook rice and oatmeal in skim or low-fat milk. When you make canned soups, substitute milk for water. Have a smoothie instead of plain orange juice.

Some foods interfere with calcium absorption. Salt, tea, coffee, protein and unleavened bread lower the amount of calcium absorbed.

If you take antibiotics, read the label on your prescription. If it says not to take it with calcium-containing foods, take the antibiotic 1 hour before or 2 hours after meals.

If you're having trouble getting enough calcium into your diet, ask your healthcare provider about taking a calcium supplement. He or she can advise you.

How Much Calcium?
. . . .

It may be hard to determine how much calcium you're getting in foods you eat. Package labeling usually lists the *percentage of calcium* in a food serving. This may be confusing because it's hard to know how much that is.

The solution is to understand that labeling is based on the RDA recommendation for a nonpregnant woman, which is 800mg a day. If a package states "calcium 20%," just multiply 800 times 0.2, which gives you the amount of 160mg. Keep a written record of how much calcium you take in every day. You need a total of 1200mg of calcium a day.

Your body can't absorb more than 500mg of calcium at a time, so spread your intake out over the day. At breakfast, if you have calcium-fortified orange juice, calcium-fortified bread, cereal with milk and a carton of yogurt, you may be taking in a lot more than 500mg, but your body won't be able to absorb it!

. . . .

Eating yogurt supplies you with calcium. It may also help regulate blood pressure. Eating a 6-ounce serving of yogurt three or four times a week is beneficial in many ways.

. . . .

Lactose Intolerance. When lactose is not properly digested, it can cause gas, bloating, cramps and diarrhea; a person with this problem is referred to as *lactose intolerant.* If you're lactose intolerant, there are many sources of calcium available to you. Look for calcium-fortified products. Try rice milk and soy milk fortified with calcium and vitamin D. You may be able to buy lactose-free milk at your grocery store. If you like cheese, there are lactose-free brands you can buy.

The OTC medicine *Lactaid* helps the body break down lactose. There are no warnings or precautions about it for use in pregnancy, but check with your healthcare provider before you use it.

Listeriosis

Every year about 1500 cases of listeriosis, a form of food poisoning, are reported in the United States. About 500 of these cases occur in pregnant women. Babies born to moms who had listeriosis are at higher risk of developing problems.

To prevent listeriosis, avoid unpasteurized milk and any foods made from unpasteurized milk. Don't eat unpasteurized soft cheeses, such as Camembert, Brie, feta, Gorgonzola, bleu cheese and Roquefort. If they have been made with pasteurized milk, soft cheeses are OK during pregnancy. Read labels very carefully.

Undercooked poultry, red meat, seafood and hot dogs can also contain listeriosis. Cook all meat and seafood thoroughly. Be careful about cross-contamination of foods. If you put raw seafood or hot dogs on a counter or cutting board, thoroughly wash the area with soap and hot water or a disinfectant before you put other food on that surface.

Unpasteurized Milk and Juice—Is It OK for You? We've had women ask us about drinking raw milk and eating products made from raw milk that comes from cows, sheep and goats to help increase their calcium needs. Our advice is *not* to drink raw milk or eat products made from it! One study by the CDC showed some people in the United States became ill after drinking and/or eating raw-milk products.

Unpasteurized raw milk can contain harmful microorganisms. With pasteurization, milk is heated to a specific temperature and kept at that temperature for a set time to kill harmful organisms. Unpasteurized food products can be especially harmful to people with weakened immune systems, which occurs in pregnant women.

What about juice? Pasteurization kills harmful bacteria and organisms found in juice. Most refrigerated and frozen juices sold at grocery stores are pasteurized. Avoid buying apple juice or cider at a farmers' market or roadside stand, which could be unpasteurized. Beverages made from ground-tagged fruits (fruit that fell to the ground and lay there awhile) might be polluted by dirt or manure. With unpasteurized juice, you could be consuming dangerous germs along with your juice.

You Should Also Know

Sexual Intimacy during Pregnancy

Many couples want to know if it's all right to have sexual intercourse during pregnancy. Many men wonder if sex can harm a growing baby. Sexual relations are usually OK for a healthy pregnant woman and her partner, and frequent sexual activity shouldn't hurt a healthy pregnancy. Neither intercourse nor orgasm should be a problem if you have a low-risk pregnancy. The baby is well protected inside the amniotic sac.

If you have questions, bring them up at a prenatal visit. If your partner goes with you to your appointments, he may benefit from hearing your healthcare provider's advice. If he doesn't go with you, assure him there should be no problems if your healthcare provider gives you the go-ahead.

Sex doesn't just mean sexual intercourse. There are other ways for couples to be sensual together, including giving each other a massage, bathing together and talking about sex. Whatever you do, be honest with your partner about how you feel—and keep a sense of humor!

Your Prenatal Vitamin

Taking a prenatal vitamin can be very important for you and baby. Be sure your prenatal vitamin contains iodine—it's important for baby's brain development. One study showed only about half of all prenatal vitamins have it. Omega-3 fatty acids and DHA are also good for baby's brain development. Ask your pharmacist

A Look at Prenatal Vitamins
· · · · · · · · · · ·

Prenatal vitamins contain many needed substances for you and baby, so take one each day until baby is born. A typical prenatal vitamin contains the following:

- calcium to build baby's teeth and bones, and to help strengthen your own
- copper to help prevent anemia and to help in bone formation
- folic acid to reduce the risk of neural-tube defects and to help in blood-cell production
- iodine to help control metabolism
- iron to prevent anemia and to help baby's blood development
- vitamin A for general health and body metabolism
- vitamin B_1 for general health and body metabolism
- vitamin B_2 for general health and body metabolism
- vitamin B_3 for general health and body metabolism
- vitamin B_6 for general health and body metabolism
- vitamin B_{12} to promote blood formation
- vitamin C to aid in your body's absorption of iron
- vitamin D to strengthen baby's bones and teeth, and to help your body use phosphorus and calcium
- vitamin E for general health and body metabolism
- zinc to help balance fluids in your body, and to aid nerve and muscle function

if your prenatal vitamin contains these important substances.

Don't drink coffee or tea for 1 hour after taking your prenatal vitamin. These drinks prevent iron absorption.

Do You Need Extra Iron?

Nearly all diets that supply enough calories for you to gain weight during pregnancy have enough minerals to prevent mineral deficiency. However, few women have iron stores to meet pregnancy demands. The recommended dose is 27mg a day.

During pregnancy, your iron needs increase. Most women don't need iron supplements during the first trimester. If you take iron then, it can worsen symptoms of nausea and vomiting. Iron intake is most important in the second half of pregnancy. Be careful with antacid use—it can interfere with iron absorption.

Other Supplementation

Zinc may help you if you are thin or underweight. We believe zinc helps a thin woman increase her chances of giving birth to a bigger, healthier baby. If you have used zinc to reduce the length and severity of a cold, talk to your healthcare provider before using it during pregnancy. We don't know how it could affect a pregnant woman. Better to be safe than sorry.

The value of *fluoride* and fluoride supplementation in a pregnant woman is unclear. Some researchers believe fluoride supplementation during pregnancy results in improved teeth in the child, but not everyone agrees. Fluoride supplementation in a pregnant woman has not been proved harmful to her baby. Some prenatal vitamins contain fluoride.

Overactive Bladder and Incontinence Medications

Do you take medicine to treat an overactive bladder? If you do, talk to your healthcare provider before pregnancy or as soon as you find out you're pregnant. He or she can advise you about continued use of your medicine during pregnancy. Some commonly prescribed medications include Ditropan, Detrol LA, Sanctura and Enablex.

Exercise for Week 7

• • • • • • •

Stand with your right side next to the sofa or a sturdy chair. Holding onto the sofa or chair with your right hand, lift your right foot and place it on the arm of the piece of furniture. Bend forward until you feel a stretch in your leg. Hold for 10 seconds. Repeat for your left leg. *Stretches hamstrings, and strengthens thigh muscles.*

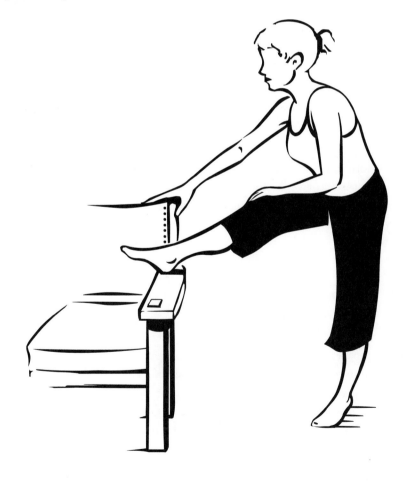

• • • • • • •

Week 8

Age of Fetus—6 Weeks

If you've just found out you're pregnant, you might want to begin by reading the previous chapters.

How Big Is Your Baby?

By this week of pregnancy, the crown-to-rump length of baby is ½ to ¾ inch (1.4 to 2cm). This is about the size of a pinto bean.

How Big Are You?

Your uterus is getting bigger, so you should be noticing a change in your waistline and the fit of your clothes. If you have a pelvic exam, your healthcare provider will be able to feel your enlarged uterus.

How Your Baby Is Growing and Developing

Your baby continues to grow and to change. Compare the illustration on page 82 with illustrations in the previous weeks. Can you see the changes?

Eyes are moving toward the middle of the face. Eyelid folds appear on the face, and nerve cells in the eye are beginning to develop. The tip of the nose is present. Internal and external ears are forming. The body's trunk area is getting longer and straightening out. Arms are longer. Elbows are present, and arms now bend at the elbows and curve slightly over the heart. Arms and legs extend forward. The beginning of fingers and toes can be seen.

Changes in You

As your uterus grows, you may feel cramping or even pain in your lower abdomen or at your sides. Some women feel tightening of the uterus throughout pregnancy. If you don't feel it, don't worry. But if you also have bleeding from the vagina, call your healthcare provider immediately.

Headaches and Migraines
Some pregnant women have various types of headaches during pregnancy. *Tension headaches* can be caused by stress, fatigue, heat, noise, thirst, hunger, loud music and bright lights. Some foods can trigger a headache, including peanuts, chocolate, cheese and some meats. If your sinuses are clogged, that may also increase headaches. *Cluster*

headaches come in groups, last about an hour and can continue for weeks or months.

. . . .

A headache or migraine that doesn't go away in late pregnancy could signal problems. Call your healthcare provider immediately!

. . . .

If you don't want to take medicine for a pounding headache, there are other things you can try. Exercise may help. Massage your neck and shoulders to help relax tight muscles. If you have a sinus headache, put a warm washcloth over your nose and eyes or a cold pack on the base of your neck. Fold a scarf lengthwise to make a 2-inch-wide band, tie it around your head and knot it at the point where pain is most intense.

Migraines. Migraine headaches are often an inherited problem. Nearly 20% of all pregnant women have a migraine at some point in pregnancy. A migraine can last for a few hours or up to 3 days. Some women suffer more during pregnancy because of their changing hormone levels.

. . . .

If you're getting a headache, try to stop it in its tracks with olive oil. Use 2 teaspoons of olive oil as a dip for bread or put it on your salad. Research shows this amount of olive oil contains the right amount of an antioxidant necessary to help control enzymes that cause headache pain.

. . . .

Ginger may help with migraines—a pinch of powdered ginger in water may be as good as prescription medicine. When you first feel symptoms, mix 1/3

teaspoon of powdered ginger in a cup of water. Drink this three or four times a day for 3 days.

Sciatic-Nerve Pain and Sacroiliac-Joint Pain

Many women experience an occasional excruciating pain in their buttocks and down their legs as pregnancy progresses. It is called *sciatic-nerve pain* or *sciatica*. Some people may mistakenly refer to it as sacroiliac pain, but they're not the same thing.

Sciatica is a sharp, searing pain that travels down your buttocks, legs and thighs. The best treatment is to lie on your opposite side to help relieve pressure on the nerve. Sitting on a tennis ball on a hard surface may also help.

Sacroiliac-joint pain (SJP) is joint related and feels like a sharp jolt of pain on either side of the back or hips. It may extend down your legs. Warm baths (not hot) and acetaminophen may help.

. . . .

Screening tests provide odds of a problem occurring. Diagnostic tests determine if a problem is present.

. . . .

How Your Actions Affect Your Baby's Development

Acne during Pregnancy

Some women notice an improvement in their acne during pregnancy, but it doesn't happen for everyone. Some women find that acne becomes a problem for them during pregnancy, even if it hasn't bothered them in the past.

Acne can range from whiteheads and blackheads to inflamed red bumps.

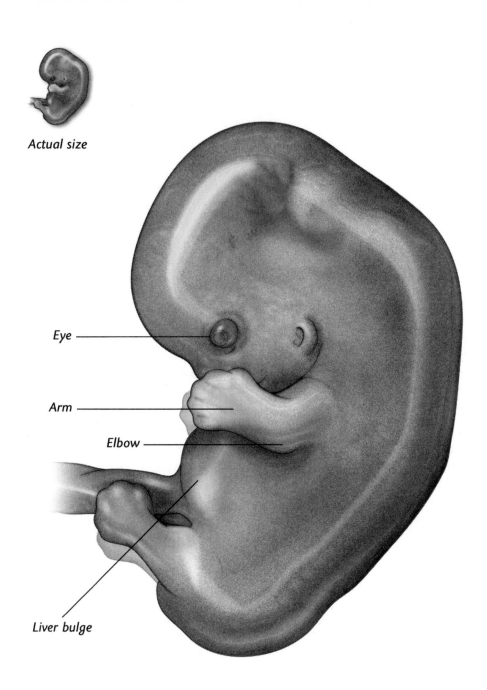

Actual size

Eye

Arm

Elbow

Liver bulge

Embryo at 8 weeks (fetal age—6 weeks).
Crown-to-rump length is about ¾ inch (20mm).
Arms are longer and bend at the elbows.

Tip for Week 8
· · · · · · · · · · ·

Wash your hands thoroughly throughout the day, especially after handling raw meat or using the bathroom. This simple act can help prevent the spread of many bacteria and viruses that cause infection.

Flare-ups in the first trimester are fairly common because of changing hormones. Pimples can appear on your neck, shoulders, back and face.

To treat acne, use a mild cleanser, followed by a mild, nonclogging moisturizer with sunscreen. Drinking lots of water also seems to help. Don't use products that contain salicylic acid; we don't know about safety during pregnancy.

Talk to your healthcare provider before using over-the-counter treatments. Avoid using any prepregnancy prescription skin products until you talk to your healthcare provider. It's safe to use azelaic acid gel 15% (Finacea) twice a day.

Accutane (isotretinoin) is commonly prescribed to treat acne. Do *not* take Accutane during pregnancy! If taken during the first trimester, it may increase your chances of miscarriage or birth defects in baby.

Miscarriage and Stillbirth
Nearly every pregnant woman thinks about miscarriage during pregnancy, but it occurs in only about 20% of all pregnancies. *Miscarriage* occurs when a pregnancy ends before the embryo or fetus can survive on its own outside the uterus, usually within the first 3 months. After 20 weeks, loss of a pregnancy is

called a *stillbirth*. Many causes of miscarriage also apply to stillbirth, and in this discussion, we will use the term "miscarriage" to apply to both. A discussion of stillbirth follows.

Some signs of miscarriage include vaginal bleeding, cramps, pain that comes and goes, pain that begins in the small of the back and moves to the lower abdomen and loss of tissue. If you experience any of these symptoms, call your healthcare provider immediately.

What Causes a Miscarriage? We don't usually know, and are often unable to find out, what causes a miscarriage. The most common reason in early miscarriages is abnormal development of the embryo, but experts believe there may be many other reasons miscarriage occurs.

Use of aspirin and nonsteroidal anti-inflammatories (NSAIDs) may increase the risk of miscarriage. Caffeine use before and during pregnancy may also increase risk. Some experts believe a father-to-be's age may play a role. When a man is over age 35, there may be a greater risk of miscarriage than for younger men, no matter what the woman's age is.

Below is a discussion of different types of miscarriage. It is included to alert you about what to watch for if you have any symptoms of a miscarriage. If you have questions, discuss them with your healthcare provider.

Different Types of Miscarriage. If you have a *threatened miscarriage*, it appears as a bloody discharge from the vagina during the first half of pregnancy. Bleeding may last for days or even weeks. There may not be any cramping or pain. If there is pain, it may feel like a menstrual cramp or a mild backache. Resting in bed is about all you can do, but being active does not cause miscarriage. No procedure or medication can keep a woman from miscarrying.

An *inevitable miscarriage* occurs when the bag of water breaks (rupture of membranes), the cervix dilates and you pass blood clots and/or tissue. Miscarriage is almost certain under these circumstances. The uterus usually expels the fetus or products of conception.

With an *incomplete miscarriage*, part of the pregnancy is passed while part of it remains in the uterus. Bleeding may be heavy and continues until the uterus is empty. A *missed miscarriage* can occur if the body retains an embryo that died earlier. There may be no symptoms or bleeding. The time period from when the pregnancy failed to the time the miscarriage is discovered is usually weeks.

About 1 to 2% of all couples will experience a *recurrent* or *habitual miscarriage*. This usually refers to three or more consecutive miscarriages. Studies show 60 to 70% of couples who have recurrent miscarriages eventually have a successful pregnancy.

A *chemical pregnancy* occurs when tissue forms that produces the hormone (HCG) that makes a pregnancy test positive. However, the tissue embryo dies very soon, so there actually is no pregnancy.

. . . .
If you suffer a miscarriage, research shows you have a 90% chance of having a healthy pregnancy the next time you get pregnant.
. . . .

If You Have Problems. If you have problems, notify your healthcare provider immediately! Bleeding often appears first, followed by cramping. Ectopic pregnancy must also be considered. A quantitative-HCG test may be useful in identifying a normal pregnancy, but a single test report doesn't usually help. Your healthcare provider needs to repeat the test over a period of several days.

Ultrasound may help if you are more than 5 gestational weeks into your pregnancy. You may continue to bleed, but seeing your baby's heartbeat may be reassuring. If the first ultrasound is not reassuring, you may be asked to wait a week or 10 days, then repeat the test.

The longer you bleed and cramp, the more likely you are having a miscarriage. If you pass all of the pregnancy and bleeding stops and cramping goes away, you may be done with it. However, if everything is not expelled, it may be necessary to perform a dilatation and curettage (D&C) to empty the uterus. It's better to do this so you won't bleed for a long time, risking anemia and infection.

Some women are given progesterone in an effort to help them keep a pregnancy. Medical experts do not agree on its use or effectiveness.

If you're Rh-negative and you have a miscarriage, you will need to receive RhoGAM. This applies only if you are Rh-negative. RhoGAM is given to protect you from making antibodies to Rh-positive blood.

* *

If you have a miscarriage, take heart in the fact that you did get pregnant, and you may not have to deal with fertility issues in the future.

* *

Stillbirth. Stillbirth is the death of a fetus after 20 weeks of pregnancy. Various reasons are cited for stillbirth, but nearly 50% of all unexplained stillbirths may be related to problems in the fetus.

If you're obese before pregnancy, it increases your risk of stillbirth. Other causes may include high blood pressure, diabetes, lupus, renal disease, thrombophilia, multiples, some infections and placenta and cord accidents.

Having a stillborn baby can be a traumatic experience for you, and it can take time to recover from it. You and your partner will probably have many questions and concerns. To help you find answers to your questions, discuss them with your healthcare provider.

If You Have a Miscarriage or Stillbirth. Having a miscarriage or stillbirth can be difficult. Some couples experience more than one miscarriage, which can be very difficult. In most cases, repeated miscarriages occur due to chance or "bad luck." Most healthcare providers don't recommend testing to find a reason for miscarriage unless you have three or more pregnancy losses in a row.

Don't blame yourself or your partner for loss of a pregnancy. It's usually impossible to determine a cause.

If a miscarriage or stillbirth occurs, give yourselves plenty of time to recover physically and emotionally. In the past, we advised a couple not to try to get pregnant immediately and to allow 3 or 4 months for a woman's body to return to its normal cycle and for hormone levels to return to normal. However, some experts now believe it's safe for a woman to try to get pregnant again as soon as she has a menstrual period. Talk to your healthcare provider if you have questions.

As a couple, you might want to allow yourselves time to recover emotionally. This may take longer than the actual physical recovery.

Your Nutrition

It's hard to eat nutritiously for every meal. You may not always get the nutrients you need in the amounts you need. On page 86 is a chart showing where you can get the various nutrients you should be eating every day. In each meal during pregnancy, try to include a whole-grain product, fruits and/or veggies, a lean protein and a healthy fat.

Your prenatal vitamin is not a substitute for food, so don't count on it to supply you with all the essential

Sources of Food Nutrients
· · · · · · · · · · ·

Nutrient	Food Sources (Daily Requirement)
Calcium (1200mg)	dairy products, dark leafy vegetables, dried beans and peas, tofu
Folic acid (0.4mg)	liver, dried beans and peas, eggs, broccoli, whole-grain products, oranges, orange juice
Iron (30mg)	fish, liver, meat, poultry, egg yolks, nuts, dried beans and peas, dark leafy vegetables, dried fruit
Magnesium (320mg)	dried beans and peas, cocoa, seafood, whole-grain products, nuts
Vitamin B$_6$ (2.2mg)	whole-grain products, liver, meat
Vitamin E (10mg)	milk, eggs, meat, fish, cereals, dark leafy vegetables, vegetable oils
Zinc (15mg)	seafood, meat, nuts, milk, dried beans and peas

vitamins and minerals you need. Food is your most important source of nutrients!

You Should Also Know

Braces during Pregnancy?

It seems people of all ages have braces these days. We've been asked about braces on teeth during pregnancy. Is it OK to continue wearing them during pregnancy? Can braces be put on during pregnancy?

If you already have braces, some things could make treatment a bit more taxing for you. If you have morning sickness and vomit a lot, you'll need to take very good care of your teeth. Brushing is important to clean acid off teeth. When braces are tightened, you may want to eat soft foods; that's acceptable for a few days.

If you're scheduled to have your braces put on then discover you're pregnant, contact your orthodontist, and tell him or her you're pregnant. Discuss any plans regarding braces with your pregnancy healthcare provider and your orthodontist before any action is taken!

Concern comes if you need dental X-rays; they may be an essential part of the treatment plan. However, with modern equipment and use of digital radiography, these risks can be reduced.

You may need to have one or more teeth pulled. Tooth extraction by itself may not be dangerous, but the anesthesia necessary to pull a tooth may not be good for you or baby. Your treatment plan must be discussed and agreed upon by your pregnancy healthcare provider and your orthodontist before you begin.

Dad Tip

· · · · · · · · · · ·

If you have pets, take over their care during your partner's pregnancy. Change the cat's litter box (she shouldn't do this while pregnant). Walk the dog (the pull on the leash might hurt her back). Buy food and other pet supplies (to save her back from the strain of lifting big food bags). Make and keep vet appointments.

Lab Tests Your Healthcare Provider May Order

When you go for your first or second prenatal visit, your healthcare provider may order a lot of tests, including blood tests. You may also have a urinalysis and urine culture as well as cervical cultures to test for STDs. A Pap smear may also be done. Other tests are done as required.

Most of the tests are done on your blood—usually only a vial or two is needed to perform all the tests. If you have difficulty with a blood draw, you might want to ask your partner to accompany you to the test. Blood tests that may be ordered include:

- complete blood count (CBC) to check your iron stores and to check for infections
- rubella titer to see if you have immunity against rubella (German measles)
- blood type to determine if your blood type is A, B, AB or O
- an Rh-factor test to determine if you are Rh-negative
- a blood-sugar-level test to check for diabetes
- test for varicella (chicken pox) to see if you have had this disease in the past

- test for hepatitis-B antibodies to determine whether you have ever been exposed to hepatitis-B
- screening test for syphilis (VDRL or ART)
- test for thrombophilia
- an HIV/AIDS test to see if you have been infected with the AIDS virus

It is not routine to screen all women for HIV during pregnancy. It may be offered to you; you must decide whether you should be tested. Some experts recommend all women undergo screening during pregnancy. Discuss it with your healthcare provider.

Ask your healthcare provider about a test for hypothyroidism. Many researchers believe women should be tested for thyroid-stimulating hormone (TSH) at the beginning of pregnancy. One study showed pregnant women who had higher-than-normal levels of TSH after 16 weeks had 4 times the chance of having a miscarriage or stillbirth than women with normal levels.

Toxoplasmosis

If you have a cat, you may be concerned about toxoplasmosis. The disease is spread by eating raw, infected meat or

Medical Conditions and "Safe" Medications to Use during Pregnancy

· · · · · · · · · · · ·

Condition	Drugs of Choice that Are Safe to Use
Acne	benzoyl peroxide, clindamycin, erythromycin
Asthma inhalers	beta-adrenergic antagonists, corticosteroids, cromolyn, ipratropium
Bacterial infection	cephalosporins, clindamycin, cotrimoxazole, erythromycin, nitrofurantoin, penicillin
Bipolar disorder	chlorpromazine, haloperidol
Cough	cough lozenges, dextromethorphan, diphenhydramine, codeine (short term)
Depression	fluoxetine, tricyclic antidepressants
Headache	acetaminophen
Hypertension	hydralazine, methyldopa
Hyperthyroidism	propylthiouracil
Migraines	codeine, dimenhydrinate
Nausea and vomiting	doxylamine plus pyridoxine
Peptic ulcer disease	antacids, rantidine

by contact with infected cat feces. Usually an infection in the mother-to-be has no symptoms but can cross the placenta to the baby.

Infection during pregnancy can lead to miscarriage or an infected infant at birth. Antibiotics can be used to treat toxoplasmosis, but the best plan is prevention. Sanitary measures prevent transmission of the disease.

Get someone else to change the kitty litter. Wash your hands thoroughly after petting your cat, and keep your cat off counters and tables. Wash your hands after contact with meat and soil. Cook all meat thoroughly. Avoid cross-contamination of foods while preparing and cooking them.

Exercise for Week 8

· · · · · · ·

Sit on the floor in a comfortable position. Inhale as you raise your right arm over your head. Reach as high as you can, while stretching from the waist. Bend your elbow, and pull your arm back down to your side as you exhale. Repeat for your left side. Do 4 or 5 times on each side. *Relieves upper backache and tension in shoulders, neck and back.*

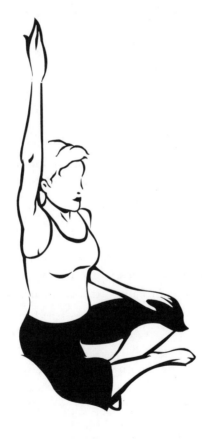

· · · · · · ·

Week 9

Age of Fetus—7 Weeks

If you've just found out you're pregnant, you might want to begin by reading the previous chapters.

How Big Is Your Baby?

The crown-to-rump length of the embryo is 1 to 1¼ inches (2.2 to 3cm). This is close to the size of a medium green olive.

How Big Are You?

Your waistline may be growing thicker. This occurs as your uterus fills your pelvic area and starts to grow up into the abdomen.

How Your Baby Is Growing and Developing

If you could look inside your uterus, you'd see many changes in your baby. The illustration on page 92 shows some of them.

Baby's arms and legs are longer. Fingers are longer, and the tips are slightly enlarged where touch pads are developing. The feet are approaching the midline of the body and may meet in front of the torso.

The head is more erect, and the neck is more developed. The pupil forms this week, and the optic nerve begins to form. Eyelids almost cover the eyes; up to this time, eyes have been uncovered. External ears are evident and well formed. Your baby now moves its body and limbs. This movement may be seen during an ultrasound exam.

The baby looks more recognizable as a human being, although it is still extremely small. But you still can't tell the difference between a boy and a girl. You won't be able to do that for another few weeks.

Changes in You

Your blood system changes a lot during pregnancy, and the amount of blood in your body, called *blood volume*, increases as much as 50%. Higher blood volume helps meet the demands of your growing baby and helps protect you both. It's also important during labor and delivery, when some blood is lost.

Increased blood volume begins during the first trimester. The greatest increase occurs in the second trimester. It continues to increase but at a slower rate during the third trimester. The increase in red blood cells increases your

How Is Pregnancy Weight Distributed?
• • • • • • • • • • •

When a baby is born, an average-weight mother should have gained between 25 and 35 pounds. A woman who has gained 30 pounds may see her weight distributed as shown below.

11 pounds	Fat, protein and other nutrients in mom
4 pounds	Increased fluid volume
2 pounds	Breast enlargement
2 pounds	Uterus
7½ pounds	Baby
2 pounds	Amniotic fluid
1½ pounds	Placenta

body's need for iron and can cause anemia. If you're anemic during pregnancy, you may get tired easily or feel ill.

How Your Actions Affect Your Baby's Development

Celiac Disease

Celiac disease, also called *celiac sprue, nontropical sprue* and *gluten-sensitive enteropathy,* is a digestive disease that affects the small intestine. If you have celiac disease, you are allergic to gluten, which causes your immune system to attack your intestines so you absorb fewer nutrients. Symptoms include diarrhea, abdominal pain, bloating, irritability and depression.

The condition is hereditary and occurs more often in women than men. It's most common in Western Europeans and rare in Africans and Asians. We believe celiac disease affects 1 in 100 people worldwide and 1 in every 133 Americans. It may be overlooked during pregnancy because symptoms can be the same as for other problems. Many healthcare providers don't know much about the disease, and it can be difficult to diagnose. A blood test can determine if you have celiac disease. A biopsy of the small intestine can confirm it.

If you have celiac disease, it's important to have it under control *before* pregnancy by eating a gluten-free diet. Because folic acid is found in many fortified grain products and you must avoid them, you will probably need supplements to ensure you receive enough folic acid.

Celiac disease may appear for the first time during pregnancy or after childbirth. If you have symptoms, talk to your healthcare provider. You may need to meet with a dietician to develop a nutritional meal plan.

Don't Detox during Pregnancy

Did you ever detox before you got pregnant? If you did, you probably did it in an effort to release toxins stored in your cells and "cleanse" your system. However, you want to avoid detoxing during pregnancy for many reasons.

When toxins are released from your cells they enter your bloodstream. When

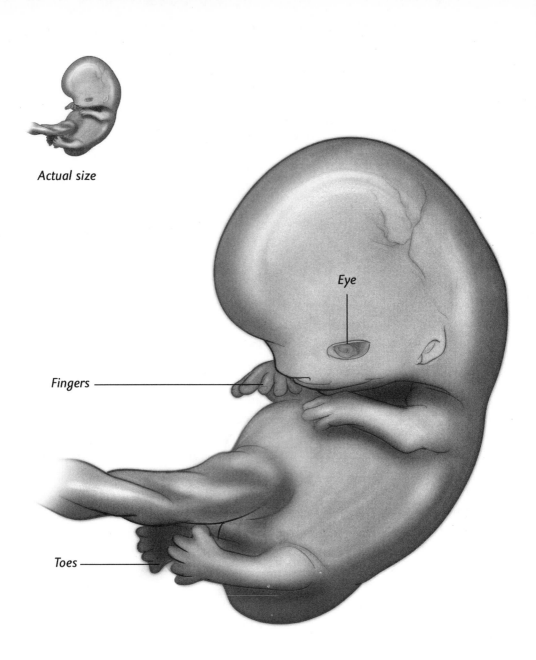

Actual size

Eye

Fingers —————

Toes ———

Embryo at 9 weeks of pregnancy (fetal age—46 to 49 days).
Toes are formed and feet are more recognizable.
Crown-to-rump length is about 1 inch (25mm).

Tip for Week 9
• • • • • • • • • •

It's an old wives' tale that you shouldn't color your hair or your hair won't curl if you have a permanent during pregnancy. Our only precaution is that if odors affect you, the fumes from a permanent or hair coloring could make you feel ill.

you're not pregnant, that's OK. During pregnancy, any toxins released into the blood could pass to the fetus through the placenta.

You risk dehydration during a detox, which isn't good for a pregnant woman, and it can affect the fetus. When you're dehydrated, nutrients baby receives from you may be reduced because your blood becomes thicker, making it more difficult to pass nutrients to baby.

You probably won't get the nutrients you need from a detox meal plan. You need a well-balanced meal plan during pregnancy; you don't get that when you're detoxing.

You often need to take many different herbs and botanicals during a detox. Many of them could be harmful to the fetus.

Instead of detoxing, enhance your nutrition. Don't cut out foods—add fresh food to your meal plan. Wait until you're back on your feet after baby's birth to think about detoxing.

Some General Lifestyle Precautions
Some women have questions about using saunas, hot tubs and spas during pregnancy. They want to know if it is OK to relax this way. We recommend you don't take a chance with a sauna,

hot tub or spa. Your baby relies on you to maintain correct body temperature. If your body temperature gets high enough and stays there for a while, it might hurt the baby.

There is disagreement about using electric blankets and electric warming pads to keep you warm in bed. Some experts question whether they can cause health problems. Electric blankets and warming pads produce a low-level electromagnetic field. The fetus may be more sensitive than an adult to these electromagnetic fields. Because we have no "acceptable level" of exposure for you or baby, it's probably best not to use them during pregnancy. There are other ways to keep warm, such as down comforters and wool blankets or snuggling with your partner. Any of these may be a better choice.

• •

Experts recommend all pregnant women be screened for diabetes at their first prenatal appointment. They believe the test should be done before the end of the first trimester. If that's not possible, it should be done as soon as possible after 13 weeks of pregnancy. If a woman has never been diagnosed with diabetes, she should still take the glucose-tolerance test between 24 and 28 weeks of pregnancy.

• •

The FDA is updating labels on prescription medicine to include a fetal-risk summary. This will tell you the possible drug effects on a fetus. It is also updating labels to include information on the amount of a medicine that may be present in breast milk after you take it. Ask your pharmacist about it if you're interested.

Your Nutrition

Fruits and vegetables are important during pregnancy. Because different kinds of produce are available in different seasons, they are a great way to add variety to your diet. They are excellent sources of vitamins, minerals and fiber. Eating a variety of fruits and vegetables can supply you with iron, folate, calcium and vitamin C.

When you eat raw veggies, to help absorb nutrients from vegetables include a little fat, such as salad dressing, a piece of avocado or some nuts. When you don't feel like eating your vegetables, soups can add variety and substance to your meal plan. Broth-based vegetable soups may provide more nutrients and fewer calories than a sandwich or a plate of pasta. To add veggies to your meal plan, grill, bake or broil them. Stir-fry veggies with a little bit of meat, or add beans to stews and soups. Make tabbouleh, and flavor it with herbs.

Vitamin C Is Important

Vitamin C can be very important during pregnancy and can help you and baby in many different ways. The recommended daily dose of vitamin C is 85mg—a bit more than what is contained in a prenatal vitamin. You can get some of the extra vitamin C you need by eating fruits and vegetables rich in the vitamin.

Each day, eat one or two servings of fruit high in vitamin C and at least one dark-green or deep-yellow vegetable for extra iron, fiber and folate. Fruits and vegetables you may choose, and their serving sizes, include the following:

- grapes or cantaloupe—¾ cup
- banana, orange, apple, kiwi—1 medium
- dried fruit—¼ cup
- fruit juice—½ cup
- canned or cooked fruit—½ cup
- broccoli, carrots, red bell pepper or other vegetables—½ cup
- potato—1 medium
- leafy green vegetables—1 cup
- vegetable juice—¼ cup

Don't take in more than the recommended dose of vitamin C; too much may cause stomach cramps and diarrhea. It can also negatively affect baby's metabolism.

When buying vitamins, look for the U.S.P. verified symbol, which means the vitamins are usually good quality.

You Should Also Know

Vscan

A test recently received FDA approval; you may see it in your healthcare provider's office. It's called *Vscan*, and it's a portable ultrasound machine about the size of your cell phone! It provides a high-quality image when the wand is passed

Eyelash-Growth Enhancers

· · · · · · · · · · ·

Prescription eyelash-growth enhancers, such as Latisse, and over-the-counter products, such as Revitalash, are used to help make eyelashes grow longer and thicker. If you normally use these products, it may be best to stop using them during pregnancy. Better to be safe than sorry.

over your abdomen. It's a benefit to your healthcare provider because he or she can see your growing baby with greater ease. This helps when you have problems that need to be closely watched.

Avoid Anxiety-Producing TV Programs

Some women get anxious after watching television programs dealing with labor and delivery. These programs may be interesting to watch, but we want you to be aware they may be "worst-case scenarios." By that we mean they may deal with situations that are not the norm for a large percentage of deliveries in the United States.

Most labor/delivery experiences are not as critical or as sensational as what is shown on TV. Think about it—who wants to watch an ordinary labor and delivery? There's no real drama in it, so these programs often focus on some kind of unusual problem a woman could face.

Even when the content is not sensational, we have found pregnant women who watch these programs often get anxious. If you haven't experienced labor and delivery before, you may be a little scared about what will happen during your own labor and delivery. That's normal.

Labor and delivery is an unknown— no one can tell you what will happen to

you until it happens. When your labor begins, your healthcare team will take care of you, in the best way they can, to ensure the safe delivery of your baby and your good health.

Be Careful of What You Read on the Internet

We have had pregnant women ask us the most bizarre questions or present us with information that is totally incorrect or only partially correct. When we ask them where they found these facts, they often tell us "the Internet."

Just because you read it on the Internet does *not* make it true. Some people think if they find it on the Internet, it's a fact. That's often not the case.

We know you can find a lot of good information on the Internet, but then again, you can also find a lot of misinformation. If you're searching for advice or facts about something, read what you find *very carefully*. If you have questions about something you find, print out the piece and take it with you to a prenatal visit so you can discuss it with your healthcare provider.

Do *not* change anything your healthcare provider has told you. Do address your questions and concerns at a prenatal appointment. Your healthcare provider knows about your unique

Dad Tip

· · · · · · · · · · ·

Ask your partner which prenatal visits she'd like you to attend. Some couples attend every visit together, when possible. Ask her to let you know the date and time of each appointment.

pregnancy situation. If you disagree or question what you're told, ask for a second opinion.

Freekeh

Freekeh is gaining popularity with people looking for new, nutritious grains to add to their meal plans. Also called *farik*, it is a ricelike grain made from green wheat that is roasted and cracked. It is related to bulgur wheat; some compare it to a cross between brown rice and barley. When harvested early, the grain retains more proteins, vitamins and minerals. After the roasting process, it has a smoky aroma and nutty flavor, and it is chewy and firm.

Freekeh is high in nutritional value and low on the glycemic index. It contains 4 times the fiber of brown rice and may help balance blood-sugar levels. It may also help healthy bacteria in your gastrointestinal tract grow and multiply to help keep you healthy. In addition, it may help with constipation, especially during pregnancy. The grain contains little gluten and may be added to diets low in gluten. But if you need to avoid gluten, as do sufferers of celiac disease, avoid freekeh.

If you want to add freekeh to your meals, you can substitute the grain in recipes that call for pasta, rice or barley.

You can also add it to foods such as puddings, pilaf, soup and risotto. Give it a try if you want to add some variety to your meals *and* get great nutrition for you and baby.

Tuberculosis (TB)

Tuberculosis in the United States primarily affects the elderly, the poor, minority groups and those with AIDS. Immigration of women from other countries has resulted in an increase of TB in pregnant women. But even with an increase in the number of TB cases, the risk to you is probably very low. Many drugs used to treat tuberculosis are safe during pregnancy.

The most common site of TB infection is the lungs, but infection can also occur in other parts of the body. You get it by breathing in the bacteria; it's passed to others through coughing and sneezing. Tuberculosis is diagnosed with skin testing; the TB skin test is safe during pregnancy.

A baby can become infected with TB from its mother's blood or from breathing bacteria after birth. If a woman has tuberculosis, the baby's pediatrician should be involved immediately after birth. If a woman is contagious, her baby may need to be separated from her for a short time. Most people aren't

Grandma's Remedy
· · · · · · · · · · ·

If you want to avoid using medication, try a folk remedy. Chew a combination of fresh mint and parsley leaves to help deal with bad breath and intestinal gas.

contagious after 2 weeks of treatment. After that time, it's safe to breastfeed.

Having a Baby Costs Money!

Every couple wants to know what it will cost to have a baby. There are really two answers to that question—it costs a lot, and cost varies from one part of the country to another. From prenatal care to baby's birth, the average cost of having a baby today is around $8000 in the United States.

Insurance makes a big difference in the cost to you. If you don't have it, you'll pay for everything. If you do have insurance, you need to check out some things. Don't be embarrassed to ask questions. You'll be happier if you get answers. Ask your employer or insurance agent the following questions.

- What type of coverage do I have? What percentage of my costs are covered? Is there a cap (limit) on total coverage?
- Are there maternity benefits? What are they?
- Do I have to pay a deductible? If so, how much is it?
- If my pregnancy lasts into a new year, will I have to pay a deductible for 2 years?
- How do I submit claims?
- Do maternity benefits cover Cesarean deliveries?

- What kind of coverage is there for a high-risk pregnancy?
- Is the cost of taking childbirth-education classes covered?
- What kind of hospital accommodations may I choose, such as a birthing center or a birthing room?
- What procedures must I follow before entering the hospital?
- Does my policy cover a nurse-midwife (if this is of interest to you)?
- Does coverage include medications? What tests during pregnancy are covered? What tests during labor and delivery are covered?
- What types of anesthesia are covered during labor and delivery?
- How long can I stay in the hospital?
- What conditions or services are not covered?
- What kind of coverage is there for the baby after it is born? How long can the baby stay in the hospital?
- Is there an additional cost to add the baby to the policy? How do I add the baby to the policy? How soon do we need to add the baby to the policy?

Much of the covered cost for the hospital is determined by how long you stay and the "services" you use. Having an epidural or Cesarean delivery may add to the bill. Your healthcare provider's bill is separate, except under some plans. Another cost is the pediatrician, who usually examines the baby, does a physical and sees baby each day in the hospital.

Pregnancy is not the time to cut corners to save money. Sometimes it's worth spending a little more to get what you want. Call around so you can compare hospitals and prices. Some hospitals and medical centers offer "pregnancy packages." A package can cover many services for one fee.

The Cost of Multiple Births. The medical costs for a multiple birth are much higher than the cost for a single baby.

When the number of babies in a pregnancy goes up, so do the costs.

One study looked at the cost of having a baby or babies over a 6-year period—results are startling! The costs we are discussing include 27 weeks during pregnancy and up to 30 days after birth. For a singleton birth, the cost averages $21,000. For triplets or more, that cost was over 20 times higher—the average cost for three or more babies was over $400,000! For a singleton birth, nearly 60% of the costs incurred were for treatment for the mom-to-be. In multiple pregnancies, up to 85% of the costs were for treatment of the babies. In addition, mothers of multiples incurred higher medical costs because they often had longer hospital stays before and after the births.

Exercise for Week 9

• • • • • • •

Hold onto a door jamb or the back of a sturdy chair. Beginning with your right leg, point your toe and lift your leg forward to 90°, then lower it to the floor. Without stopping, lift the same leg to the side, as far as you can but not beyond 90°. Return to the starting position. Repeat 10 times for each leg. *Tones leg muscles and buttocks muscles.*

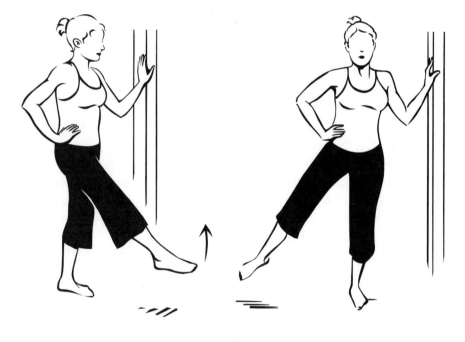

• • • • • • •

Week 10

Age of Fetus—8 Weeks

How Big Is Your Baby?

By this week, crown-to-rump length of baby is about 1¼ to 1¾ inches (3.1 to 4.2cm). Baby is starting to put on a little weight, so we'll add weight in this section. Before this week, weight was too small to measure weekly differences. The baby weighs close to 0.18 ounce (5g) and is the size of a small plum.

How Big Are You?

A condition that can make you grow too big too fast is a *molar pregnancy*, sometimes called *gestational trophoblastic neoplasia (GTN)* or *hydatidiform mole*. A molar pregnancy develops from an abnormally fertilized egg, but an embryo does not usually develop. Abnormal placental tissue grows instead.

The most common symptom is bleeding during the first trimester. A woman may have a lot of nausea and vomiting. Another symptom is the size of the mother-to-be and how far along she is supposed to be in pregnancy. Half the time, a woman is too large. Twenty-five percent of the time, she is too small.

The most effective way to diagnose molar pregnancy is by ultrasound. The ultrasound picture has a "snowflake" appearance. The problem is usually found when the test is done to find the cause of bleeding or rapid growth of the uterus.

A molar pregnancy can become cancerous. When it is diagnosed, surgery (dilatation and curettage [D&C]) is usually done as soon as possible.

After a molar pregnancy, effective birth control is important to be sure the molar pregnancy is completely gone. Most healthcare providers recommend using reliable birth control for at least 1 year before trying to get pregnant again.

How Your Baby Is Growing and Developing

The end of this week is the end of the embryonic period. During the embryonic period, the baby has been most susceptible to things that could harm it. Most birth defects occur then. It's good to know a vital part of your baby's development is behind you. Few birth defects happen after this time. However, drugs and other harmful exposures, such as radiation (X-ray), can hurt the baby at any time during pregnancy. Continue to avoid them.

Changes in You

Emotional Changes

When pregnancy is confirmed, it can affect you in many ways. Some consider it a blessing, while others feel it's a problem. If you aren't excited about pregnancy, don't feel alone; it's common.

When and how you begin to regard the fetus as a person is different for everyone. Some women say it's when their pregnancy test is positive. Others say it occurs when they hear the fetal heartbeat, usually around 12 weeks. For still others, it happens when they first feel their baby move, at between 16 and 20 weeks.

You may find you are emotional about many things. You may feel moody, cry at the slightest thing or drift off in daydreams. Emotional swings are normal and continue to some degree throughout your pregnancy. We believe emotional changes occur because of pregnancy hormones.

Some emotions may be caused by other things. For example, if you cry and feel down for longer than 2 weeks, feel worthless or hopeless, or don't take pleasure in most things, you may be depressed. Be sure you discuss how you feel emotionally with your healthcare provider.

Help yourself by getting good prenatal care and following your healthcare provider's advice. Keep all prenatal appointments. Establish good communication with your healthcare provider and the office staff. Ask questions. If something bothers you or worries you, discuss it with someone reliable.

How Your Actions Affect Your Baby's Development

When You're Underweight

If you are underweight when you begin pregnancy, you face special challenges. You may need to gain between 28 and 40 pounds during your pregnancy. Weight loss can occur during the first trimester if you have morning sickness. If you're underweight and lose weight, talk to your healthcare provider.

Gaining weight gives your baby the nutrients it needs to grow and to develop. If you need to gain extra weight during pregnancy, there are ways to accomplish this. Don't drink diet sodas or eat low-calorie foods. Choose nutritious foods to help you gain weight, such as cheeses, dried fruits, nuts, avocados, whole milk and ice cream. Eat higher-calorie foods. Add nutritious, calorie-rich snacks to your daily menu. Avoid junk food with lots of empty calories.

You may need to exercise less if you burn too many calories when you work out. Eating small, frequent meals may help. Make a good nutrition plan at the beginning of pregnancy. Ask your healthcare provider about seeing a dietician to help you.

. . . .

You should be gaining weight slowly; it can be harmful to baby if you don't. Although pregnancy is not the time to experiment with different diets or cut down on calories, it doesn't mean you have the go-ahead to eat anything you want, any time you want. Exercise and a proper nutrition plan, without junk food, will help you manage your weight. Be smart about food choices.

. . . .

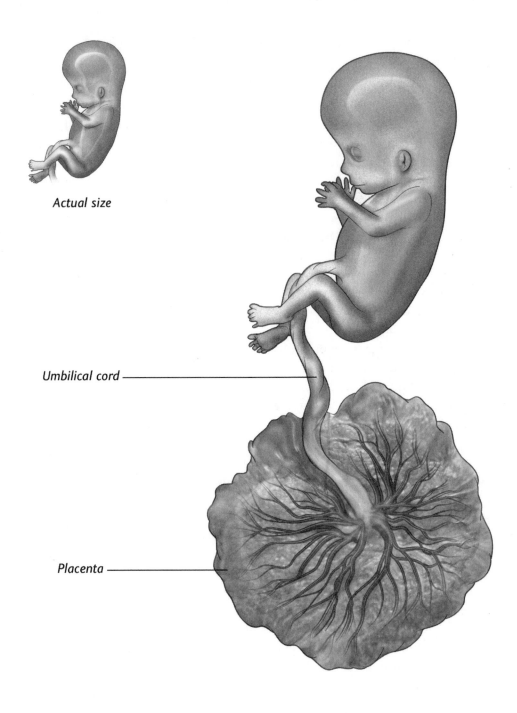

Actual size

Umbilical cord —————

Placenta —————

Baby is shown attached to the placenta by its
umbilical cord. Eyelids are fused and remain closed
until week 27 (fetal age—25 weeks).

> ## Tip for Week 10
> . . . .
> It's common for your breasts to tingle and to feel sore early in pregnancy. In fact, it may be one of the first signs of pregnancy.

Vaccinations and Immunizations

Immunizations and vaccinations protect you from diseases. A vaccine is usually given by injection or taken orally. Each vaccine dose contains a very small amount of a weakened form of the disease. When you receive a vaccine, your immune system makes antibodies to fight the disease in the future. In most cases, this is enough to keep you from getting a disease. However, in some cases, it doesn't prevent the disease entirely but lessens the symptoms.

Vaccines come in three forms—*live* virus, *killed* (dead) virus and *toxoids* (chemically altered proteins from harmless bacteria). Most vaccines are made from killed viruses; it's nearly impossible to get the disease after receiving this type of vaccine. With a live-virus vaccine, the virus is so weakened that if your immune system is normal, you probably won't get sick from it.

Many women of childbearing age have been immunized against measles, mumps, rubella, tetanus and diphtheria. A blood test for measles and rubella is necessary to determine immunity. Physician-diagnosed mumps or a mumps vaccination is necessary to know you're immune.

Risk of Exposure. During pregnancy, try to reduce your chance of exposure to disease and illness. If you're exposed or if exposure is unavoidable, the risk of the disease must be balanced against the likely effects of vaccination.

The vaccine must be measured in terms of its effectiveness and its expected effect on a pregnancy. There's not a lot of information on harmful effects of a vaccine on a developing baby. However, live-measles vaccine should never be given to a pregnant woman.

. . . .

The night before you get your flu shot, go to bed extra early. When you're well rested, your body produces twice as many infection-fighting antibodies.

. . . .

Vaccinations You Should Have during Pregnancy. The only immunizing agents recommended for use during pregnancy are the Tdap (or DPT) vaccine and the flu vaccine. The Tdap vaccine (tetanus, diphtheria, pertussis) can help you avoid whooping cough. Be sure to get a Tdap booster if it's been 10 years since your last one. If you work in the garden, with your hands in dirt, you need a booster.

It is recommended that all women who will be pregnant during flu season get a flu shot. A flu shot can protect you against three strains of influenza and can be given safely during all three trimesters. It usually takes about 2 weeks before you are protected. In some cases, you may get the flu after receiving the flu vaccine; however, you usually won't be as sick.

Other Vaccines during Pregnancy. As many as 35% of all pregnant women are at risk of getting measles, mumps or rubella because they haven't been vaccinated or they have been vaccinated but their immunity has weakened. The MMR vaccine should be given before pregnancy or after delivery; wait at least 1 month to get pregnant after receiving the vaccine.

A pregnant woman should receive a vaccination against polio only if her risk of exposure to the disease is high. Only inactivated polio vaccine should be used. If your healthcare provider believes you may be at risk for getting hepatitis B, it's safe to take the vaccine during pregnancy.

Ask about receiving the pneumococcal vaccine if you have a chronic medical condition. This vaccine protects you against bacteria that can cause pneumonia, meningitis and ear infections. Antibodies you make after taking the vaccine pass to your baby and may protect him or her from ear infections for up to 6 months!

Human papillomavirus (HPV) vaccine is a series of shots over 6 months to protect against HPV. HPV is responsible for 70% of cervical cancers and 90% of genital-warts cases. Don't have this vaccine during pregnancy. If a woman discovers she's pregnant while receiving the vaccine, she should delay finishing the series until after she gives birth. Women who are breastfeeding can receive the vaccine.

Thimerosal Use during Pregnancy. Thimerosal is a preservative used in some vaccines; it contains ethyl mercury. It was barred from childhood vaccines several years ago but is still used in most flu vaccines. Some experts recommend pregnant women ask for a thimerosal-free flu vaccine. However, the CDC states it believes it's OK for pregnant women to receive these flu vaccines. They state the benefits of flu vaccine with thimerosal outweigh the risk. The American Congress of Obstetricians and Gynecologists (ACOG) has issued a similar statement.

Influenza (Flu)

The flu seems to be a problem every year because different flu viruses come and go. One year, the H1N1 flu affected many people. When an outbreak of influenza occurs, it can impact a pregnant woman more greatly because of her altered immune system. If you're pregnant when a breakout occurs, you should receive the specific flu vaccine *and* the seasonal flu vaccine. You can be vaccinated any time during pregnancy.

There are ways to protect yourself in addition to getting a seasonal flu shot. Use "social distancing." Avoid crowded areas, use a mask and wash your hands frequently.

Follow your healthcare provider's guidelines about using medicine you are advised to take. The benefits of taking a medicine outweigh any risk to baby. Treatment should begin as soon as possible; don't wait for lab results to confirm the type of flu.

Rubella Immunity

It's a good idea to get checked to see if you are immune to rubella before you get pregnant. Rubella (German measles)

Effects of Infections on Your Baby
. . . .

Some infections and illnesses a woman contracts can affect her baby's development. The chart below cites a type of infection or disease and the effects each may have on a developing baby.

Infections	Effects on Fetus
Cytomegalovirus (CMV)	microcephaly, brain damage, hearing loss
Rubella (German measles)	cataracts, deafness, heart lesions, can involve all organs
Syphilis	fetal death, skin defects
Toxoplasmosis	possible effects on all organs
Varicella	possible effects on all organs

during pregnancy can cause various pregnancy problems. Because there's no known treatment for rubella, the best approach is prevention.

If you're not immune, you can receive a vaccination after delivery while you take reliable birth control. Don't have a vaccination shortly before or during pregnancy because of the possibility of exposing baby to the rubella virus.

Chicken Pox during Pregnancy

Did you have chicken pox when you were a child? Ninety percent of women today are immune to chicken pox. If you didn't have chicken pox, you may be one of the 1 in 2000 women who will develop it during pregnancy. Chicken pox is more serious during the first 10 weeks of pregnancy. If you get it during the third trimester, it could affect baby's brain development.

Chicken pox usually affects kids; only 2% of all cases occur in the 15-to-49 age group. The CDC, the American Academy of Pediatrics and the American Academy of Family Physicians all recommend healthy children age 1 year and older receive the chicken-pox vaccine; it is usually given at 12 to 18 months of age.

If you get chicken pox during pregnancy, take good care of yourself. About 15% of those who get chicken pox also develop a form of pneumonia, which can be very serious for a pregnant woman. If you get chicken pox 5 days before or 2 days after delivery, baby can also develop a severe chicken-pox infection.

If you're exposed to chicken pox, contact your healthcare provider immediately! A pregnant woman should receive varicella-zoster immune globulin (VZIG). If you receive it within 72 hours of exposure, it can help prevent infection or lessen symptoms. If you do get chicken pox, you will probably be treated with acyclovir.

Your Nutrition

Pregnancy increases your protein needs, which is important for you and baby. Try to eat 6 ounces of protein each day during the first trimester and 8 ounces a day during the second and third trimesters. But don't eat too much protein; it should only make up about 15% of your total calorie intake.

Many protein sources are high in fat. If you need to watch your calories, choose low-fat protein sources. Some protein foods you may choose, and their serving sizes, include the following:

- chickpeas (garbanzo beans)—1 cup
- cheese, mozzarella—1 ounce
- chicken, roasted, skinless—½ breast (about 4 ounces)
- eggs—1
- hamburger, broiled, lean—3½ ounces
- milk—8 ounces
- peanut butter—2 tablespoons
- tuna, canned in water—3 ounces
- yogurt—8 ounces

Studies suggest eating 2 cups of fresh fruit a day may help reduce your risk of getting a cold or the flu by nearly 35%. Bright-colored fruit is your best bet, such as oranges, kiwi, red grapes, strawberries and pineapple. If you do get a cold, eating nutrient-rich foods may help your body produce more white blood cells to help fight it. Eat ½ cup pineapple or ½ cup sweet potatoes to increase your resistance.

When you eat eggs or dairy products for protein, be sure to add a complementary plant protein source for a complete protein. A complete protein contains all nine essential amino acids. Rice and beans, tofu and sesame seeds or green beans with almonds are good choices. If eating protein makes you ill, look for a carbohydrate food (like crackers, cereal, pretzels) that contains protein.

Brain Builders

Choline and docosahexaenoic acid (DHA) can help build baby's brain cells. Choline is found in milk, egg yolks, chicken liver, wheat germ, cod, cooked broccoli, peanuts and peanut butter, whole-wheat bread and beef. You need at least 450mg of choline a day during pregnancy. DHA is found in fish, egg yolks, poultry, meat, canola oil, walnuts and wheat germ.

Some pregnancy nutrition bars contain DHA; others have added vitamins and minerals. If you eat a variety of foods that contain choline and DHA during pregnancy and while breastfeeding, you can help your baby obtain important nutrients.

You Should Also Know

Down Syndrome

Older women have traditionally been offered various tests to determine whether their fetus is affected by Down syndrome. Today, nearly every pregnant woman receives information on the condition.

Babies born with Down syndrome have an extra chromosome 21. The normal number of human chromosomes is 46. With Down syndrome, an individual has 47 chromosomes.

The syndrome occurs in about 1 in 800 births. Some women are at higher risk of giving birth to a child with Down syndrome, including older women. Many screening tests are available *to screen* for Down syndrome in a developing fetus, including maternal alpha-fetoprotein test, triple-screen test, quad-screen test, nuchal translucency screening, and ultrasound. Tests *to diagnose* Down syndrome include amniocentesis and chorionic villus sampling (CVS).

. . . .

Cell-free DNA (cfDNA) tests fetal DNA found in mom's blood and can be done as early as 10 weeks of pregnancy. This is not an over-the-counter test; it must be ordered by your healthcare provider. It is most commonly used in high-risk pregnancies to detect Down syndrome, trisomy 18 and trisomy 13, and other serious chromosome abnormalities. Diagnostic testing following the screening test is essential. If you have questions or concerns, discuss them with your healthcare provider.

. . . .

ACOG Recommendations. The American Congress of Obstetricians and Gynecologists recommends all pregnant women be offered Down-syndrome screening. In the past, testing for Down syndrome was offered mainly to women over age 35 and others who were at risk. Even though many women would not consider terminating a pregnancy with a Down-syndrome child, it's important to know this information before baby's birth so specialized care can be planned for delivery.

Although the condition occurs at a higher frequency in older mothers, the majority of babies born with Down syndrome are born to younger women. Younger women give birth to a larger

number of babies; therefore, a larger number of babies with Down syndrome are delivered to younger women. Eighty percent of babies born with Down syndrome are born to women under age 35.

If your healthcare provider offers Down testing, consider it. Ask any questions you may have about the condition, and, together with your partner, decide whether to have the test. It may be most useful when screening is done during the first trimester.

Down Syndrome Children Are Special. A child born with Down syndrome can bring a special, valuable quality of life into the world. Down children are well known for the love and joy they bring to their families and friends.

The average IQ for a child with Down syndrome is between 60 and 70. Most are in the mildly retarded range. Less than 5% of those with Down syndrome are severely retarded.

The average reading level of those with Down syndrome is about 3rd grade. Most people with Down syndrome are employable as adults, and most are capable of living independently or in group homes. The average life expectancy is about 55 years.

Rearing a child with Down syndrome can be challenging, but many who have faced this challenge are positive about it. If you have a child with Down syndrome, you may work harder for every small advance in your child's life. You may experience frustration and feelings of helplessness at times, but every parent has these feelings at some time.

Dad Tip
· · · · · · · · · · ·

Are you concerned about sex during pregnancy? You both may have questions, so talk about them together and with your partner's healthcare provider. Occasionally during a pregnancy you'll need to avoid intercourse. However, pregnancy is an opportunity for increased closeness and intimacy for you as a couple. Sex can be a positive part of this experience.

Fetoscopy

Fetoscopy provides a view of the baby and placenta inside your uterus so some abnormalities and problems can be detected and corrected. The goal of fetoscopy is to correct a problem before it worsens, which could keep a baby from developing normally. A physician can see some problems more clearly with fetoscopy than with ultrasound.

The test is done by placing a scope, like the one used in laparoscopy, through the abdomen. The procedure is similar to amniocentesis, but the fetoscope is larger than the needle used for amniocentesis.

If your healthcare provider suggests fetoscopy, ask about possible risks, advantages and disadvantages of the procedure. The test should be done only by someone experienced in the technique. Risk of miscarriage is 3 to 4% with this procedure. It is not available everywhere. If you have fetoscopy and are Rh-negative, you should receive RhoGAM after the procedure.

Chorionic Villus Sampling

Chorionic villus sampling (CVS) is a highly accurate diagnostic test used to detect genetic abnormalities. Sampling is done early in pregnancy, usually between the 9th and 11th weeks. The test offers an advantage over amniocentesis because it is done much earlier, and results are available in about 1 week. If a pregnancy will be terminated, it can be done earlier and may carry fewer risks to the woman.

Chorionic villus sampling involves placing an instrument through the cervix or abdomen to remove fetal tissue from the placenta, which is tested for abnormalities. Over 95% of women who have CVS learn their baby does *not* have the disorder for which the test was done.

If your healthcare provider recommends CVS, ask about its risks. The test should be performed only by someone experienced in the technique. The risk of miscarriage is small—between 1 and 2%—and the test is considered as safe as amniocentesis. If you have CVS and are Rh-negative, you should receive RhoGAM after the procedure.

Find Out Baby's Sex This Week?

You may have seen over-the-counter gender tests advertised that use your blood or a urine sample to determine baby's sex. Be aware that these tests may not offer accurate results.

One test claims it can predict your baby's sex as early as this week. Called the *IntelliGender's Gender Prediction Test*, it tests a pregnant woman's urine to provide immediate results that indicate baby's gender, based on a color match. Green indicates boy, and orange indicates girl. However, before you rush off to buy the test, realize test results are actually only about 80% accurate. They only indicate the *possibility* of determining whether baby is a girl or a boy.

The *Pink or Blue* test is another at-home test that examines DNA in the blood of the mom-to-be. Fetal DNA can be found in a mother's bloodstream.

A woman sends a small sample of her blood to their lab, and results of the test (boy or girl) are sent to the parents-to-be. The makers of the product claim the test is 95% accurate and can predict a baby's sex as early as 6 weeks after conception.

Some medical authorities are concerned some couples may consider ending a pregnancy because of baby's sex, based on the result of these tests. If you have questions or concerns, discuss them with your healthcare provider.

Exercise for Week 10

• • • • • • •

Kneel on your hands and knees, with your hands directly below your shoulders and your knees directly under your hips. Inhale as you raise your head and gaze forward. Then exhale as you slowly bring your head down, round your back and shoulders and tuck in your tummy. Do 4 times. *Stretches back and tummy muscles, and increases flexibility.*

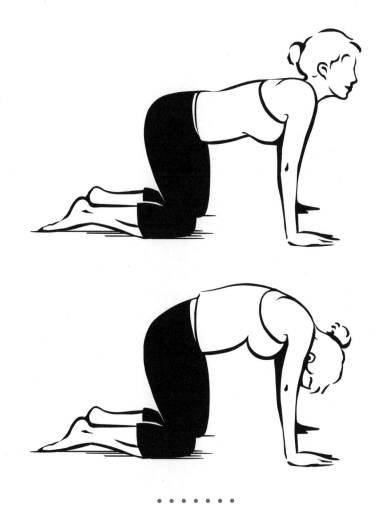

• • • • • • •

Week 11

Age of Fetus—9 Weeks

How Big Is Your Baby?

Crown-to-rump length of baby is 1½ to 2½ inches (4.4 to 6cm). Fetal weight is about 0.3 ounce (8g). Your baby is about the size of a large lime.

How Big Are You?

You're near the end of the first trimester! Your uterus is almost big enough to fill your pelvis and may be felt in your lower abdomen, above the middle of your pubic bone.

How Your Baby Is Growing and Developing

Fetal growth is rapid now. As you can see in the illustration on page 112, the head is almost half the baby's entire length. As the head moves backward toward the spine, the chin rises from the chest, and the neck develops and lengthens. Fingernails appear.

External genitalia are beginning to show distinguishing features. Development into a male or female is complete in another 3 weeks. All embryos begin life looking the same as far as outward appearances go. Whether the embryo develops into a boy or girl is determined by the genetic information contained within it.

By this time, the small intestine begins to contract and relax, which pushes substances through it. The small intestine is capable of passing sugar from inside itself into the baby's body.

Changes in You

Some women notice changes in their hair, fingernails or toenails during pregnancy. Some lucky pregnant women see an increase in hair and nail growth. Others find they lose some hair during this time, or their nails break more easily. This doesn't happen to everyone, but if it happens to you, don't worry about it.

Some experts believe these changes happen because of increased circulation in your body. Others credit the hormone changes in you. In any event, these changes are rarely permanent.

Pregnancy May Reveal Future Problems

Your body goes through many changes during pregnancy to allow it to accept and to tolerate the genetically "different" fetus. Changes also help your body adapt

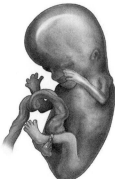

Actual size

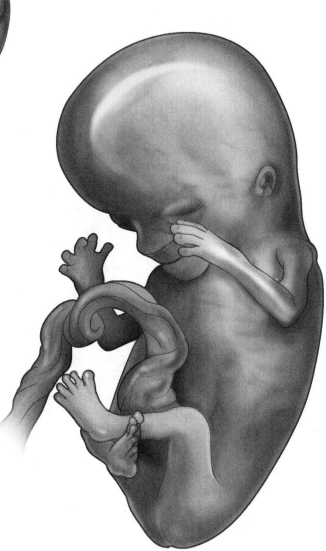

By week 11 of gestation (fetal age—9 weeks),
fingernails are beginning to appear.

to nourish and to support the fetus and to prepare you for delivery. In some women, these changes result in pregnancy problems and provide clue, as to what long-term health problems might lie ahead. You may be able to take steps now to help prevent serious problems later.

One example is gestational diabetes. Women who have pregnancy-induced diabetes are more likely to have diabetes later in life. Another example is women who have pre-eclampsia; they are at greater risk for stroke in later life.

Talk to your healthcare provider about any changes you experience during your pregnancy. Discuss steps you can take now and after pregnancy to help reduce your risk of problems in later life.

How Your Actions Affect Your Baby's Development

Traveling during Pregnancy

Pregnant women frequently ask whether travel can hurt their baby. If your pregnancy is uncomplicated and you aren't at high risk, travel is usually OK. Ask your healthcare provider about any travel you're considering *before* making firm plans or buying tickets.

The biggest risk of traveling during pregnancy is developing a problem while you're away from those who know your medical and pregnancy history. Signs you shouldn't travel include:

- severe swelling of the face, arms, legs, hands or feet
- bleeding
- severe nausea and vomiting
- cramping
- severe headaches
- fever

If you do decide to take a trip, be sensible in your planning. Don't overdo it. Take it easy!

Traveling by Air. Air travel is safe for most pregnant women. Most U.S. airlines let women fly up to 36 weeks of pregnancy. For international travel, the cutoff is usually 35 weeks of pregnancy.

Pregnant women who are at high risk should avoid all air travel. High-altitude flights (nonstop cross-country or overseas flights) cruise at a higher altitude, and oxygen levels can be lower. This increases your heart rate as well as your baby's; baby also receives less oxygen.

If you have problems with swelling, wear loose-fitting shoes and clothes. (This is good advice for every traveler.) Avoid pantyhose, tight clothes, knee socks or stockings, and tight waistlines.

If you know your flight serves a meal, order special meals. If your flight is long and doesn't serve food, bring along nutritious snacks. Drink lots of water to keep you hydrated. Take along an empty bottle, and fill it after you go through security.

Get up and move around when you can during the flight. Try to walk at least 10 minutes every hour. Sometimes just standing up helps your circulation. Try to get an aisle seat, close to the bathroom. If you have to go to the bathroom a lot, it's easier if you don't have to crawl over someone to get out.

Auto Safety during Pregnancy

Many women are concerned about driving and using seat belts and shoulder harnesses during pregnancy. There's no reason not to drive while you're pregnant

Dad Tip

• • • • • • • • • • •

Remember that despite morning sickness, headaches and a changing waistline, pregnancy is a miracle! Pregnancy and childbirth happen only a few times in your life. Enjoy this special time together. You'll look back fondly at the challenge of becoming parents and probably even say, "That wasn't so bad." We know that because couples get pregnant again and have more kids!

if your pregnancy is normal and you feel OK (and you know how to drive).

Wear safety restraints during pregnancy to lower the chance of getting hurt in an accident. If you don't wear a seat belt, you could cause a serious injury to your baby if you're in an accident.

Seat belts do *not* increase the risk of injury to you or your baby; they actually protect you both from life-threatening injuries. Don't skip wearing seat belts as you get bigger because you're uncomfortable. Studies show pregnant women who weren't wearing seat belts when they were in an accident were twice as likely to have excessive bleeding and were nearly three times more likely to lose their babies.

Below are some common excuses (and our responses) for not using seat belts and shoulder harnesses in pregnancy.

- "Using a safety belt will hurt my baby." There's no evidence seat-belt use increases the chance of injury to a baby. Your chance of survival with a seat belt is better than without one. Your survival is important to your unborn baby.
- "I don't want to be trapped in my car if there is a fire." Few automobile accidents result in fires. Even if a fire did occur, you could probably undo the restraint and escape if you were conscious. Ejection from a car accounts for about 25% of all deaths in automobile accidents. Seat-belt use prevents this.
- "I'm a good driver." Defensive driving doesn't prevent an accident.
- "I don't need to use a safety belt; I'm just going a short distance." Most accidents occur within 25 miles of home.

We know the lap/shoulder seat-belt system is safe to wear during pregnancy, so buckle up for you and your baby. Move your seat as far away from the air bag as possible—10 inches is a good distance. You might want to consider riding in the back seat when you're not driving. The middle of the back seat is the safest place in the car.

Biotin Use in Pregnancy

Biotin, also called *vitamin H* or *vitamin B7*, is an important water-soluble vitamin your body needs during pregnancy because the fetus requires large amounts of it for growth. However, studies show that as many as half of all pregnant women may not have enough biotin to meet baby's needs.

The Proper Way to Wear a Lap Belt and Shoulder Harness
· · · · · · · · · · ·

The proper way for you to wear a seat belt during pregnancy is to place the lap-belt portion under your abdomen and across your upper thighs. The shoulder portion of the belt should rest between your breasts and over the middle of your collarbone. Don't slip the belt off your shoulder. Both the shoulder belt and lap belt should be snug but comfortable. Adjust your position so the belt crosses your shoulder without cutting into your neck. You might want to check out a seat-belt extender or a maternity seat belt to help keep the seat belt from riding up on your tummy.

Causes of a biotin deficiency include not getting enough biotin in your diet, malabsorption of enzymes in the small intestine, prolonged use of antibiotics and being diabetic. Symptoms of a biotin deficiency include dry skin, brittle nails, muscle pain, anemia, hair loss, fatigue and nausea. Because many of these symptoms are common to pregnancy—without a biotin deficiency—if you experience any of them, don't panic. Bring up the subject at a prenatal appointment, and discuss it with your healthcare provider.

You can reduce your risk of a biotin deficiency by eating a healthful diet that includes cooked egg yolks, cooked oats, bananas, soybeans, rice bran, nuts, milk, wheat, meat, grapefruit, Swiss chard and romaine. Supplementation with 30mcg of biotin each day for pregnant women may also be a solution.

Medication Classification for Pregnancy

Medication a pregnant woman might use has been classified by the Food and Drug Administration (FDA) to show the risk to the baby if a mother-to-be takes it.

For nearly 40 years, healthcare providers caring for pregnant and breastfeeding women have relied on the FDA's categories for drugs—categories A, B, C, D, X. Labeling was created in the 1970s when we learned thalidomide was a human teratogen. Medical professionals felt safe recommending medicines in categories A and B. They were concerned about C and stayed away from those categorized as D and X.

In 2015, the FDA released the *Pregnancy and Lactation Labeling Rule (PLLR)*. New drugs use the new format; older drugs will be phased in. Important elements of the rule include:

- prominently listed contact information for pregnancy exposure
- risk summaries, clinical consideration and supporting data
- a subsection with information about use of the drug while breastfeeding
- subsection on females' and males' reproductive potential

The new format is designed to give the provider and user more comprehensive information to make decisions about medication use. This requires good communication between caregivers and patients. We need more information regarding drugs and pregnancy. It is hoped the pregnancy exposure registry will aid us in gathering this information.

Your Nutrition

Carbohydrate foods provide the primary source of energy for your growing baby. These foods also help your body use protein efficiently. Foods from this group are almost interchangeable, so it should be easy to get all the servings you need. Some carbohydrate foods you may choose, and their serving sizes, include the following:

- tortilla—1 large
- pasta, cereal or rice, cooked—½ cup
- cereal, ready-to-eat—1 ounce
- bagel—½ small
- bread—1 slice
- roll—1 medium

. . . .

If you're feeling down, look at your carbohydrate intake. Complex carbohydrates that are used slowly by the body result in more stable blood-sugar levels in you, which is better for baby. It may also help a bit with mood swings. Complex carbohydrates to choose from include fruits and vegetables as well as beans, lentils and oats.

. . . .

Is There Arsenic in Your Food?

There's been some discussion in the media about the safety of rice. Studies indicate it contains small amounts of arsenic. Additional research suggests other foods also contain small, measurable amounts of arsenic. These foods include cruciferous vegetables, such as broccoli, cauliflower and Brussels sprouts, kale, nonorganic chicken, dark-meat fish, such as salmon and tuna, and apple juice and grape juice.

Does this mean you need to avoid these foods during pregnancy? Experts propose moderation. It's OK for pregnant women to eat these foods occasionally. You can have a serving of these foods once or twice a week—you won't be putting yourself or your baby at risk. Just don't go overboard and make them the only foods you eat!

. . . .

You're at greater risk of food poisoning when you're pregnant. Avoid raw oysters and raw clams. Don't eat smoked or cured seafood unless it's been cooked. Limit your liver consumption, and avoid refrigerated meat spreads and pâtés.

. . . .

You Should Also Know

Instant Risk Assessment (IRA)

A screening test for Down syndrome called *IRA (Instant Risk Assessment)* offers women faster results at an earlier stage in pregnancy with a 91% accuracy rate. IRA has two parts—a blood test and an ultrasound. Women receive a collection kit from a healthcare provider or the hospital.

The woman pricks her finger and marks a card in the kit with her blood, which is sent to the lab for analysis. It is tested for levels of HCG (human chorionic gonadotropin) and a substance called *pregnancy-associated plasma protein A (PAPP-A)*. Elevated levels have been associated with Down syndrome.

The second part of the test, the ultrasound, is a nuchal translucency exam, in which an ultrasound measures the space on the back of the baby's neck. See Week 13. The larger the space in this area, the higher the chance of the baby having Down syndrome. Your healthcare provider can schedule the ultrasound.

Ultrasound in Pregnancy

By this point, you may have discussed ultrasound with your healthcare provider. Or you may already have had an ultrasound test. Ultrasound (also called *sonography* or *sonogram*) is one of our most valuable tools for evaluating a pregnancy. Healthcare providers, hospitals and insurance companies (yes, they get involved in this too) don't agree whether ultrasound should be done or if every pregnant woman needs an ultrasound test during pregnancy. It is a noninvasive test, and there are no known risks associated with it. In the United States, millions of obstetrical ultrasounds are performed each year!

With ultrasound, a lubricant is rubbed on the skin to improve contact with a transducer, which passes over the tummy, above the uterus. Sound waves pass through the tummy, into the pelvis. As sound waves bounce off tissues, they travel back to the transducer. The reflection of sound waves can be compared to "radar" used by airplanes or ships.

Different tissues of the body reflect ultrasound signals differently, and we can distinguish among them. Motion can also be seen, so we can detect motion of the baby or parts of the baby, such as the heart. With ultrasound, a fetal heart can be seen beating as early as 5 or 6 weeks into a pregnancy. Your baby's body and limbs can be seen moving as early as 4 weeks of embryonic growth (6th week of pregnancy).

Your healthcare provider uses ultrasound in many ways in relation to your pregnancy, such as:

- helping in the early identification of pregnancy
- showing the size and growth rate of baby
- identifying the presence of two or more babies
- measuring the fetal head, abdomen or femur to determine the stage of pregnancy
- identifying some fetuses with Down syndrome
- identifying some birth defects or internal-organ problems
- measuring the amount of amniotic fluid
- identifying the location, size and maturity of the placenta
- identifying placental abnormalities, uterine abnormalities or tumors
- differentiating between miscarriage, ectopic pregnancy and normal pregnancy
- in connection with various tests, such as amniocentesis, percutaneous umbilical-cord blood sampling (PUBS) and chorionic villus sampling (CVS), to select a safe place to do each test

Tip for Week 11
· · · · · · · · · · ·

You may be able to get a "picture" of your baby before birth from an ultrasound test. Some facilities can even make a visual recording you can take with you. Ask about it before the test if you're scheduled to have one.

You may be asked to drink a lot of water before an ultrasound examination. Your bladder is in front of your uterus. When your bladder is empty, your uterus is harder to see because it's farther down inside the pelvic bones. Bones disrupt ultrasound signals and make the picture harder to interpret. With your bladder full, your uterus rises out of the pelvis and can be seen more easily. The bladder acts as a window to look through to see the uterus and the fetus inside.

Other Ultrasound Tests. The *ultrasound vaginal probe*, also called a *transvaginal ultrasound*, can be used in early pregnancy for a better view of the baby and placenta. A probe is placed inside the vagina, and the pregnancy is viewed from this angle.

The *UltraScreen* test identifies babies at increased risk of having certain birth defects. The test combines maternal blood tests and an ultrasound measurement at 11 to 13 weeks. The UltraScreen test is fairly effective in detecting Down syndrome.

Fetal nasal-bone evaluation is another type of ultrasound exam that increases Down syndrome detection accuracy to 95%, with a small percentage of false-positives. The benefit of first-trimester screening is earlier diagnosis.

Three-dimensional ultrasound is also available in many areas. It is discussed in Week 17.

Can Ultrasound Determine Baby's Sex? Some couples ask for ultrasound to determine whether they are going to have a boy or girl. If the baby is in a good position and it's old enough for the genitals to have developed and they can be seen clearly, determination may be possible. However, many healthcare providers feel this reason alone is not a good reason to do an ultrasound exam. Discuss it with your healthcare provider. Understand ultrasound is a test, and test results can occasionally be wrong.

· ·

Fragile-X syndrome is one of the most common inherited causes of mental retardation. The condition can occur in both boys and girls. Testing for the gene that causes it is done with amniocentesis. Prenatal testing should be offered to known carriers of the fragile-X gene and to families with a history of mental retardation.

· ·

Fetal MRI

One test healthcare providers use has fewer limitations than ultrasound—*fetal MRI*. Fetal MRI (magnetic resonance imaging) is most helpful when findings from ultrasound are unclear or cannot be seen clearly. Ultrasound is more

Relax and Have a Great Pregnancy!
· · · · · · · · · · ·

It's natural to feel nervous about being pregnant and what lies ahead—labor and delivery, and going home with baby. It's important to deal with any anxieties you may have, and focus on having a great pregnancy. Below are some guidelines to help you do just that.

- Don't panic if someone bumps your tummy. Your baby is well protected.
- It's OK to lift things—just don't lift heavy objects. Sacks from the market or lifting a young child won't hurt you.
- You don't have to worry about using a computer, a cell phone, a microwave oven or going through airport security. None of the machines involved in these procedures produce enough "bad vibes" to hurt you or baby.
- Coloring or perming your hair is OK. The chemicals used in these preparations aren't harmful. However, if the fumes make you sick, wait until you aren't bothered so much by smells to have a perm or color your hair.
- Ask your partner to take pictures of you as you move through pregnancy. It's fun to look back at them and remember how big you were when.
- Even though you may not feel sexy, wear a beautiful, supportive bra made for expecting moms. It can help you feel pretty and desirable (which you are anyway!). For added comfort for your breasts, check out sleep bras. They can add support to sore breasts while you sleep.
- Pamper your feet. Wear good, comfortable shoes. Get a pedicure or foot massage. Soak your feet when they're sore. Use foot cream to help keep skin soft.

widely available and lower in cost than MRI and is still the first choice for discovering problems. However, MRI can be helpful in special situations.

MRI does not use radiation. Several studies have shown MRI is safe to use during pregnancy. To be cautious, MRI is still not advised during the first trimester. The test is most useful in diagnosing babies with specific birth defects.

Exercise for Week 11

· · · · · · ·

Place your left hand on the back of a chair or against the wall. Lift your right knee up, and put your right hand under your thigh. Round your back, and bring your head and pelvis forward. Hold position for count of 4, straighten up, then lower your leg. Repeat with your left leg. Do 5 or 8 times with each leg. *Reduces back tension, and increases blood flow to the feet.*

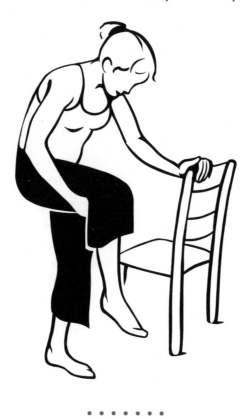

· · · · · · ·

Week 12

Age of Fetus—10 Weeks

How Big Is Your Baby?

Your baby weighs between ⅓ and ½ ounce (8 to 14g), and crown-to-rump length is almost 2½ inches (6.1cm). As you can see on page 122, your baby's size has almost doubled in the past 3 weeks!

How Big Are You?

Around this time, you may be able to feel your uterus above your pubic bone (pubic symphysis). Before pregnancy, your uterus holds ⅓ ounce (10ml) or less. During pregnancy, it becomes a muscular container big enough to hold the baby, placenta and amniotic fluid. The uterus increases its capacity 500 to 1000 times during pregnancy! By the time baby is born, it's grown to the size of a medium-size watermelon. The weight of the uterus also changes. When your baby is born, your uterus weighs almost 40 ounces (1.1kg), compared to 2½ ounces (70g) before pregnancy.

How Your Baby Is Growing and Developing

Few structures in the baby are formed after this week, but the structures already formed continue to grow and to develop. At your 12-week visit (or near then), you'll probably be able to hear your baby's heartbeat! It can be heard with Doppler, a special listening machine (not a stethoscope) that magnifies the sound of baby's heartbeat so you can hear it.

Bones are forming. Fingers and toes have separated, and nails are growing. Bits of hair begin to appear on the body.

The small intestine is capable of pushing food through the bowels. It is also able to absorb sugar.

Baby's pituitary gland is beginning to work. The nervous system has developed further. Stimulating baby may cause it to squint, open its mouth and move its fingers or toes.

The amount of amniotic fluid is increasing. Total volume is now about 1½ ounces (50ml).

Changes in You

Around this time, morning sickness often begins to improve—that's always a plus. You aren't very big and are probably still quite comfortable. If it's your first pregnancy, you may still be wearing

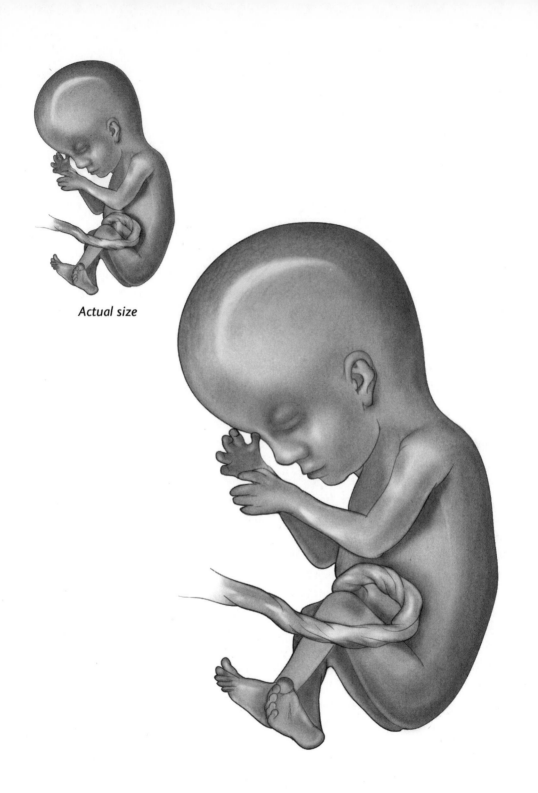

Actual size

Your baby is growing rapidly. It has doubled
its length in the past 3 weeks.

> ## Dad Tip
> • • • • • • • • • • •
> At this prenatal visit, it may be possible to hear baby's heartbeat. If you can't be there, ask your partner to record it for you to listen to later.

regular clothes. If you've had other pregnancies, you may start to show earlier and to feel more comfortable in looser clothing, such as maternity clothes.

You may be getting bigger in places besides your tummy. Your breasts are probably growing, and you may notice weight gain in your hips, legs and at your sides.

Changes in Your Skin

During pregnancy, many things can cause changes in your skin, such as hormones and stretching skin. Below we discuss some of the changes you may experience.

Skin-Color Changes. Melanin cells in your skin produce pigment; hormones can cause your body to produce more pigment. These may lead to a variety of skin-color changes. Women of color may be at increased risk for changes in skin color, which may leave the skin darker or lighter than it was before.

Itchy Skin. Pregnant women often have dry, itchy skin. Moisturizers can help, but you can also help your skin by eating omega-3 fatty acids. They're good for you and baby. Olive oil, almonds, walnuts, canola oil, flaxseed and macadamia nuts contain omega-3 fatty acids, so eat these if you do not eat fish.

If you have sensitive skin and experience itchy hives, try rubbing milk of magnesia on the affected area. Rubbing it into the skin helps reduce itching.

Cholestasis of Pregnancy. Cholestasis of pregnancy, also called *intrahepatic cholestasis of pregnancy (ICP)* or *prurigo gravidarum*, is a rare condition in which a woman has severe itching on palms and soles. Itching then spreads to the rest of the body, but there's no rash. Intense itching all over begins in the third trimester and may be much worse at night. Other symptoms include jaundice, light-colored stools and dark urine. Treatment includes anti-itch creams and UVB-light treatments. Symptoms generally disappear a few days after baby's birth.

Chloasma. Occasionally irregular brown patches appear on the face and neck, called *chloasma* or *mask of pregnancy*. These disappear or get lighter after delivery. Birth-control pills may cause similar changes. Up to 70% of all pregnant women develop chloasma after sun exposure. Women of color are more prone to developing the condition.

The best way to prevent chloasma is to stay out of the sun, especially between 10am and 3pm. Wear sunscreen and hats, long-sleeved shirts and long pants to protect you. Brown patches usually fade in the months after delivery. If they don't, ask your healthcare provider about using Retin-A after pregnancy.

Plaques of Pregnancy (PUPP). Some women have a severe, itchy rash of red bumps that begins on the tummy and spreads to the lower body, then to the arms and legs. This is called *plaques of pregnancy, toxemic rash, polymorphic eruption of pregnancy* or *pruritic urticaria pappules (PUPP).* With plaques of pregnancy, your healthcare provider may first rule out scabies.

PUPP is the most common skin problem pregnant women experience. It may be caused by skin stretching rapidly, which damages tissue, resulting in bumps and inflammation. The condition usually appears in first pregnancies during the third trimester. It often affects women who gain a lot of weight or those expecting multiples.

The good news is that PUPP won't harm the baby. The bad news is the itching can be so severe that relief may be all you think about, especially at night, which may cause you to lose sleep. PUPP usually resolves within a week after delivery and doesn't usually come back with future pregnancies.

Many treatments have been recommended for relief, including Benadryl, powders, creams, calamine lotion, soaking in cold tubs, oatmeal baths, witch hazel, going without clothes and UVB-light therapy. If you can't find relief, talk to your healthcare provider. He or she may have some recommendations for home remedies that have worked for other women. If all else fails, a prescription for oral antihistamines, topical steroids or cortisone cream may be needed.

Pemphigoid Gestationis (PG; Herpes Gestationis). Pemphigoid gestationis (PG) usually begins with blisters around the bellybutton. It may occur in the second or third trimester or immediately after birth. Despite its name, PG has no relationship to the herpes simplex virus. The name came about because the blisters appear similar to herpes infections.

The problem begins with sudden onset of intensely itchy blisters on the tummy in about 50% of cases; for the other 50%, blisters can appear anywhere on the body. It often resolves during the last part of pregnancy. More than 60% of the time, it can flare up at delivery or immediately after baby's birth.

The goal of treatment is to relieve itching and to limit blister formation. Oatmeal baths, mild creams and steroids are used. PG usually eases a few weeks after delivery and can recur in your next pregnancies or with oral-contraceptive use. Infants are not at risk.

Other Skin Changes. *Vascular spiders,* called *telangiectasias* or *angiomas,* are small red elevations on the skin, with branches extending outward. A similar condition is redness of the palms, called *palmar erythema.* Vascular spiders and palmar erythema often occur together. Symptoms are temporary and disappear shortly after delivery.

In many pregnant women, skin down the middle of the abdomen becomes markedly darker or pigmented with a brown-black color. It forms a vertical line called the *linea nigra.* It causes no problems and may be permanent.

Atopic eruption of pregnancy (AEP) covers three different pregnancy skin conditions that cause itching—eczema of pregnancy, prurigo of pregnancy and pruritic folliculitis of pregnancy. If you experience *eczema*, you may need prescription skin cream.

Prurigo of pregnancy is a poorly understood pregnancy skin condition. It may look like insect bites, and it itches. Treatment includes anti-itch creams and steroid creams. The condition usually resolves after delivery. There's no risk to you or baby.

Pruritic folliculitis of pregnancy (PFP) occurs in the second and third trimesters. It usually appears as an elevated, red area in hair follicles on the chest and back. Usually some mild itching is involved; the problem resolves 2 to 3 weeks after delivery.

It's very important to discuss psoriasis treatment options with your healthcare provider before you get pregnant. Some medications you may take can cause birth defects; others may need to be considered if your psoriasis is severe.

Psoriasis

Over 7 million people in the United States have psoriasis. It causes red, scaly, inflamed patches on the skin. It is a highly manageable condition caused by a hyperactive immune system; psoriasis can develop anywhere on the body. Researchers believe it is a genetic disorder. A child has a 10% chance of inheriting the disease if one parent is affected. If both parents are affected, chances are higher.

This skin condition can be itchy, painful, unsightly and uncomfortable. The most common form of psoriasis, called *plaque psoriasis*, occurs when the body produces new skin cells too rapidly. The normal process of skin-cell development usually takes many weeks, but in those with psoriasis, new skin cells are produced in days. Cells begin to build up on the skin because they can't be shed fast enough and appear as red, scaly patches.

Nearly a third of those with psoriasis also develop *psoriatic arthritis (PA)*, which affects joints, causing them to become stiff, painful and swollen. It's important to diagnose PA as soon as possible. Left untreated, it can damage joints within a few years.

Various lifestyle practices can trigger psoriasis, including obesity, smoking cigarettes, alcohol use, stress and certain medications. In addition, close to 15% of all psoriasis sufferers are sensitive to gluten.

Treatment. There is no cure for psoriasis. Some treatments work for a while then stop working. Others don't seem to work at all. Some treatments are very successful in treating the symptoms and may send the condition into remission. You and your healthcare provider will work together to develop a treatment plan for you.

Research indicates an anti-inflammatory diet and lifestyle changes can help many people. Phototherapy and fish-oil supplementation have also been successful in treating the condition.

Psoriasis and Pregnancy. Psoriasis does not seem to affect the reproductive system. However, it is considered a chronic condition, so you should discuss pregnancy with your healthcare provider *before* you become pregnant. Most experts agree women should stop taking all medications, including over-the-counter products, before pregnancy. In some cases, a particular medication may need to be avoided for a few *years* before pregnancy is attempted. You will need to discuss these concerns with your healthcare provider.

Pregnancy may or may not affect your psoriasis. Some women experience improvement in their condition, some see no change and others get worse. Many women experience flare-ups after delivery. And the severity of symptoms can vary from pregnancy to pregnancy.

Psoriasis can appear in the genital area; this is called *genital psoriasis*. If you suffer from genital psoriasis, be sure to tell your healthcare provider, especially if you are planning a vaginal delivery.

If you have psoriatic arthritis, some medications can be used safely during pregnancy. Discuss all prescription and nonprescription medications you use to treat this problem with your healthcare provider.

. . . .

If your psoriasis improves during pregnancy, it may be due to increased estrogen levels.

. . . .

Psoriasis Treatment during Pregnancy. Some treatments are not used during pregnancy. *Alternative nonmedication approaches* may be used, including sun and water therapy, meditation, yoga and over-the-counter topical treatments.

Managing stress and losing weight (before pregnancy) may be two options for women contemplating pregnancy. Exercising regularly before and during pregnancy may also help improve the condition. Getting enough rest and sleep—7 to 8 hours of sleep at night—can also be beneficial.

During pregnancy, topical treatments are the first choice to treat the condition. Moisturizers and emollients, such as petroleum jelly, can be used. Your healthcare provider may also OK limited use of topical steroids if they are low- to moderate dosages. Lanolin can be an irritant to people with psoriasis.

Narrow-band UVB-light therapy may also be considered to treat psoriasis during pregnancy. If this treatment is not available in your area, broad-band UVB phototherapy may be used.

If symptoms are severe, discuss the use of adalimumab (Humira), etanercept (Enbrel), infliximab (Remicade) and ustekinumab (Stelara) with your healthcare provider. It is recommended you avoid acitretin, oral retinoids, tazarotene, methotrexate and cyclosporin while preparing for and during pregnancy. These medications are known to cause birth defects.

Entering Pregnancy with High Blood Pressure

Blood pressure is the amount of force exerted by blood against arterial walls. If you've had high blood pressure before pregnancy, you have *chronic hypertension.* Your condition will not go away during pregnancy and must be controlled to avoid problems.

If you have chronic high blood pressure, you have a greater chance of having complications during pregnancy. You may have more ultrasounds to monitor baby's growth. You may want to purchase a blood-pressure monitor to use at home so you can check your pressure any time.

Most blood-pressure medications are safe to use during pregnancy. However, avoid ACE inhibitors.

. . . .

Chew each mouthful of food for 10 seconds to break it down and make it easier for your body to absorb vitamins and minerals.

. . . .

How Your Actions Affect Your Baby's Development

Physical Injury during Pregnancy

Physical injury occurs in 6 to 7% of all pregnancies. Motor-vehicle accidents account for 65% of these cases; falls and assaults account for the remaining 35%. More than 90% of these are minor injuries.

If you are injured, you may be taken care of by emergency-medicine personnel, trauma surgeons, general surgeons and your obstetrician. Most experts recommend observing a pregnant woman for a few hours after an accident to provide adequate time to monitor the baby. Longer monitoring may be necessary in a more serious accident.

It's important to take care during pregnancy so you don't get hurt. There

are many ways to do this; it just takes practice and awareness. Use the tips below.

- Keep your eyes open, and pay attention to your surroundings.
- Slow down. Don't be in a rush to get someplace—that's how many accidents occur, whether you're walking, driving or just making your way.
- Don't try to do too much—it can divert your attention from safety.
- Wear clothes and shoes that are comfortable and safe. Avoid long skirts that can trip you, carry a smaller purse, put away high heels and opt for comfortable shoes. During pregnancy, comfort and safety go hand in hand.
- Use handrails when available, such as on stairs, escalators, buses and other places.
- Wear your seat belt every time you ride in a car.

Your Nutrition

Some women don't understand the concept of increasing their caloric intake during pregnancy. Don't fall into this trap! It's unhealthy for you and baby if you gain too much weight, especially early in pregnancy. It makes carrying your baby more uncomfortable, and delivery may be more difficult. It may also be hard to shed the extra pounds after pregnancy.

After baby's birth, most women are anxious to return to "normal" clothes and to look the way they did before pregnancy. Having to deal with extra weight can interfere with reaching that goal.

. . . .

Late-night nutritious snacks are beneficial for some women. However, for many women, snacking at night is unnecessary. If you're used to ice cream or other goodies before bed, you may pay for it during pregnancy with excessive weight gain. Food in your stomach late at night may also cause heartburn or indigestion.

. . . .

Junk Food

Is junk food your kind of food? Do you eat it several times a day? Pregnancy is the time to break that habit!

Snack foods account for nearly 20% of the average American's daily calorie intake. Now that you're pregnant, you may need to do away with junk food. What you eat affects someone besides just yourself—your growing baby. If you're used to skipping breakfast, getting something "from a machine" for lunch, then eating dinner at a fast-food restaurant, it doesn't help your pregnancy.

What and when you eat become more important when you realize how your actions affect your baby. Good nutrition takes planning on your part, but you can do it. Avoid foods that contain a lot of sugar and/or fat. Choose healthful alternatives. If you work, take healthy foods with you for lunches and snacks. Stay away from fast food and junk food.

Fats and Sweets

You may need to be cautious with fats and sweets, unless you're underweight and need to gain some weight. Many of these foods are high in calories and low in nutritional value. Eat them sparingly.

Instead of selecting a food with little nutritional value, like potato chips or cookies, choose a piece of fruit, some cheese or a slice of whole-wheat bread with a little peanut butter. You'll satisfy your hunger and your nutritional needs at the same time! Some fats and sweets you may choose, and their serving sizes, include the following:

- sugar or honey—1 tablespoon
- oil—1 tablespoon
- margarine or butter—1 pat
- jam or jelly—1 tablespoon
- salad dressing—1 tablespoon

You Should Also Know

Fifth Disease

Fifth disease, also called *parvo virus B19*, was the fifth disease to be described with a certain kind of rash. (It is not related to the parvo virus common in dogs.) It is a mild, moderately contagious airborne infection and spreads easily through groups, such as classrooms or daycare centers. About 60% of pregnant women have previously had fifth disease. However, you have only a 10% chance of being infected after exposure.

The rash looks like reddened skin caused by a slap. The reddening fades and recurs, and lasts from 2 to 34 days. Joint pains are another symptom. There is no treatment. Fifth disease is most harmful to baby during the first trimester.

If you believe you have been exposed to fifth disease, contact your healthcare provider. A blood test can determine whether you previously had the virus. If you haven't, your healthcare provider can monitor you to detect problems in the baby. Some problems can be dealt with before baby is born.

Cystic Fibrosis

Cystic fibrosis (CF) is a genetic disorder that causes digestive and breathing problems. It causes the body to produce sticky mucus that builds up in the lungs, pancreas and other organs. Those with the disorder are usually diagnosed early in life.

You and your partner can be tested before pregnancy to determine if either of you are carriers. A test can also be done in the first and/or second trimester of pregnancy to see if the baby has cystic fibrosis. Medical experts urge Caucasians to have the CF test; it's the most common birth defect in this group. Screening is also recommended for others at higher risk, such as Ashkenazi Jews. The screening test uses a blood sample or a saliva sample.

For baby to have cystic fibrosis, both parents must be carriers. If only one parent is a carrier, the baby will not have CF.

Screening for Cystic Fibrosis. Screening for cystic fibrosis may be offered to couples as part of genetic counseling. One test, the *Cystic Fibrosis (CF) Complete Test*, can identify more than 1000 mutations of the CF gene. A panel that screens for 23 CF mutations is the recommended test.

If both parents carry the CF gene, the baby will have a 25% chance of having cystic fibrosis. Your developing baby can be tested during your pregnancy with chorionic villus sampling around the 10th or 11th week of pregnancy. Amniocentesis may also be used to test the baby.

Some CF gene mutations cannot be detected by the current test. This means you could be told you don't carry the gene when in fact you do. The test cannot detect all CF mutations because researchers don't know all of them at this time. However, unknown CF gene mutations are rare.

If you believe cystic fibrosis is a serious concern or if you have a family history of the disease, talk to your healthcare provider. Testing is a personal decision you and your partner must make.

Many couples choose not to have the test because it would not change what they would do during the pregnancy. In addition, they do not want to expose the mother-to-be or the developing fetus to the risks of CVS or amniocentesis. However, testing is recommended so care can be provided to baby after birth.

Exercise for Week 12

· · · · · · ·

Lie on your left side, with your body in alignment. Support your head with your left hand, and place your right hand on the floor in front of you for balance. Inhale and relax. While exhaling, slowly raise your right leg as high as you can without bending your knee or your body. Keep your foot flexed. Inhale and slowly lower your leg. Repeat on your right side. Do 10 times on each side. *Tones and strengthens hip, buttock and thigh muscles.*

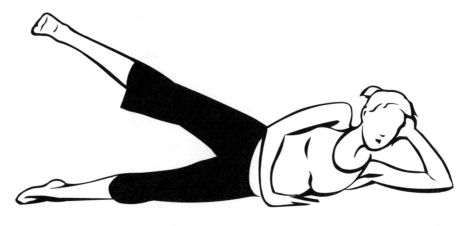

· · · · · · ·

Week 13

Age of Fetus—11 Weeks

How Big Is Your Baby?

Your baby continues to grow rapidly! Its crown-to-rump length is 2½ to 3 inches (6.5 to 7.8cm), and it weighs between ½ and ¾ ounce (13 to 20g). It is about the size of a peach.

How Big Are You?

You can probably feel the upper edge of your uterus about 4 inches (10cm) below your bellybutton. Your uterus fills your pelvis and is growing upward into your abdomen. It feels like a soft, smooth ball.

You have probably gained some weight by now. If morning sickness has been a problem, you may not have gained much. As you feel better and as your baby starts to gain weight rapidly, you'll also gain weight.

How Your Baby Is Growing and Developing

Fetal growth is particularly striking from now through about 24 weeks of pregnancy. The baby has doubled in length since the 7th week. Changes in fetal weight have also been dramatic.

There is a relative slowdown in the growth of your baby's head compared to the rest of its body. In week 13, the head is about half the crown-to-rump length. By week 21, the head is about ⅓ of baby's body. At birth, your baby's head is only ¼ the size of its body. Body growth speeds up as head growth slows down.

Eyes are moving closer together on the face. The ears move to their normal position on the sides of the head. Sex organs have developed enough so a male can be distinguished from a female if examined outside the womb.

Intestines began to develop within a large swelling in the umbilical cord outside the body. About this time, they draw back into the abdominal cavity. If this doesn't occur and the intestines remain outside the abdomen at birth, a condition called an *omphalocele* occurs. It is rare, and the condition can usually be repaired with surgery. Babies do well afterward.

Changes in You
Stretch Marks

Many women notice stretch marks, called *striae distensae*, appear during

Grandma's Remedy
· · · · · · · · · · ·

If you want to avoid using medication, try a folk remedy. If you get a paper cut, apply some lip balm to help heal the cut and reduce skin irritation.

pregnancy. They occur when the elastic fibers and collagen in deeper layers of skin are pulled apart to make room for baby. When skin tears, collagen breaks down and shows through the top layer of your skin as a pink, red or purple indented streak.

Nearly 9 out of 10 pregnant women develop stretch marks on their breasts, tummy, hips, buttocks and/or arms. They may appear any time during pregnancy. After birth, they may fade to the same color as the rest of your skin, but they won't go away.

You can help yourself by gaining weight slowly and steadily during pregnancy. Any large increase in weight can cause stretch marks to appear more readily.

Drink lots of water, and eat healthy foods. Foods high in antioxidants provide nutrients you need to repair and heal tissue. Eating enough protein and smaller amounts of "good" fats, such as flaxseed, flaxseed oil and fish oils, may also help you. Stay out of the sun! Keep up with your exercise program.

Ask your healthcare provider about using creams with alpha-hydroxy acid, citric acid or lactic acid. Some of these creams and lotions improve the quality of the skin's elastic fibers.

Don't use steroid creams, such as hydrocortisone or topicort, to treat stretch marks during pregnancy without first checking with your healthcare provider. You absorb some of the steroid into your system, and the steroid can pass to baby. And stretch creams really can't penetrate deeply enough to repair damage to your skin.

· ·

Although you'd like to think you can keep stretch marks from happening to you, there really isn't much you can do to prevent them. Creams and lotions you see advertised on TV and in magazines don't really work. You'll get stretch marks if you're going to get them. (Some lucky women get very few, if any!) They're just a part of being pregnant.

· ·

Treatment after Pregnancy. After pregnancy, you have quite a few treatment options. Some treatments hold promise. If you're left with lots of stretch marks, you may want to ask about prescription creams, such as Retin-A or Renova, or laser treatments.

Retin-A, in combination with glycolic acid, has been shown to be fairly effective. Prescriptions are needed for Retin-A and Renova; you can get glycolic acid from your dermatologist. Cellex-C, with glycolic acid, also helps with stretch marks.

The most effective treatment is laser treatment, but it can be costly. It's often done in combination with the medication methods described above. However, lasers don't work for everyone.

Massage may help—it increases blood flow to the area, which helps get rid of dead surface cells. Discuss treatment with your healthcare provider if stretch marks bother you after pregnancy.

Changes in Your Breasts

Your breasts are changing. See the illustration on page 134. Before pregnancy, your breasts may weigh about 7 ounces (200g) each. During pregnancy, they increase in size and weight as you add fat in your breast tissue. Near the end of pregnancy, each breast may weigh 14 to 28 ounces (400 to 800g). During nursing, each breast can weigh 28 ounces (800g) or more!

A breast is made up of glands, tissue to provide support and fatty tissue for protection. Each nipple contains nerve endings, muscle fibers, sebaceous glands, sweat glands and about 20 milk ducts. Milk-producing sacs connect with the ducts leading to the nipple.

From the beginning of pregnancy, your body is getting ready to breastfeed. Soon after pregnancy begins, the alveoli begin to increase in number and grow larger. Milk sinuses, located close to the nipple, begin forming; they hold the milk you will produce. By as early as 20 weeks of pregnancy, your breasts will begin to produce milk. Even if you give birth weeks earlier than your due date, your breast milk will be nutritious enough to nourish a premature baby.

You may notice veins appear just beneath the skin and nipples get larger and more sensitive. The nipple is surrounded by the areola, a circular, pigmented area.

During pregnancy, the areola darkens and grows larger. A darkened areola may act as a visual signal to baby. Bumps on your nipples, called *Montgomery glands*, secrete fluid to lubricate and protect your nipples if you breastfeed.

During the second trimester, a thin yellow fluid called *colostrum* begins to form. It can sometimes be pressed from the nipple by gentle massage. You may also notice stretch marks on your breasts. During the third trimester, your breasts may itch as skin is stretched. An alcohol-free, perfume-free moisturizer may help. Your breasts will reach their maximum size a few days after baby's birth.

. . . .

You may be wondering about taking some medicine you normally use now that you're pregnant. Zicam is an over-the-counter product to help lessen cold symptoms. Amitiza is a prescription medication taken for constipation. Ambien and Rozerem are medications to help you sleep. If you're considering using any of these medications, check first with your healthcare provider, who will determine whether you should use it.

. . . .

How Your Actions Affect Your Baby's Development

Working during Pregnancy

Today, many women work outside the home, and many continue to work during pregnancy. Most pregnant women can work until they deliver if they choose.

In the United States, millions of babies are born to women who have been employed at some time during

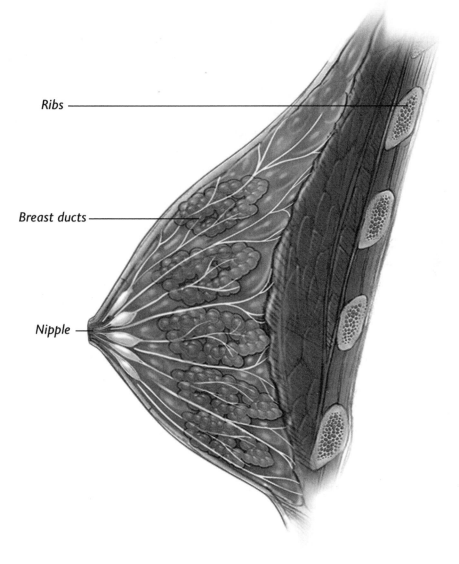

Ribs

Breast ducts

Nipple

Development of the maternal breast by the end of
the first trimester (13 weeks of pregnancy).

pregnancy. These women often have concerns about safety at work. It's common for women and their employers to have questions.

- Is it safe to work while I'm pregnant?
- Can I work my entire pregnancy?
- Am I in danger of harming my baby if I work?

You may feel anxious when you have to tell your boss you're pregnant, but it's something you must do. It's better if he or she hears it from you, not someone else.

Find out your company's maternity leave policy and what benefits it provides to pregnant women and new mothers. Be sure to document everything as you progress through pregnancy.

Legislation that May Affect You. The *U.S. Pregnancy Discrimination Act* prohibits job discrimination on the basis of pregnancy or childbirth. It states pregnancy and related conditions should be treated the same as any other disability or medical condition. A healthcare provider may be asked to certify a pregnant woman can work without endangering herself or her baby.

You may experience a pregnancy-related disability. It can come from the pregnancy itself, complications of pregnancy or a job situation, such as standing for a long time or exposure to various substances.

If you have worked for your present employer for at least 1 year, the *Family and Medical Leave Act (FMLA)* may apply to you. The law allows a new parent (mom or dad) to take up to 12 weeks of unpaid leave in any 12-month period

for the birth of a baby. Any time taken off before the birth of a baby is counted toward the 12 weeks a person is entitled to in any given year. (You might have to take time off if you have health or medical problems.) Leave may be taken intermittently or all at the same time. Check with your company's HR person to see if you are covered.

If you work for a company with fewer than 15 people, you aren't covered by the FMLA or the Pregnancy Discrimination Act. You'll probably want to find out what your company's policy is regarding pregnancy leave well in advance of your due date. Check state laws and any other local laws that apply to you to determine what kind of leave you can take.

The *Health Insurance Portability and Accountability Act (HIPAA;* pronounced hip-ah) may also apply to you. This law protects most women who change health plans or enroll in a new plan after they become pregnant. The law states that if you change jobs and insurance plans during pregnancy, you can't be denied insurance coverage if you had insurance in your former job. And your baby can't be denied coverage if you sign him or her up within a certain period after birth.

State Laws and Parental Leave. Many states in the United States have passed legislation that deals with parental leave. Some states provide disability insurance if you have to leave work because of pregnancy or birth. If you're self-employed, you aren't qualified to receive state disability payments. You may want to consider a private disability policy to cover you during the time your healthcare provider says you can't work. The glitch here is the policy must be in place *before* you become pregnant.

State laws about parental leave differ, so check with your state labor office or consult the personnel director in your company's human resources department. A summary of state laws on family leave is also available from:

Women's Bureau
U.S. Department of Labor
200 Constitution Avenue NW,
Room S-3311
Washington, DC 20210

Some Risks If You Work during Pregnancy. It can be hard to know the exact risk of a particular job. In most cases, we don't have enough information to know about everything that can harm a developing baby.

The goal is to minimize the risk to mom and baby while still allowing a woman to work. A normal woman with a normal job should be able to work throughout her pregnancy. However, she may need to change some things about her job.

If your job involves lifting, climbing, carrying or standing for a long time, you may need to make some changes. If you're exposed to any hazardous substances, you will want to make changes.

If you have any type of health problem, your healthcare provider may want you to limit activities on and off the job. He or she may also certify you have a pregnancy-related disability, meaning you have a health problem caused by your pregnancy that keeps you from doing your normal duties.

Work with your healthcare provider and your employer. If problems arise, listen to your healthcare provider. If bed rest at home is suggested, follow that advice. As your pregnancy progresses, you may have to work fewer hours or do lighter work. Be flexible. It doesn't help you or your baby if you wear yourself out and make things worse.

Take Care of Yourself. If you work, be smart! Don't participate in anything that is dangerous for you or baby. Don't stand for long periods. Don't wear clothes that are tight around the waist, especially if you sit most of the day.

Rest at breaks and during lunch. Get up and walk a little every 30 minutes. Going to the bathroom may be a good reason to get up and move around. Drink lots of water. Bring a healthy lunch and snack foods to help you keep tabs on your calorie intake; fast foods can be loaded with empty calories.

Try to keep stress to a minimum. Don't take on new projects or those that take a lot of time and attention.

Your Nutrition

Caffeine is a stimulant found in many beverages and foods, including coffee, tea, various soft drinks and chocolate. It may also be found in some medicine, such as headache remedies.

. . . .

If a woman takes in a lot of caffeine, it may affect her baby's respiratory system. One study showed exposure before birth might be linked to sudden infant death syndrome (SIDS).

. . . .

Tip for Week 13
. . . .
When cutting down on caffeine during pregnancy, read labels. More than 200 foods, beverages and over-the-counter medicines contain caffeine!

You may be more sensitive to caffeine during pregnancy. For over 25 years, the Food and Drug Administration (FDA) has recommended pregnant women avoid caffeine. It isn't good for you or baby. If you drink as little as two 8-ounce cups of coffee a day, you may be doubling your risk of early miscarriage. In addition, research shows for every 100mg of caffeine you consume each day (on a regular basis), your baby's birthweight may be lowered by 1 ounce. For example, if you consume 300mg of caffeine each day, your baby's birthweight could be reduced by 3 ounces. It's an important consideration when deciding whether to have another cup of coffee.

Cut down on caffeine, or eliminate it from your diet. Caffeine crosses the placenta to the baby—if you're jittery, baby may suffer the same effects. And caffeine passes into breast milk, which can cause irritability and sleeplessness if you breastfeed baby.

Do you know caffeine is now added to some foods? We found it added to some potato chips, candy and cereal. Be sure to read labels because caffeine must be listed as an ingredient; however, the amount may not be listed.

The list below details the amounts of caffeine from various sources:

- coffee, 5 ounces—from 60 to 140mg and higher
- tea, 5 ounces—from 30 to 65mg
- cocoa, 8 ounces—5mg
- 1½-ounce chocolate bar—10 to 30mg
- baking chocolate, 1 ounce—25mg
- soft drinks, 12 ounces—from 35 to 55mg
- pain-relief tablets, standard dose—40mg
- allergy and cold remedies, standard dose—25mg

Be careful when choosing bottled waters— some contain caffeine.

You Should Also Know
Lyme Disease

Lyme disease is transmitted to humans by ticks. About 80% of those bitten have a bite with a distinctive look, called a *bull's eye*. There may also be flulike symptoms. After 4 to 6 weeks, symptoms may become more serious.

There is evidence that Lyme disease may be transmitted sexually, putting it under the STD label. Studies show the same strain of the bacteria in married couples who had unprotected sex. If your partner has had Lyme disease, talk to your healthcare provider about it. Early on, blood tests may not diagnose Lyme disease. A blood test done later can establish the diagnosis.

Dad Tip

· · · · · · · · · · ·

Exercise is important for a pregnant woman. If there are no complications to forbid it, nearly all pregnant women are advised to exercise at least 5 times a week. Ask your partner's healthcare provider if there's some exercise you can do together on a regular basis, such as walking, swimming or playing golf or tennis. It can help you get in shape, too.

We know Lyme disease can cross the placenta. However, we don't know whether it is dangerous to the baby. Treatment requires long-term antibiotic therapy. Many medications used to treat Lyme disease are safe to use during pregnancy.

Avoid exposure if you can. Stay out of areas with ticks, especially heavily wooded areas. If you can't, wear long-sleeved shirts, long pants, a hat or scarf, socks and boots or closed shoes. Check your hair when you come in; ticks often attach themselves there. Check your clothing to make sure no ticks remain in folds, cuffs or pockets.

Probiotics

Your digestive system contains more than 500 different types of bacteria. These bacteria help digest food and keep intestines healthy. Researchers believe they may also help bolster your immune system.

Some studies indicate if the balance of good bacteria is disturbed, such as after an infection or the use of antibiotics, intestinal problems can result. Taking *probiotics* in these cases might help restore balance in the digestive tract.

Probiotics are health-promoting, live bacteria found in yogurt, supplements and some fortified foods. They are considered *good bacteria* that support the healthy bacteria that live in our digestive tracts. These good bacteria aid in digestion and vitamin absorption. They may also help fight various diseases and may help lower blood pressure, reduce LDL (bad) cholesterol and help with psoriasis and chronic fatigue syndrome.

During pregnancy, probiotics may help protect you against bacterial infection and listeriosis. However, more research on probiotics needs to be done for these claims to be proved.

If you now take probiotics or if you're interested in taking them during pregnancy, talk with your healthcare provider. Eating yogurt fortified with probiotics is probably OK because it can supply you with needed calcium. Just don't go overboard and eat too much— three or four times a week is good. However, don't take supplements without first getting the OK of your healthcare provider.

Gas (Flatulence)

Are you experiencing more gas (flatulence) than normal? It's not uncommon. What you eat definitely has an impact on gas production. And foods that trigger gas may change each trimester.

Eating slowly may help reduce the amount of air you take in, which in turn helps reduce gas. Keep exercising—it can help break up gas pockets. Stay away from certain foods, including sugar, some dairy and bread products. Sorbitol, a sugar substitute found in many "lite" foods, can also cause gas.

Nuchal Translucency Screening

Nuchal translucency screening is a test to help healthcare providers and pregnant women find answers about whether a baby has Down syndrome. Test results are available in the first trimester, so a couple may make earlier decisions regarding the pregnancy, if they choose to do so.

A detailed ultrasound allows the healthcare provider to measure the space behind baby's neck. When combined with a blood test, the results of the two tests (ultrasound and blood test) can be used to predict a woman's risk of having a baby with Down syndrome.

Exercise for Week 13

· · · · · · ·

Stand with your feet apart and your knees relaxed. Holding a light weight in your right hand (a 16-ounce can will do fine), extend your right arm straight over your head. Contract your tummy muscles, bend slightly at the waist, then swing your arm down and over your left foot. Complete the exercise by making a complete circle and returning your arm to the original position, above your right shoulder. Repeat 8 times on each side. *Strengthens back and shoulder muscles.*

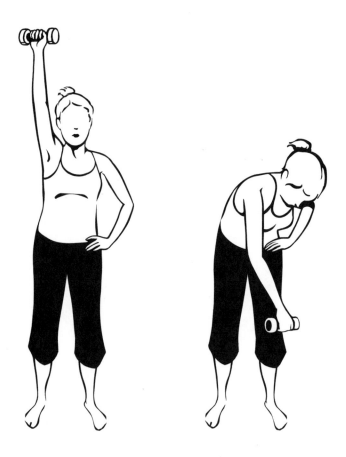

· · · · · · ·

Week 14

Age of Fetus—12 Weeks

How Big Is Your Baby?

Crown-to-rump length is 3¼ to 4 inches (8 to 9.3cm). Your baby is about the size of your fist and weighs almost 1 ounce (25g).

How Big Are You?

Maternity clothes may be a "must" by now. Some women try to get by for a while by not buttoning or zipping their pants all the way or using rubber bands or safety pins to increase the size of their waistbands. Others wear their partner's clothing, but that usually works for only a short time. You'll enjoy your pregnancy more and feel better with clothing that fits comfortably and provides you room to grow.

How Your Baby Is Growing and Developing

As you can see in the illustration on page 142, baby's ears have moved to the sides of its head. The neck has grown, so the chin no longer rests on the chest.

Changes in You

Skin Tags and Moles

Pregnancy can make skin tags and moles change and grow. *Skin tags* are small tags of skin that may appear for the first time or may grow larger during pregnancy. *Moles* may appear for the first time during pregnancy, or existing moles may grow larger and darken. If you notice any changes in a mole, show it to your healthcare provider!

Do You Have Hemorrhoids?

Hemorrhoids are dilated blood vessels around or inside the anus and are a common problem during or after pregnancy. Pregnant women often develop hemorrhoids during the second and third trimesters. Hormone changes and the growing baby are contributing factors. Hemorrhoids may worsen toward the end of pregnancy and may get worse with each succeeding pregnancy.

Eat lots of fiber, and drink lots of fluid. Stool softeners and bulk-fiber products may also help. Fiber tablets, wafers or fiber products you can add to

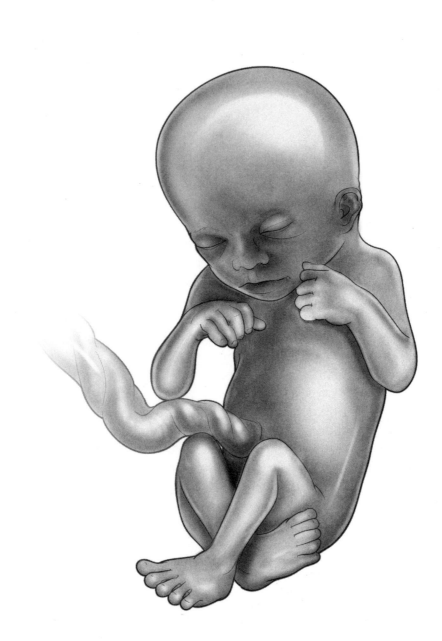

Your baby continues to change. Ears and eyes move
to a more normal position by this week.

any food or drink without adding texture may also be good remedies.

If hemorrhoids cause a lot of discomfort, discuss it with your healthcare provider. He or she will know what treatment method is best for you. Try the following for relief.

- Don't sit or stand for long periods. Rest at least 1 hour every day with your feet and hips elevated.
- Lie with legs elevated and knees slightly bent when you sleep at night.
- Take warm (not hot) baths for relief.
- Suppository medications, available without a prescription, may help. Over-the-counter products that contain hydrocortisone may help relieve itching and swelling. Ask your healthcare provider about them.
- Apply ice packs, cold compresses or cotton balls soaked in witch hazel to the affected area.
- Get up and walk often to relieve pressure on the anus.

After pregnancy, hemorrhoids usually improve, but they may not go away completely. Use the above treatment methods when pregnancy is over.

How Your Actions Affect Your Baby's Development
X-Rays, CT Scans and MRIs during Pregnancy

Some women are concerned about tests that use radiation during pregnancy. Can these tests hurt baby? Can you have them at any time in pregnancy? Unfortunately, we do not know of any "safe"

amount of radiation for a developing baby.

Some problems may require an X-ray for diagnosis and treatment; discuss the need for X-rays with your healthcare provider. It's your responsibility to let your healthcare provider and others know you're pregnant, or may be pregnant, before you have any medical test. It's easier to deal with the questions of safety and risk *before* a test is performed.

If you enjoy listening to baby's heartbeat, devices are available so you can listen at home! Some people believe doing this helps a couple bond with baby. If you're interested in a use-at-home Doppler device, check with your healthcare provider at an office visit. Or check out these devices on the Internet.

If you have an X-ray or a series of X-rays, then discover you're pregnant, ask your healthcare provider about the possible risk to your baby. He or she will be able to advise you.

Computerized tomographic scans, also called *CT* or *CAT scans*, are a form of specialized X-ray. This technique combines X-ray with computer analysis. Many researchers believe the amount of radiation received by a fetus from a CT scan is much lower than that from a regular X-ray. However, use caution when having these tests until we know more about the effects of even this small amount of radiation on a baby.

Magnetic resonance imaging, also called *MRI*, is another test widely used today. At this time, no harmful effects in pregnancy have been reported from the use of MRI. However, it may be best to avoid MRI during the first trimester.

Dental Care

See your dentist at least once during pregnancy, and tell your dentist you're pregnant. If you need dental work, postpone it until after the first 13 weeks, if possible. You may not be able to wait if you have an infection; an untreated infection could be harmful to you and your baby.

Antibiotics or pain medicine may be necessary. If you need medication, consult your pregnancy healthcare provider before taking anything. Many antibiotics and pain medications are OK to take during pregnancy.

Be careful about anesthesia for dental work during pregnancy. Local anesthesia is OK. Avoid gas and general anesthesia when possible. If general anesthesia is necessary, make sure an experienced anesthesiologist who knows you're pregnant administers it.

. . . .

If brushing your teeth makes you nauseous, try a different toothpaste or use plain baking soda. Avoid mouthwashes that contain alcohol.

. . . .

Gum Disease. During pregnancy, hormones and increased blood volume can make existing gum problems worse. *Gingivitis*, the first stage of periodontal disease, appears as swollen, bleeding, reddened gums. It's caused by bacteria growing in the spaces between the gums and teeth. Experts believe these bacteria can enter the bloodstream, travel to other parts of the body and cause infections in you.

Regular flossing and brushing help prevent gingivitis. Brushing with a power toothbrush, especially one with a 2-minute timer, may help clean teeth more thoroughly and may help toughen gums.

Oil Pulling. *Oil pulling* may be another way to achieve dental health. Studies show this alternative-medicine technique may help prevent tooth decay and bad breath as well as help improve gum health.

Once a day you swish 1 tablespoon of an edible oil, such as olive oil or sesame oil, around in your mouth for 10 to 15 minutes to help reduce plaque and germs that cause gum disease. Spit out the oil at the end of this time, then brush your teeth. When combined with brushing and flossing, oil pulling may help improve gum and tooth health.

. . . .

If you have a condition during pregnancy that causes severe pain, such as a root canal or a severe sprain, ask your healthcare provider about using analgesic codeine. It's considered safe during the first and second trimesters.

. . . .

Dental Emergencies. Dental emergencies do occur. Emergencies you might face include root canal, pulling a tooth, a large cavity, an abscessed tooth or problems resulting from an accident or injury. A serious dental problem must be treated. Problems that could result from not treating it are more serious than the risks you might be exposed to with treatment. Dental X-rays are sometimes necessary and can be done during pregnancy if your abdomen is shielded with a lead apron before X-rays are taken.

Some Tips for Whiter Teeth
· · · · · · · · · · ·

Want to have whiter teeth without using a bleaching kit or having your dentist whiten your teeth? There are some things you can do on your own to help keep teeth bright and shining. Try the following.

1. Drink through a straw. This helps keep what you're drinking away from teeth.
2. Limit coffee, tea or colas. They can stain your teeth.
3. Grab a strawberry, and rub it on your teeth. Strawberries contain an enzyme that acts like a whitener. Rub it on, then rinse well.
4. Eat crunchy raw veggies to help remove plaque.
5. Dark leafy green veggies, such as spinach and kale, create a film that can help keep stains on your teeth from recurring.
6. When brushing your teeth, dip your toothbrush head in baking soda, then brush.
7. Change your toothbrush often.
8. Don't brush too hard or you may reduce the amount of enamel on your teeth and cause gums to recede.

Your Nutrition

Being overweight when pregnancy begins may present special problems for you. Your healthcare provider may advise you to gain less weight than the average 25 to 35 pounds recommended for a normal-weight woman. You will probably have to choose lower-calorie, lower-fat foods to eat. A visit with a nutritionist may be necessary to help you develop a healthful food plan. You will be advised not to diet during pregnancy. See the following discussion dealing with obesity during pregnancy.

· ·

Don't take flax oil (it's not the same as flaxseed oil); it's often recommended as an herbal treatment for constipation. If taken during the second and third trimesters, it may increase your risk of premature birth.

· ·

You Should Also Know

Overweight/Obesity Bring Special Precautions

If you are overweight when you get pregnant, you're not alone. Statistics show up to 38% of all pregnant women are overweight; 8% of pregnant women are obese.

A new category has been added to pregnancy weight-gain guidelines. The category is for *obese women*, and the recommendation is a weight gain of between 11 and 20 pounds for an entire pregnancy. Some experts also cite *morbid obesity* as a subcategory of obesity; experts suggest weight gain should be determined on an individual basis for women in this category.

You're considered overweight if your body mass index (BMI) is between 25 and 29; over 30, you are considered obese. If

Calculation of BMI (Body Mass Index)

· · · · · · · · · · · ·

BMI is determined from the measurement of height and weight. Be sure you use your prepregnancy weight for this calculation. It is calculated as shown below:

$$BMI = \frac{weight\ (pounds) \times 703}{height\ squared\ (inches)}$$

For example, the BMI of a woman who is 5'4" tall who weighs 152 pounds would be calculated as follows:

$$\frac{152 \times 703}{64 \times 64} = BMI\ of\ 26$$

you have a BMI of 40 or over, you are considered morbidly obese.

Ask your healthcare provider to help you figure out your BMI at a prenatal appointment, or do it yourself using the formula above. When figuring your BMI, use your *prepregnancy weight*. For example, a woman who is 5'4" tall who weighs 158 pounds has a BMI of 27 and is considered overweight. A woman who is 5'4" tall who weighs 184 pounds has a BMI of 32 and is considered obese. A woman who is 5'4" tall who weighs 239 pounds has a BMI of 41 and is considered morbidly obese.

If you're overweight, it can contribute to a variety of problems. Research shows over 65% of all overweight women gain more weight than their healthcare provider recommends during pregnancy. Gaining more weight than the amount advised by your healthcare provider may increase your chances of a Cesarean delivery. It can also make carrying baby more uncomfortable, and vaginal delivery may be more difficult. And it may be harder to lose any weight you

gain during pregnancy after baby is born.

Women who are overweight may need to see their healthcare provider more often. Ultrasound may be needed to pinpoint a due date, and you may need other tests.

Take Care of Yourself. Gain your total-pregnancy weight slowly. Weigh yourself weekly, and watch your food intake. Eat nutritious, healthful foods, and eliminate those with empty calories. A visit with a nutritionist may help you develop a healthful food plan.

Don't diet during pregnancy. Choose nonfat or low-fat products, meats, grain products, fruits and vegetables. Many supply a variety of nutrients. Take your prenatal vitamin every day throughout your entire pregnancy.

Talk to your healthcare provider about exercising. Discuss swimming and walking, which are good exercises for any pregnant woman.

Eat regular meals—5 to 6 small meals a day is a good goal. Your total calorie intake should be between 1800 and 2400 calories a day. Keep a daily food diary to help you track how much you're eating and when you're eating. It can help you identify where to make changes if necessary.

. . . .

Eating raisins can inhibit the growth of bacteria that cause gum disease and tooth decay. Be sure to rinse your mouth out after eating raisins to get rid of excess sugar.

. . . .

Maternity Clothes

Every pregnant woman makes some mistakes during her pregnancy. After all, if this is your first pregnancy, you'll probably be learning the ropes as you make this 9-month journey. But knowing in advance about some common mistakes pregnant women make with maternity clothes may help you avoid them. Let's look at some we've seen all too often.

We know you're excited to let the world know you're pregnant, but don't start wearing your maternity clothes too early. Wear your regular clothes as long as you can. From experience, we know you will probably be very sick of maternity clothes by the time baby arrives.

When you buy maternity clothes, buy outfits and pieces you can wear in many ways. A top that can be worn with pants and skirts or over your bathing suit is a good example. A dress you can wear during the day then dress up for a night out is another good choice.

Don't overbuy. As much fun as it is to buy these clothes that let the world know you're pregnant, you may not need as many as you think you will. Try to borrow clothes from friends or relatives. And check out resale and thrift shops for gently worn maternity clothes.

Be sure you buy a couple of pairs of good shoes. Good choices include ones that expand if your feet swell and get bigger. Some flats with a strap you can loosen as feet swell might fit the bill. Avoid high heels, especially toward the end of pregnancy. Keep the heel height to 1½ inches or less.

Another must is supportive undergarments. Buy some good pregnancy bras. You might also want some sleep bras. Maternity hose might be a necessity. And consider underpants with a cotton crotch. Avoid thong underwear because wearing them could lead to UTIs—the thong portion of the underpants is a direct line for carrying feces from the anus to the vaginal area.

Is a Belly Band for You?

Have you heard of a belly band to wear during pregnancy and after baby's birth? It can be a very versatile piece of clothing for you. A *belly band* is like a tube top or elastic band of fabric that goes around your middle. Belly bands are popular and can be purchased in many colors and styles. Some of the belly bands we have seen come with Velcro fasteners so they are adjustable. Other belly bands are more like a T-shirt or a blouse.

Wearing a belly band during pregnancy can help you in many ways and has a variety of uses. Your body changes a great deal during your pregnancy, and your prepregnancy clothes won't fit after awhile. A belly band can hide the unzipped fly of your pants or jeans and help you extend the length of time you wear your prepregnancy clothes. Just slide the belly band up over your pants until it covers the zipper, the buttons and your tummy. The band should hold your pants in place, even if you can't fasten them!

Some belly bands are designed only to cover your baby bump and help with clothes issues. Others are designed to support your back and growing abdomen. Some belly bands are designed specifically to give you extra support during pregnancy and ease some pregnancy discomforts. A belly band can cost from $20 to $100. You may need to buy more than one to fit you as you grow larger.

In addition to a belly band, you may hear about *hip bands*. A hip band is worn under your shirt or top, and over the top of your pants or jeans. It can really be a boon in later pregnancy when shirts are too short to cover the top of pants. A *belly bra* provides support to your stomach, back and breasts while your pregnancy is growing. It can be especially beneficial during the third trimester.

For a discussion of belly bands after pregnancy, see the after-pregnancy chapter that begins on page 401.

Pregnancy in the Military

Are you pregnant and currently on active duty in the military? If you are, you have made the decision to stay in the Armed Forces. Before 1972, if you were on active duty and became pregnant, you were automatically separated from the military, whether you wanted to be or not!

Today, if you want to stay in the service, you can. Each branch of the service

has particular policies regarding pregnancy. Below is a summary of those policies for the Army, Navy, Air Force, Marines and Coast Guard.

Army Policies. During pregnancy, you are exempt from body composition and fitness testing. You cannot be deployed overseas. At 20 weeks, you're required to stand at parade rest or attention for no longer than 15 minutes. At 28 weeks, your work week is limited to 40 hours a week, 8 hours a day.

Navy Policies. During pregnancy, you are exempt from body composition and fitness testing. You are not allowed to serve on a ship after 20 weeks of pregnancy. You're limited to serving duty in places within 6 hours of medical care. Your work week is limited to 40 hours, and you're required to stand at parade rest or attention for no longer than 20 minutes.

Air Force Policies. During pregnancy, you are exempt from body composition and fitness testing. Restrictions are based on your work environment. If you are assigned to an area without obstetrical care, your assignment will be curtailed by week 24.

Marine Corps Policies. You will be on full-duty status until a medical doctor certifies full duty is not medically advised. You may not participate in contingency operations nor may you be deployed aboard a Navy vessel. Flight personnel are grounded, unless cleared by a medical waiver. If a medical doctor deems you are unfit for physical training

Tip for Week 14
· · · · · · · · · · ·

If you must have dental work or diagnostic tests, tell your dentist or your health-care provider you're pregnant so they can take extra care with you. It may be helpful for your dentist and healthcare provider to talk before any decisions are made.

or you cannot stand in formation, you will be excused from these activities. However, you will remain available for worldwide assignments.

Pregnant Marines will not be detached from Hawaii aboard a ship after their 26th week. If serving aboard a ship, a pregnant woman will be reassigned at the first opportunity but no later than by 20 weeks.

U.S. Coast Guard. During pregnancy, you are exempt from body composition and fitness testing. After 28 weeks of pregnancy, your work week will be limited to 40 hours. You will not be assigned overseas. Other duty restrictions are based on your job; however, you will not be assigned to any rescue-swimmer duties during your pregnancy.

You may not be deployed from the 20th week of your pregnancy through 6 months postpartum. You will not be assigned to any flight duties after your second trimester (26 weeks), and you are limited to serving duty in places within 3 hours of medical care.

Some General Cautions. We know women who get pregnant while they're on active duty face many challenges. The pressure to meet military body-weight standards can have an effect on your

health; that's the reason these requirements are relaxed during pregnancy.

Work hard to eat healthy foods so you have adequate levels of iron and folic acid. Examine your job for any hazards you may be exposed to, such as standing for long periods, heavy lifting or exposure to toxic chemicals. Before receiving any vaccinations or inoculations, discuss them with your healthcare provider. Any of these factors can impact your pregnancy.

If you are concerned about any of the above, discuss it with a superior. Changes beyond those described above may have to be made.

Taking Others to Prenatal Visits
Take your partner with you to as many prenatal appointments as possible. It's nice for your partner and healthcare provider to meet before labor begins. Maybe your mother or the other grandmother-to-be would like to go with you to hear the baby's heartbeat. Or you may want to record the heartbeat for others to hear. Things have changed since your mother carried you; many grandmothers-to-be enjoy this type of visit.

It's a good idea to wait until you have heard baby's heartbeat before bringing other people. You don't always hear it the first time, which can be frustrating and disappointing.

> ### Dad Tip
> · · · · · · · · · · ·
>
> Be thoughtful about staying in touch. If you have to go out of town, call your partner at least once a day. Let her know you're thinking about her and the baby. You can also ask friends and family members to check on her and be available to help out.

Some women bring their children with them to a prenatal appointment. Most office personnel don't mind if you bring your children occasionally. They understand it isn't always possible to find someone to watch them. However, if you have problems or have a lot to discuss with your healthcare provider, don't bring your child or children.

If a child is sick, has just gotten over chicken pox or is getting a cold, leave him or her at home. Don't expose everyone else in the waiting room.

Some women like to bring one child at a time to a visit if they have more than one. That makes it special for mom and the child. Crying or complaining children can create a difficult situation, however, so ask your healthcare provider when it's good to bring family members with you before you come in with them.

Exercise for Week 14

• • • • • • •

Kegel exercises strengthen pelvic muscles; practicing it helps relax your muscles for delivery. The exercise can also be helpful in getting vaginal muscles back in shape after delivery of your baby. You can do it anywhere, anytime, without anyone knowing you're doing it!

While sitting, contract the lowest muscles of your pelvis as tightly as you can. Tighten the muscles higher in the pelvis in stages until you reach the muscles at the top. Count to 10 slowly as you move up the pelvis. Hold briefly, then release slowly in stages, counting to 10 again. Repeat 2 or 3 times a day. You can also do Kegel exercises by tightening the pelvic muscles first, then tightening the anal muscle. Hold for a few seconds, then release slowly, in reverse order. To see if you're doing the exercise correctly, stop the flow of urine while you're going to the bathroom.

Week 15

Age of Fetus—13 Weeks

How Big Is Your Baby?

The fetal crown-to-rump length by this week is 4 to 4½ inches (9.3 to 10.3cm). The fetus weighs about 1¾ ounces (50g). It's close to the size of a softball.

How Big Are You?

Changes in your lower abdomen change the way your clothes fit. Your pregnancy may not be obvious to other people when you wear regular clothes. But it may become obvious if you start wearing maternity clothes or put on a swimsuit. You may be able to feel your uterus about 3 or 4 inches (7.6 to 10cm) below your bellybutton.

How Your Baby Is Growing and Developing

It's still a little early to feel movement, although you should feel your baby move in the next few weeks!

Baby's skin is thin, and you can see blood vessels through the skin. Baby may be sucking its thumb. This has been seen with ultrasound examination.

As you can see in the illustration on page 154, ears now look more normal. In fact, your baby looks more human every day. Bones that have already formed are getting harder. If an X-ray were done at this time, the baby's skeleton would be visible.

Alpha-Fetoprotein (AFP) Testing

As baby grows, it produces alpha-fetoprotein (AFP) in its liver and passes some of it into your bloodstream. It's possible to measure AFP by drawing your blood; too much or not enough of the protein in your blood can be a sign of problems.

An AFP test is usually done between 16 and 18 weeks of gestation. Timing is important and must be tied to the gestational age of your pregnancy and to your weight.

An elevated AFP level can indicate problems in baby. A connection has been found between a low level of AFP and Down syndrome. If your AFP level is abnormal, your healthcare provider may choose to do other tests to look for problems.

The AFP test is not done on all pregnant women, although it is required in some states. AFP is often used with other tests. One use of the test is to help a woman decide whether to have amniocentesis. If the test isn't offered, ask about it. There's little risk, and it helps your healthcare provider determine how baby is growing and developing.

. . . .

Ultrasound during the second trimester can diagnose multiple fetuses, is used with amniocentesis, investigates bleeding related to placenta previa or placental abruption, diagnoses intrauterine-growth restriction (IUGR) and evaluates baby's well-being. Done around 20 weeks, it may help determine if the placenta has attached normally and is healthy.

. . . .

Changes in You

During your first prenatal visit, you probably had a Pap smear; one is usually done at the beginning of pregnancy. A Pap smear identifies cancerous or precancerous cells coming from the cervix. This test has helped decrease the number of deaths from cervical cancer because of early detection and treatment.

An abnormal Pap smear during pregnancy must be handled individually. When abnormal cells are "not too bad" (premalignant or not as serious), it may be possible to watch them during pregnancy.

If your healthcare provider is concerned, he or she may do a *colposcopy*, a procedure to examine the cervix. Abnormal areas can be seen so biopsies can be taken after pregnancy. Most obstetricians/gynecologists can do this procedure in the office. There are several ways to treat abnormal cells on the cervix; most treatment methods are done after pregnancy.

How Your Actions Affect Your Baby's Development

Change Sleeping Positions Now

Some women have questions about their sleeping positions and sleep habits while they're pregnant. Some want to know if they can sleep on their stomachs. Lying on your stomach puts extra pressure on your growing uterus. Others want to know if they should stop sleeping on their waterbed. (It's OK to continue to sleep on a waterbed.)

As you get bigger, finding comfortable sleeping positions gets harder. Don't lie on your back when you sleep. As your uterus gets larger, lying on your back can decrease circulation to your baby and parts of your body. Some pregnant women also find it harder to breathe when lying on their backs.

It's important to learn to sleep on your side. For some women, their favorite thing after delivery is to be able to sleep on their stomach again!

. . . .

Start now to learn to sleep on your side; it will pay off later as you get bigger.

. . . .

Communicating with Your Healthcare Provider

Communication between you and your healthcare provider is critical. Being able to communicate effectively will help you deal more easily with personal issues. It's worth the effort to find a provider you're comfortable with and with whom you can talk easily and effectively. Miscommunication can be a source of conflict.

If language is a barrier, try to find a healthcare provider who speaks your

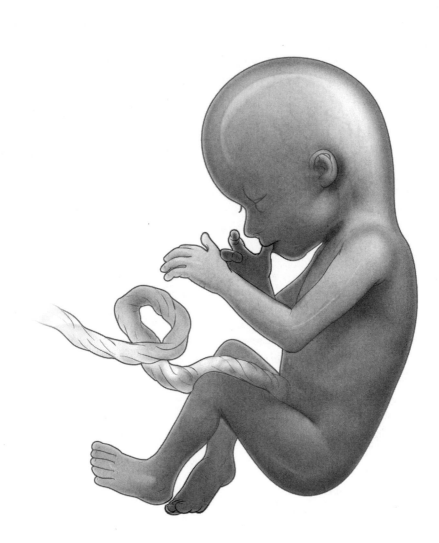

By week 15 of pregnancy (fetal age—13 weeks),
your baby may suck its thumb. Eyes are at the front of
the face but are still widely separated.

Dad Tip
· · · · · · · · · · ·

Having a baby can mean a lot of financial changes in your life. Examine your wills and update them if necessary. Name a guardian for your child in case something happens to both of you. Other important tasks include checking life insurance and medical-health insurance to be sure coverage is enough for your family. You also need to consider child-care costs, if one of you is not going to be a stay-at-home parent.

language fluently. If this isn't possible, ask if someone on the staff speaks your language. If language is still a barrier, find someone (a friend or even a professional interpreter) to attend every office visit with you so you can ask questions and get accurate answers. You'll be better able to understand advice and instructions, treatment plans or directions.

You must be the best patient you can be. Follow your healthcare provider's instructions; if you have questions or disagree with something, discuss it. Speak up when you're confused or dissatisfied. When a test or procedure is ordered, ask why it is being done. And be sure you get test results.

Don't withhold information, even if it's embarrassing. Tell your healthcare provider everything he or she needs to know about you. In this way, your healthcare team will have all the information they need to provide you and baby the best care possible.

Go to visits prepared with your questions and concerns written down. Then write down answers you receive or have someone come with you to help you remember important instructions or suggestions. Be an active participant in your health care for your good health and the good health of your baby.

Changing Healthcare Providers. If these suggestions don't work, it's OK to change healthcare providers—it happens all the time. If you need to find someone new, start as soon as possible.

When you find a new healthcare provider, be sure he or she is accepting new patients. Also check whether your insurance plan covers this healthcare provider. Tell your current healthcare provider you're leaving, and explain why. Ask for your records. It's better to take them with you instead of having them sent, which can take some time. Be sure also to request copies of all tests and test results.

Take your records to your first office visit. Bring a list of all prescription and over-the-counter medications you take. Be prepared to cover your health and pregnancy history in detail to provide your new healthcare provider a complete picture of your health care to date.

Your Nutrition

About this time, you may need to start adding extra calories to your meal plan to meet the needs of your growing baby and your changing body. If you're a normal-weight woman, eat between 2200 and 2500 calories a day during the first trimester. During the second trimester, increase that amount by about 300 calories a day. In the third trimester, add only an additional 100 calories (beyond the 300 calories you added during the second trimester). By the end of pregnancy, you should be eating between 2600 and 2900 calories a day. If you are overweight or obese, your healthcare provider will give you a daily calorie goal.

Below are some choices of extra food for one day to get additional calories. Be careful—300 calories is *not* a lot of food.

- Choice 1: 2 thin slices pork, ½ cup cabbage, 1 carrot
- Choice 2: ½ cup cooked brown rice, ¾ cup strawberries, 1 cup orange juice, 1 slice fresh pineapple
- Choice 3: 4 ounces salmon steak, 1 cup asparagus, 2 cups Romaine lettuce
- Choice 4: 1 cup cooked pasta, 1 slice fresh tomato, 1 cup 1% milk, ½ cup cooked green beans, ¼ cantaloupe
- Choice 5: 1 container of yogurt, 1 medium apple

. . . .

If you eat a lot of high-fat food during the day, you may pay for it at night by tossing and turning. Pastas and other complex carbohydrates may help relax you.

. . . .

You Should Also Know

Getting a Good Night's Sleep

Discomforts of pregnancy may impact your sleep, and sleeping soundly may be difficult for you. Research shows if a woman has difficulty sleeping during pregnancy, she may be at higher risk of some pregnancy problems. If you're exhausted when you begin labor, you may be at a higher risk for a Cesarean delivery. Studies show if you get less than 6 hours of sleep a night during the last few weeks of pregnancy, your labor may be longer. Less sleep may also increase your risk of postpartum depression.

Sleep disturbances are common in pregnancy; between 65 and 95% of all pregnant women experience some sleep changes. There are ways to get a good night's sleep. Develop a nighttime ritual. Go to bed and wake up at the same time each day. Even if you feel exhausted, don't nap close to bedtime.

Don't drink much after 4pm so you don't have to get up to go to the bathroom all night long. Avoid caffeine after late afternoon. Slowly drink a glass of milk before bed.

Keep your bedroom dark and cool. Record favorite late-night TV shows, and watch them the next day.

If you get heartburn at night, sleep propped up or sitting in a comfortable chair. Studies show listening to soothing sounds before bedtime can help you fall asleep faster and sleep longer. If you experience shortness of breath due to your bigger tummy, it can interfere with sleep. Lie on your left side. Prop up your head and shoulders with extra pillows. If this doesn't help, try a warm shower or a soak in a warm (not hot) tub.

Get regular exercise. Stretching during the day may help you sleep better; it eases muscle tension so you're more relaxed when you go to bed.

Tip for Week 15

· · · · · · · · · · ·

Sometimes it helps to use a few extra pillows when you go to bed. Put one behind you so if you roll onto your back, you won't lie flat. Put another between your legs, or rest your top leg on a pillow. Consider using a "pregnancy pillow" to support your entire body.

If you still have trouble sleeping after trying these suggestions, talk with your healthcare provider. He or she may prescribe a medication for you. You may ask your healthcare provider to check your iron levels, which can impact sleep.

Domestic Violence

Domestic violence is an epidemic problem in the United States; every year almost 5 million women experience a serious assault by someone who says they love them. We have evidence that nearly one in three women has suffered abuse from a spouse or partner.

The term *domestic violence* refers to violence against adolescent and adult females within a family or intimate relationship. It can take the form of physical, sexual, emotional, economic or psychological abuse. *Physical violence* is defined as punching, slapping, pushing or choking a person; being attacked with a weapon also falls into this category. *Sexual violence* is described as feeling mentally or physically forced into having sex. Being compelled to perform or engage in humiliating or degrading sexual acts are also characterized as sexual violence.

Unfortunately, abuse does not usually stop during pregnancy. Research shows most women who experience violence during pregnancy may have experienced it before.

Domestic abuse occurs in 4 to 8% of all pregnancies and kills more pregnant women than any medical complication of pregnancy, accounting for 20% of all pregnancy-related deaths. Studies indicate abuse may begin or escalate during pregnancy.

Abuse can be an obstacle to prenatal care. Some abused pregnant women do not seek prenatal care until later in pregnancy and may miss more prenatal appointments. Women at risk may not gain enough weight, or they may suffer more injuries during pregnancy.

If you're unsure if you are in an abusive relationship, ask yourself the following questions.

- Does my partner threaten me or throw things when he's angry?
- Does he make jokes at my expense and put me down?
- Has he physically hurt me in the past year?
- Has he forced me to perform a sexual act?
- Does he say it's my fault when he hits me?
- Does he promise me it won't happen again, but it does?
- Does he keep me away from family and friends?

If you answered "yes" to any of these questions, your relationship may be abusive.

If you're being abused, we encourage you to seek help immediately. Intervention can be lifesaving for you and your unborn child. Talk to someone—a friend, relative, someone at your church or your healthcare provider are good resources. There are many domestic-violence programs, crisis hotlines, shelters and legal-aid services available to help you. Call the 24-hour National Domestic Violence Hotline at 800-799-7233 for help and advice.

Plan for your safety. This may include a "fast exit." A recommended safety plan includes packing a suitcase and arranging for a safe place to stay, regardless of the time of day or night. Know where to go for help if you are hurt.

Hide some cash, and keep needed items in a safe place, such as prescription medicines, health insurance cards, credit cards, checkbook, driver's license and medical records. Be prepared to call the police.

If you're hurt before you can leave permanently, go to the nearest emergency room. Tell personnel there how you were hurt. Ask for a copy of your medical records, and give them to your own healthcare provider.

These steps may seem drastic, but remember—domestic violence is a serious problem with serious consequences. Protect yourself and your unborn baby!

Old Wives' Tales

Now that you're pregnant, you may receive all sorts of information—whether or not you welcome it. Some may be useful, some may be frightening and some may be laughable. Should you believe everything you hear? Probably not.

Here are some old wives' tales you can definitely ignore. When you hear one of them, smile and nod. You'll know the truth and not worry this will happen to you!

- You need calcium if you crave ice cream. Craving spinach means you need iron.
- Cold feet and/or dry hands mean you're going to have a boy.
- Dangling a wedding ring over your tummy indicates baby's sex.
- Your baby will be born with a hairy birthmark if you see a mouse.
- If you carry out in front, it's a boy; carrying around your middle means it's a girl. Or if you carry high, it's a boy; carrying low means it's a girl.
- Eating berries causes red splotches on baby's skin.
- If you perspire a lot, refuse to eat the heel on a loaf of bread or crave orange juice, it's a girl.
- Taking a bath can hurt, or even drown, a fetus. (But do be careful of soaking for a long time in hot water, like in a spa—that could harm the fetus.)
- Stretching your arms over your head can cause the umbilical cord to wrap around baby's neck.
- Craving greasy foods means your labor will be short.
- Your baby will be cross-eyed if you wear high heels.

Were You Hard to Live with When You Had Morning Sickness?
· · · · · · · · · · ·

If you suffered with morning sickness and you're starting to feel better, you may want to take stock of your relationship with your partner. Were you hard to get along with when you weren't feeling good? Your partner needs your support as pregnancy progresses, just as you need his support. You may need to make an effort to work very hard at treating each other well—you're both in this together!

- Using various techniques or substances will start labor. Do not try to induce labor by walking, exercising, drinking castor oil, going on a bumpy ride (not a good idea during pregnancy anyway) or using laxatives.

There are some old wives' tales that are true. If you've heard that if you suffer from heartburn, baby will have a full head of hair, it's true! Studies show over 80% of women who experienced moderate to severe heartburn during pregnancy had babies with lots of hair! Hormones that cause heartburn also control hair growth. Who knew?

Another tale to believe is that if you have sex during late pregnancy, it may cause labor to start. If you have sex after 36 weeks of pregnancy, you're more likely to deliver sooner than women who don't have sex. Semen contains prostaglandin, and when combined with your hormones, it may cause contractions to begin.

Tay-Sachs Disease

Tay-Sachs disease is an inherited disease of the central nervous system. The most common form of the disease affects babies, who appear healthy at birth and seem to develop normally for the first few months, then development slows and symptoms begin to appear. There is no treatment and no cure for Tay-Sachs disease at this time, and death usually occurs before age 5.

The disease occurs most frequently in descendants of Ashkenazi Jews from Central and Eastern Europe. About one in every 30 American Jews carries the Tay-Sachs gene. Some non-Jewish people of French-Canadian ancestry (from the East St. Lawrence River Valley of Quebec) and members of the Cajun population in Louisiana are also at increased risk. These groups have about 100 times the rate of occurrence as other ethnic groups.

The disease is hereditary; babies born with Tay-Sachs disease lack a protein called *hexosaminidase A*, or *hex-A*, which is necessary to break down certain fatty substances in brain and nerve cells. When hex-A isn't available, substances build up and gradually destroy brain and nerve cells until the central-nervous system stops working.

Tay-Sachs disease can be diagnosed before birth with amniocentesis and chorionic villus sampling (CVS). If prenatal testing shows hex-A is present, the baby will not have Tay-Sachs.

When two carriers become parents, there is a one-in-four chance any child they have will have the disease. If only one parent is a carrier, each child has a 50–50 chance of being a carrier.

There are various types of Tay-Sachs disease. The classic type, which affects babies, is the most common. Other rare deficiencies of the hex-A enzyme are sometimes included under the umbrella of Tay-Sachs disease and are referred to as juvenile, chronic and adult-onset forms of hex-A deficiency.

Exercise for Week 15

• • • • • • •

Place a chair in the corner so it won't slide when you push against it. Place your right foot on the chair seat; support yourself against the wall with your hand, if necessary. Stretch your left leg behind you, lift your chest and arch your back. Turn your shoulders, and lean your torso to the right. Hold 25 to 30 seconds. Do 3 stretches for each side. Do this stretch before beginning tummy exercises. *Tones back muscles.*

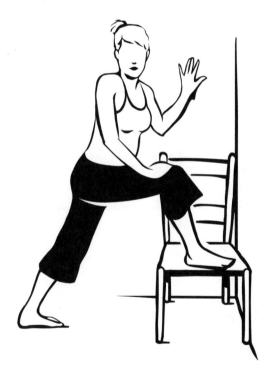

• • • • • • •

Week 16

Age of Fetus—14 Weeks

How Big Is Your Baby?

Baby's crown-to-rump length by this week is 4⅓ to 4⅔ inches (10.8 to 11.6cm). Weight is about 2¾ ounces (80g).

How Big Are You?

Six weeks ago, your uterus weighed about 5 ounces (140g). It weighs about 8¾ ounces (250g) now. The amount of amniotic fluid around the baby has increased to about 7½ ounces (250ml) of fluid. You can easily feel your uterus about 3 inches (7.6cm) below your bellybutton.

How Your Baby Is Growing and Developing

Fine hair covers baby's head. The illustration on page 164 shows soft hair, called *lanugo*. The umbilical cord is attached to the abdomen; this attachment has moved lower on the body of the fetus. Fingernails are well formed.

Arms and legs are moving; you can see movement on an ultrasound exam. You may also be able to feel baby move; many women describe feelings of movement as a "gas bubble" or "fluttering." Often, it's something you may notice for

a few days but didn't realize what you were feeling. Then you realize you're feeling baby moving inside you!

Changes in You

If you haven't felt your baby move yet, don't worry. Fetal movement, also called *quickening*, is usually felt between 16 and 20 weeks of pregnancy. The time is different for every woman and can be different from one pregnancy to another. One baby may be more active than another. The size of the baby or the number of fetuses can also affect what you feel.

Multiple-Marker Tests

Multiple-marker tests, such as the *triple-screen* and *quad-screen* tests, are usually done 15 to 18 weeks after your last menstrual period. These tests measure levels of certain substances in your blood and are based on your age, weight, race and whether you smoke or have diabetes requiring insulin. The triple-screen test is discussed below. The quad-screen test is discussed in Week 17.

Triple-Screen Test. This screening blood test is used to find possible problems. A diagnostic test may be done to confirm any diagnosis.

The triple-screen test can go beyond alpha-fetoprotein testing in helping your healthcare provider determine if you might be carrying a child with Down syndrome. The test checks your alpha-fetoprotein level along with the amounts of human chorionic gonadotropin (HCG) and unconjugated estriol (a form of estrogen produced by the placenta). Abnormal levels can indicate baby has a problem.

This test has a higher level of false-positives, which means the test says there's a problem when there really isn't one. One reason for this is a wrong due date. If you believe you're 16 weeks pregnant but are actually 18 weeks pregnant, hormone levels will be off, which could make test results incorrect. If you're carrying more than one baby, it can also cause inaccurate test results. If you have an abnormal result, ultrasound and amniocentesis may be recommended.

How Your Actions Affect Your Baby's Development

Amniocentesis

Amniocentesis is a test in which amniotic fluid is removed from the amniotic sac to test for some genetic defects and for fetal lung maturity. It is often performed around 16 to 18 weeks of pregnancy. By this point, your uterus is large enough and there is enough fluid surrounding the baby to make the test possible.

Fetal cells that float in amniotic fluid can be grown in cultures and used to identify some birth defects. We know of more than 400 abnormalities a child can be born with—amniocentesis identifies about 40 (10%) of them, including the following:

- chromosomal problems, particularly Down syndrome
- fetal sex, if sex-specific problems, such as hemophilia or Duchenne muscular dystrophy, must be identified
- fetal infections
- central-nervous-system diseases, skeletal diseases and blood diseases
- chemical problems or enzyme deficiencies

Ultrasound is used to locate a pocket of fluid where the baby and placenta are out of the way. Abdomen skin is numbed, and a needle is passed through the abdominal wall into the uterus. About 1 ounce of fluid is withdrawn from the area around the baby with a syringe; if you are carrying twins, fluid may be taken from each sac.

Risks from amniocentesis include injury to the baby, placenta or umbilical cord, infection, miscarriage or premature labor. The use of ultrasound to guide the needle helps avoid problems but doesn't eliminate all risk.

Bleeding from the baby to the mother can occur, which can be a problem. An Rh-negative woman should receive RhoGAM after the test to prevent isoimmunization.

Over 95% of women who have amniocentesis learn their baby does *not* have the disorder the test was done for. Fetal loss from amniocentesis is estimated to

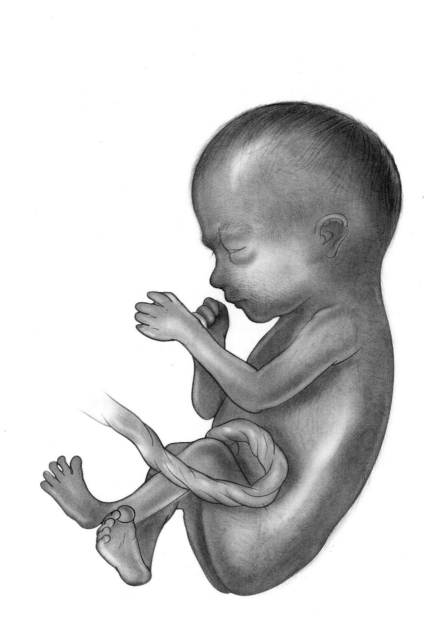

By this week, soft lanugo hair covers
the baby's body and head.

Dad Tip
· · · · · · · · · · ·

Do you have concerns you haven't shared with anyone? Are you concerned about your partner's health or the baby's? Do you wonder about your role in labor and delivery? Are you worried about being a good father? Share your thoughts with your partner. You won't burden her. In fact, she'll probably be relieved to know she's not alone in feeling a little overwhelmed by this monumental life change.

be less than 3%. The procedure should be done only by someone who has experience doing it.

Are You an Older Mother-to-Be?

More women are getting pregnant in their 30s or 40s. If you waited to start a family, you're not alone. Close to 15% of new mothers are now 35 or older. You may have waited to get married, or you may be in a second marriage and starting a new family. Some couples have experienced infertility and do not achieve a pregnancy until they have gone through testing or surgery. Or you may be a single mother who has chosen donor insemination to achieve pregnancy.

Today, many healthcare professionals gauge pregnancy risk by the pregnant woman's health status, not her age. Pre-existing medical conditions have the greatest impact on a woman's well-being during pregnancy. For example, a healthy 39-year-old is less likely to develop problems than a diabetic woman in her 20s. A woman's fitness can also have a greater effect on her pregnancy than her age.

An older woman in good physical condition who has exercised regularly may go through pregnancy as easily as a woman 15 to 20 years younger. An exception—women in a first pregnancy who are over 40 may have more problems than women the same age who have previously had children. But most healthy women will have a safe delivery.

Some health problems can be age related, and the risk of developing a condition increases with age. You may not know you have a problem unless you see your healthcare provider regularly.

Genetic Counseling May Be a Wise Choice. If either you or your partner is over 35, genetic counseling may be recommended; this can raise many questions for you. The risk of chromosome problems exceeds 5% for the over-35 age group.

Genetic counseling brings together a couple and professionals who are trained to deal with questions about the occurrence, or risk of occurrence, of a genetic problem. With genetic counseling, information about human genetics is applied to a particular couple's situation. Information is interpreted so the couple can make informed decisions.

Will Your Pregnancy Be Different If You're Older? Your healthcare provider may see you more often or you may have more tests. You may be advised to

> *Tip for Week 16*
> . . . .
> Some of the foods you normally love may make you sick to your stomach during pregnancy. You may need to substitute other nutritious foods you tolerate better.

have amniocentesis or CVS to find out whether your child has Down syndrome. Even if you would never terminate a pregnancy, this information helps you and your healthcare team prepare for the birth of your baby.

If you're over 35, you have a greater chance of having problems, so you may be watched more closely during pregnancy. Some issues can be troublesome, but with good medical care, they can usually be handled fairly well.

Pregnancy when you're older can take its toll. You may gain more weight, see stretch marks where there were none before, notice your breasts sag lower and feel a lack of tone in your muscles. Attention to nutrition, exercise and rest can help a great deal.

Fatigue may be one of your greatest problems—it's a common complaint. Rest is essential to your health and baby's. Rest and nap when possible. Don't take on more tasks or new roles. Don't volunteer for big projects. Learn to say "No." You'll feel better!

Moderate exercise can help boost energy levels and may ease some discomforts. However, check first with your healthcare provider before starting any exercise program.

Stress may be relieved by exercise, eating healthfully and getting as much rest as possible. Take time for yourself. Some women find a pregnancy support group is an excellent way to deal with difficulties they may experience. Ask your healthcare provider for further information.

We know labor and delivery for an older woman may be different. Labor may last longer. Older women also have a higher rate of Cesarean deliveries. After baby's birth, your uterus may not contract as quickly; postpartum bleeding may last longer and be heavier.

For an in-depth look at pregnancy for women over age 35, we suggest you read our book *Your Pregnancy after 35.*

Your Nutrition

Good news—pregnant women should snack often, particularly during the second half of pregnancy! You should have three or four snacks a day, in addition to your regular meals. There are a couple of catches, though. First, snacks must be nutritious. Second, meals may need to be smaller so you can eat those snacks. One nutritional goal in pregnancy is to eat enough food so nutrients are always available for your body's use and for use by the growing fetus.

Usually you want a snack to be quick and easy. It may take some planning and effort on your part to make sure nutritious foods are available for snacking. Prepare things in advance. Cut up fresh vegetables for later use in salads and for munching with low-cal dip. Keep some hard-boiled eggs on hand. Low-fat cheese and cottage cheese provide calcium. Peanut butter, pretzels and plain popcorn are good choices. Replace soda with fruit juice. If juice has more sugar than you need, cut it with water.

You Should Also Know

No More Lying on Your Back

Week 16 is the turning point—no more lying flat on your back while resting or sleeping, or lying flat on the floor while exercising or relaxing. Reclining in a chair or propped against pillows is OK. Just don't lie flat on your back!

Lying on your back puts pressure on the aorta and vena cava, which can reduce blood flow to your baby. Baby won't get all the nutrients it needs to develop and to grow. Don't endanger baby's well-being by forgetting this important action.

Have a Green Pregnancy

Today, many people are looking for ways to become "greener." They want to do what they can to help protect the environment for themselves, their children and the rest of the world. One way to begin is to have a *green pregnancy.*

Having a green pregnancy can range from being selective about the products you use to how you treat your body. We've gathered together some ideas about ways you can have a green pregnancy.

Check cosmetics and other personal products you use to see if any contain harmful chemicals. Choose ones that are good for the environment. Use green cleaning products, laundry detergents and other household products. Be sure they're safe to use during pregnancy—not all green products are.

Eat organic foods some of the time to cut down your exposure to pesticides and other harmful substances. Grow your own vegetables when possible. A garden can be a wonderful addition to your lifestyle.

Try to avoid outdoor pollutants, such as car exhaust and smog. Walk when you can instead of driving. Make recycling a part of your life every day. Donate or sell items you don't need to make room for baby and all the stuff you'll need for him or her. Buy secondhand baby clothes.

Buy a water bottle for your personal use. If you have an older home, run cold water for 30 seconds to 2 minutes to help flush out any lead in the pipes. A good water filter can also help. Take 1200mg of calcium every day while you breast-feed to help reduce the amount of lead in your milk.

When fixing up baby's room, choose no- or low-VOC paint, which has fewer pollutants. (VOC means *volatile organic compounds.*) If you install carpet, select natural fibers when possible, such as wool, jute or sisal. Or look for carpets with the Green Label Plus logo—they contain lower amounts of VOC chemicals.

Keep baby's bed and bedding natural. Many products are available that are free of dioxins, synthetic petrochemicals and formaldehyde, including crib mattresses and crib bedding.

Watch your energy consumption, and try to live light. Use energy-efficient light bulbs in your lamps and fixtures. Take shorter showers. Keep thermostats lower in winter and higher in summer.

Ask friends to give you a green baby shower. Register for eco-friendly products. Remember—if it's not good for you, it's not good for baby!

Are You Noticing Changes in Your Feet? Do your feet seem to be getting bigger during your pregnancy? It can happen! In fact, your feet can grow up to a half size with *each child* you give birth to. For some unfortunate women, this change is permanent.

If you wear too-tight shoes, various foot problems can occur. To avoid this predicament, shop for shoes at the end of the day—your feet are probably the most swollen at this time. When you try on shoes, stand up and be sure there is at least a thumb's width of space between your toe and the end of the shoe.

Foot Exercises. Doing some foot exercises may help strengthen and stretch your feet during pregnancy. Exercises can help with swelling in your feet and may improve your balance and coordination, both important during pregnancy.

For the first exercise, take off your shoes. Sit in a comfortable chair. Starting with your right foot, move your foot in circles, then move it side to side. Don't move your leg, just your foot and ankle. When you finish with the first foot, do the same exercises with your other foot.

When you've worked both feet, do toe curls. Curl your toes under, then uncurl them. If this causes foot cramps, stop

and rub your foot. If you can't reach your foot, ask your partner to do it for you. After toe curls, place both feet flat on the floor. Try to lift *only* your big toes. Then try to keep your big toes on the floor while you lift your other toes.

You can also try picking up an object with your toes, such as a pencil. Sometimes in later pregnancy, this is the only way you'll be able to get it off the floor!

Using a tennis ball or a small rubber ball, roll it around under your bare foot. It's a great way to massage your feet when your partner isn't around!

Rh Disease and Sensitivity
It's important during pregnancy to know your blood type (O, A, B, AB) and your Rh-factor. The Rh factor is a protein in your blood, determined by a genetic trait. You have either Rh-positive blood or Rh-negative blood. If you have the Rh factor in your blood, you are Rh-positive—most people are Rh-positive. If you do not have the Rh factor, you are Rh-negative. Rh-negativity affects about 15% of the white population and 8% of the Black/African-American population in the United States.

If you're Rh-positive, you don't have to worry about any of this. If you are Rh-positive and your partner is Rh-negative, you won't have a problem. If both partners are Rh-negative, there will be no problems.

However, if you are Rh-negative, you do need to know about it. An Rh-negative woman who carries an Rh-positive child could face problems, which could result in a very sick baby.

At the beginning of pregnancy, a blood test is done to determine if you are Rh-positive or Rh-negative, and if you have antibodies. If you're Rh-positive, like most people, you don't need to worry about any of this.

If you are Rh-negative, you may:

- be sensitized (already have antibodies)—you will be monitored closely for fetal anemia and other problems
- be unsensitized (do not have antibodies)—you will receive a RhoGAM injection at 28 weeks, then receive a RhoGAM injection at 40 weeks if you are still pregnant

Your baby is checked at delivery with a blood test to see if it is Rh-positive or Rh-negative. If baby is:

- Rh-negative, nothing further will be done
- Rh-positive, a test is done on your blood to determine how much RhoGAM you should receive

Rh Disease. Rh disease is a condition caused by incompatibility between a mother's blood and her baby's blood. If you are Rh-negative, you can become sensitized if baby is Rh-positive. Baby may be Rh-positive *only* if your partner is Rh-positive.

Over 4000 babies develop Rh disease before birth every year. If you're Rh-negative and your baby isn't or if you have had a blood transfusion or received blood products of some kind, you might have a problem. There's a risk you could become Rh-sensitized or isoimmunized. *Isoimmunized* means you make antibodies that circulate inside your system. The antibodies don't harm you, but they can attack the Rh-positive blood of your growing baby. (If your baby is Rh-negative, there is no problem.)

Cause of Problems. You and your fetus do not share blood systems during pregnancy. However, in some situations, blood passes from baby to mom.

Occasionally when this happens, the mother's body reacts as if she were allergic to the fetus's blood. She becomes sensitized and makes antibodies. These antibodies can cross the placenta and attack the fetus's blood. Antibodies can break down the baby's red blood cells, which results in anemia in the baby and can be very serious.

With a first baby, if fetal blood enters the mother's bloodstream, the baby may be born before the woman can become sensitized. The mom-to-be may not produce enough antibodies to harm the baby, but antibodies stay in the woman's circulation forever. In the next pregnancy, antibodies already formed in the mom could cross the placenta and attack the baby's red blood cells, resulting in anemia.

Preventing Problems. If you're Rh-negative, you'll be checked for antibodies at the beginning of pregnancy. If you have antibodies, you are already sensitized. If you don't have antibodies, you're unsensitized (this is good).

Rh-positive blood can mix with an Rh-negative woman's blood in many ways. These include miscarriage, abortion, ectopic pregnancy, amniocentesis, chorionic villus sampling, PUBS or cordocentesis, blood transfusion, bleeding during pregnancy, such as with placental abruption, or in an accident or injury, such as blunt-force trauma to the uterus in an auto accident.

If you're Rh-negative and are not sensitized, a treatment is available to prevent you from becoming sensitized. It is called *RhoGAM* or *Rh immune globulin (RhIg)*. RhoGAM is extracted from human blood. (If you have religious, ethical or personal reasons for not using blood or blood products, consult your healthcare provider or minister.) If your blood mixes with baby's blood, RhoGAM keeps you from becoming sensitized. If you're already sensitized, RhoGAM will not help and will not be given to you.

If you are not sensitized, your healthcare provider will probably suggest you receive RhoGAM around the 28th week of pregnancy to prevent sensitization. You're more likely to be exposed to baby's blood during the last 3 months of pregnancy and at delivery. If you go beyond your due date, your healthcare provider may suggest another dose of RhoGAM.

RhoGAM is given within 72 hours after delivery if your baby is Rh-positive.

If your baby is Rh-negative, you don't need RhoGAM after delivery and you didn't need the shot during pregnancy. But it's better not to take that risk and to have the RhoGAM injection during pregnancy.

After delivery, if blood tests show that a larger than normal number of Rh-positive blood cells (from baby) have entered your bloodstream, you may be given RhoGAM. The RhoGAM treatment is necessary for every pregnancy.

Rh Disease and Your Growing Baby. If your healthcare provider suspects fetal problems from Rh disease, amniocentesis and cordocentesis can help determine whether baby is developing anemia and how severe it is. These tests may need to be repeated every 2 to 4 weeks. Amniocentesis can also determine whether the fetus is Rh-negative or Rh-positive.

Ultrasound may be used to measure the speed of blood flowing through an artery in the baby's head. This can help detect moderate to severe anemia.

Your blood can be tested to determine Rh status in the fetus. This may mean you won't need amniocentesis later in pregnancy to determine this factor.

If your baby has a problem, there are procedures that can be done before birth. Babies have been treated with blood transfusions as early as 18 weeks of pregnancy.

Exercise for Week 16

· · · · · · ·

You now know why you shouldn't lie on your back to exercise after the 16th week, so no more abdominal crunches. However, you can do a modified, pregnancy-friendly crunch. Sit on the floor in a crossed-leg position. Brace your back against the wall. Use pillows for added comfort. Exhaling through your nose, pull your bellybutton in toward your spine. Hold for 5 seconds, then inhale through your nose. Begin with 5 repetitions and work up to 10. *Strengthens stomach muscles, and keeps lower back and spine strong.*

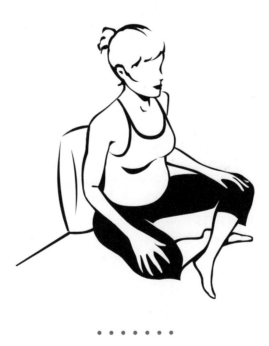

· · · · · · ·

Week 17

Age of Fetus—15 Weeks

How Big Is Your Baby?

The crown-to-rump length of your baby is 4½ to 4¾ inches (11 to 12cm). Fetal weight has doubled in 2 weeks and is now about 3½ ounces (100g). By this week, your baby is about the size of your hand spread open wide.

How Big Are You?

Your uterus is 1½ to 2 inches (3.8 to 5cm) below your bellybutton. You now have an obvious swelling in your lower abdomen. Maternity clothing is a must for comfort's sake. When your partner gives you a hug, he may feel the difference in your lower abdomen. A total 5- to 10-pound (2.25 to 4.5kg) weight gain by this point in your pregnancy is normal.

How Your Baby Is Growing and Developing

If you look at the illustration on page 174, then look at earlier weeks, you'll see the incredible changes occurring in your baby. Fat, also called *adipose tissue*, begins to form this week. It's important to baby's heat production and metabolism. At birth, fat makes up about 5¼ pounds (2.4kg) of the total average weight of 7¾ pounds (3.5kg).

You have felt your baby move, or you will soon. You may not feel it every day. As pregnancy progresses, movements become stronger and more frequent.

Changes in You

Feeling your baby move can reassure you things are going well with your pregnancy. This is especially true if you've had problems.

As pregnancy advances, the uterus becomes more oval than round as it fills the pelvis and starts to grow into the abdomen. Your intestines are pushed upward and to the sides. Your uterus eventually reaches almost to your liver.

When you stand, your uterus touches your abdominal wall in the front. You may feel it most easily in this position. When you lie on your back, it can fall backward onto your spine and blood vessels (vena cava and aorta).

Round-Ligament Pain

Round ligaments are attached to each side of the upper uterus and to the pelvic side wall. With the growth of the uterus,

Tip for Week 17
· · · · · · · · · · ·

If you experience leg cramps during pregnancy, there are some things to try. Don't stand for long periods. Rest on your side as often as possible. Do stretching exercises. You may use a heating pad on the cramped area, but don't use it for longer than 15 minutes at a time. Eat raisins and bananas—they're great sources of potassium. Inadequate calcium intake can also affect leg cramps. Be sure you take in 1200mg of calcium every day. Drinking lots of water may also help. Also try Grandma's Remedy for leg cramps; see the box in Week 25.

these ligaments stretch and pull, and become longer and thicker. Moving may cause pain or discomfort called *round-ligament pain*. Pain may occur on one side only or both sides, or it may be worse on one side than another. This pain does not harm you or your baby.

If you experience this pain, you may feel better if you lie down and rest. Talk to your healthcare provider if pain is severe or if other symptoms arise. Warning signs of serious problems include bleeding, loss of fluid from the vagina or severe pain.

How Your Actions Affect Your Baby's Development

Additional Tips for Choosing Maternity Clothes

Today's maternity clothes are more stylish than in the past. As cute as they are, the main goals in choosing maternity clothes are comfort and room to grow in your pregnancy.

A waistband shouldn't be too tight. Clothing that fits tightly at the waist can put pressure on veins in the tummy, which can cut off circulation to the legs. Adjustable-waist pants, skirts and shorts help avoid this problem.

Select a pregnancy bra with wide straps; it won't put as much pressure on the trapezius muscle in your back. If this muscle becomes tight and knotted, you may experience neck pain, a headache or tingling and/or numbness in your arms. A sports bra with a racer back evenly distributes the weight of breasts.

Choose clothes you can use for work (if you work outside your home) and for leisure. Pants and comfortable tops can often do double duty. You may want to buy one nice dress to have on hand for special occasions. Don't forget about shoes—low-heeled styles can work with pants and dresses.

Ultrasound at this Time

Ultrasound has proved very effective for diagnosing problems and giving reassurance. During the second trimester, it can be used with amniocentesis, with bleeding related to placenta previa or abruption, when there is concern about intrauterine-growth restriction (IUGR), to evaluate fetal well-being and to diagnose multiple fetuses.

3-Dimensional Ultrasound. A 3-dimensional ultrasound provides detailed, clear pictures of the baby inside you.

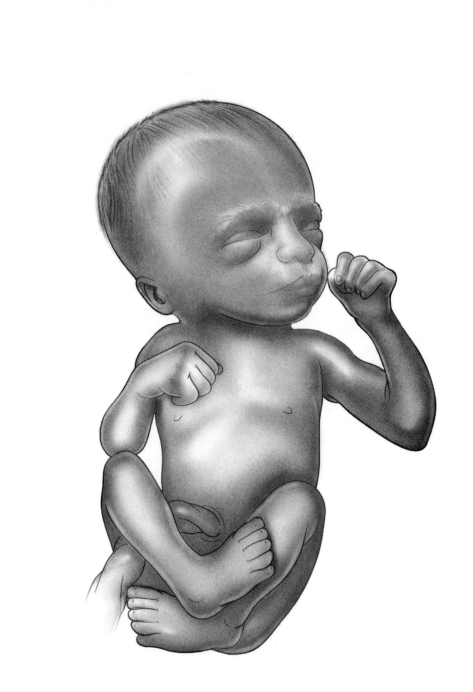

Your baby's fingernails are well formed.
The baby is beginning to accumulate a little fat.

Dad Tip

. . . .

Massage can work wonders to help relieve your partner's discomforts and tiredness. It can also help ease any anxiety she may be having. Massage can be very relaxing for her and you! Offer your partner tension-relieving, muscle-relaxing head, back and foot massages. It may make you both feel great.

Images almost look like photos. For the pregnant woman, the test is almost the same as a 2-dimensional ultrasound. The difference is computer software "translates" the picture into a 3-D image.

A 3-D ultrasound may be used when there is suspicion of problems with the baby. This test can furnish information that helps with diagnosis and treatment. It helps medical personnel understand the severity of the problem so a treatment program can be planned that can be started immediately after birth.

Testing with 3-D ultrasound helps assess babies with facial problems, hand and foot problems, spine problems and neural-tube defects. Some studies show 3-D images can be a valuable teaching aid for parents, who may have trouble visualizing defects. A 3-D ultrasound is used to identify various problems and rule out some birth defects.

Increased Vaginal Discharge

During pregnancy, it's normal to have an increase in vaginal discharge, called *leukorrhea*. This discharge is usually white or yellow and fairly thick. It's not an infection. We believe it's caused by increased blood flow to the skin and muscles around the vagina; this also causes a violet or blue coloration of the vagina. This is visible to your healthcare provider early in pregnancy and is called *Chadwick's sign*.

You may have to wear sanitary pads if you have a heavy discharge. Avoid wearing pantyhose and nylon underwear. Choose underwear with a cotton crotch to allow more air circulation.

Vaginal infections can and do occur during pregnancy. The discharge with these infections is often foul-smelling, yellow or green, and causes irritation or itching around or inside the vagina. If you have any of these symptoms, call your healthcare provider. Many creams and antibiotics are safe to use during pregnancy.

. . . .

Most healthcare providers agree you should not douche during pregnancy. Bulb-syringe douches are definitely out! Douching may cause you to bleed or may cause more serious problems. Avoid this practice.

. . . .

Your Nutrition

Are You a Vegetarian?

Some women choose to eat a vegetarian diet because of personal or religious preferences. Other women are nauseated by meat during pregnancy. Is it safe to eat a vegetarian diet while you're pregnant? It can be, if you pay close attention to the types and combinations of foods you eat.

Research shows most women who eat a vegetarian diet eat a more nutrient-rich variety of foods than those who eat meat. Vegetarians may make an extra effort to include more fruits and vegetables in their food plans when they eliminate meat products.

If you're a vegetarian by choice, and have been for a while, you may know how to get many of the nutrients you need. Discuss your vegetarian diet with your healthcare provider at your first prenatal visit. He or she may want you to see a nutritionist.

* *

If you're not eating meat because it makes you ill, ask for a referral to a nutritionist. You may need help developing a good eating plan.

* *

During pregnancy, you must eat the right kind of calories. Choose fresh foods to supply you with a variety of vitamins and minerals. Eat enough different sources of protein to provide energy for you and baby.

There are different vegetarian nutrition plans, each with unique characteristics. If you are an *ovo-lacto vegetarian*, you eat milk products and eggs. If you are a *lacto vegetarian*, your diet includes milk products. A *vegan* diet includes only foods of plant origin, such as nuts, seeds, vegetables, fruits, grains and legumes. A *macrobiotic* diet limits foods to whole grains, beans, vegetables and moderate amounts of fish and fruits. A *fruitarian* diet is the most restrictive; it allows only fruits, nuts, olive oil and honey.

Macrobiotic and fruitarian diets are too restrictive for a pregnant woman. They do not provide enough vitamins, minerals, protein and calories for baby's development.

Your goal is to eat enough calories to gain weight during pregnancy. You don't want your body to use protein for energy because you need it for your growth and your baby's growth.

By eating a wide variety of whole grains, legumes, dried fruit, beans and wheat germ, you should be able to get enough iron, zinc and other trace minerals. If you don't drink milk or include milk products in your diet, you must find other sources of vitamins D, B_2, B_{12} and calcium. Getting enough folic acid is usually not a problem for vegetarians. Folate is found in many fruits, legumes and vegetables (especially dark leafy ones).

Women who eat little or no meat are at greater risk of iron deficiency during pregnancy. To get enough iron, eat an assortment of grains, vegetables, seeds, nuts, legumes and fortified cereal every day. Spinach, prunes and sauerkraut are excellent sources of iron, as are dried fruit and dark leafy vegetables. Tofu is also a good source. Cook in cast-iron pans because traces of iron will attach to whatever you're cooking.

If you are a lacto or ovo-lacto vegetarian, do not drink milk with foods that are iron rich; calcium reduces iron absorption. Don't drink tea or coffee with meals because tannins present in those beverages inhibit iron absorption by 75%. Many breakfast foods and breads are now iron-fortified. Read labels.

To get omega-3 fatty acids, add canola oil, tofu, flaxseed, soybeans, walnuts and wheat germ to your food plan. These foods contain linolenic oil, a type of omega-3 fatty acid. You can also eat flaxseed flour and flaxseed oil—both are available in markets and health-food stores—but avoid plain flax.

Vegetarians and pregnant women who can't eat meat may have a harder time getting enough vitamin E. Vitamin E is important during pregnancy because it contributes to building muscles and red blood cells. Foods rich in the vitamin include olive oil, wheat germ, spinach and dried fruit.

. . . .
Almonds contain high levels of magnesium, vitamin E, protein and fiber.
. . . .

Vegetarians are more likely to have a zinc deficiency, so pay close attention to getting enough zinc every day. Lima beans, whole-grain products, nuts, dried beans, dried peas, wheat germ and dark leafy vegetables are good sources of zinc.

If you're a vegan, eating no animal products may make good nutrition more difficult. You may need to ask your healthcare provider about supplements for vitamin B_{12}, vitamin D, zinc, iron and calcium. Eat turnip greens, spinach, beet greens, broccoli, soy-based milk products and cheeses, and fruit juices fortified with calcium.

You Should Also Know

Quad-Screen Test

The quad-screen test can help determine if you might be carrying a baby with Down syndrome. This blood test can also help rule out other problems, such as neural-tube defects.

The quad-screen test is the same as the triple-screen test, with the addition of a fourth measurement—your inhibin-A level. The addition of inhibin-A increases the detection rate of Down syndrome and lowers the false-positive rate. The quad-screen test is able to identify 79% of those fetuses with Down syndrome. It has a false-positive result of 5%.

Complementary and Alternative Medical Techniques

There are many complementary and alternative medicine techniques that may help a woman during pregnancy. These techniques refer to treatments and products not considered part of traditional medicine. Healthcare providers don't learn about them during training nor are they usually practiced by healthcare providers. When used with traditional medicine, they are called *complementary medical techniques.* When used in place of traditional medicine, they are called *alternative medicine.*

Many complementary and alternative treatments are untested. There is no definite way to determine if a treatment is safe or effective, so it's important to talk to your healthcare provider about any of these treatments if you are interested.

The exception to the rule stated above is *osteopathy.* It uses manipulation and physical therapies to restore structural balance and improve the function of the body. Doctors of osteopathic medicine have graduated from an accredited osteopathic school of medicine and have fulfilled requirements for a medical license. Treatments by an osteopathic physician are learned in osteopathic schools of medicine and are safe.

Homeopathy uses small, highly diluted substances to alleviate symptoms. In high doses, these same substances cause these symptoms. *Chiropractic* involves manipulating the spine to relieve pain and to assist the body's ability to heal itself.

The *Alexander technique* is a gentle approach to movement that can help you rebalance faulty posture. *Electromagnetic fields*, also called *energy healing*, uses magnets, low-frequency thermal waves, electrical nerve stimulation and electromagnetic waves to relieve nerve and joint pain and to provide energy to heal the body.

Acupuncture is the practice of placing tiny needles along pathways believed to connect energy points in your body with specific organs. It is performed by trained practitioners. Research shows acupuncture has many benefits, including helping the body produce its own pain-killing substances. *Acupressure* is similar to acupuncture, except it uses pressure instead of needles on key acupoints on the body.

Biofeedback employs various devices to give you visual or audio feedback about your effort to control automatic body functions. *Guided imagery* uses imaginary mental pictures to focus on imagining yourself being well. It is useful for managing common stress-related problems, such as headaches or high blood pressure.

Therapeutic touch involves having a therapist pass his or her hands over a person's body to bring energy into balance. *Reflexology* applies pressure to specific points on the hands and feet believed to be linked to specific organs in the body.

Massage therapy employs the ancient healing art of rubbing and manipulating body tissue to help make your body, mind and spirit relax. *Meditation* relaxes your mind and helps you get in touch with deeper thoughts. *Yoga* uses postures designed to align a person's spiritual, mental, emotional and physical aspects.

Aromatherapy uses scented plant oils that are inhaled or applied to the skin. *Dietary supplements* include vitamins, minerals, herbs and supplements used as medicine to help prevent illness. *Chinese medicine* is based on the belief that balanced energy (qi) flows through the body of a healthy person, and disease causes the flow to be interrupted.

Be sure to talk to your healthcare provider about any of these treatments if you are interested in using them.

Are You Thinking about Using a Doula?

You may be wondering whether you want a doula to help you during baby's birth. A *doula* is a woman who is trained to provide support and assistance during labor and delivery. The doula supports you from the onset of labor until baby's birth.

Doulas don't deliver babies, replace a doctor or midwife, or play the role of a nurse. They are there to comfort the

Questions to Ask a Prospective Doula
. . . .

If you are considering a doula, interview more than one. Some questions you may want to ask and some perceptions you might want to analyze are listed below.

- What are your qualifications and training? Are you certified? By which organization?
- Have you had a baby yourself? What childbirth method did you use?
- Are you familiar with the childbirth method we have chosen (if you have a particular method you want to use)?
- What kind of plan would you use to help us through our labor?
- How available are you to answer our questions before the birth?
- How often will we meet before the birth?
- How do we contact you when labor begins?
- What happens if you aren't available when we go into labor? Do you work with other doulas? May we meet some of them?
- Are you experienced in helping a new mom with breastfeeding? How available are you after the birth to help with this and other postpartum issues?

Perceptions include how easy the doula is to talk to and to communicate with. Did she listen well and answer your questions? Did you feel comfortable with her? If you don't hit it off with one doula, try another!

mom-to-be, soothe her fears and help her through labor. They can provide continuous care through labor. They provide pain relief through massage, breathing techniques and water therapy. In some cases, a doula can guide partners in helping during labor and delivery. A doula may even be able to help you begin breastfeeding your baby.

One strength of a doula is to provide support to a woman who has chosen to have a drug-free labor and delivery. If you've decided you want anesthesia, no matter what, a doula may not be a good choice for you.

A doula may assist the labor coach. She does not displace a labor coach; she works with him or her. In some situations, a doula may serve as the labor coach.

The services of a doula may be expensive and can range from $250 to $1500. This usually covers meetings before birth, attendance at labor and delivery, and one or more postpartum visits.

If you and your partner choose to have a doula present during labor and birth, talk to your healthcare provider about your decision. He or she may find her presence intrusive and veto the idea. Or the healthcare provider may be able to give you the name of someone he or she often works with.

If you decide to use a doula, begin early to search for someone. Start looking as early as your 4th month of pregnancy—certainly no later than your 6th month. If you wait any longer, choices may be limited. Starting early allows you to evaluate more critically any women you interview. Visit DoulaNetwork.com to find doulas in your area.

Postpartum Doulas. *Postpartum doulas* help ease the transition into parenthood. A postpartum doula will help a new mother and her family learn to enjoy and to care for the new baby through education and hands-on experience.

These doulas provide emotional and breastfeeding support, and make sure a new mother is fed, hydrated and comfortable. She may go with mom and baby to pediatric appointments. A postpartum doula may also take care of grocery shopping, preparing meals and other household tasks. She may even help tend older children.

A postpartum doula's services are most often used in the first 2 to 4 weeks after birth, but support can last anywhere from one or two visits to visits for 3 months or longer. Some work evenings and/or overnight.

Doulas don't treat postpartum depression but can offer support to a woman who experiences it. Some postpartum doulas are trained to help women screen themselves for depression and will make referrals to healthcare providers and support groups.

If you think you may want a postpartum doula, make arrangements a few months before your due date. Even though you don't know exactly when your baby will arrive (unless you're having a scheduled Cesarean delivery),

contract with a postpartum doula in advance to be sure of her availability. Costs range between $15 and $30 an hour for this service, depending on the postpartum doula's additional training and experience.

Should You Be Concerned about Autism?

Today, many pregnant couples have questions about *autism*. Autism is a complex disorder. The problem is characterized by impaired social interaction, problems with verbal and nonverbal communication, and unusual/repetitive and/or severely limited activities and interests. Experts estimate that 3 to 6 children out of every 1000 are autistic.

At this time, we don't know what causes autism. Some researchers believe it is a combination of genetics and environment. Families with one autistic child have a 5% risk of having a second child with autism.

Research indicates children born to older fathers have a higher risk of being autistic. And if babies are born fairly close together, your second child may be at increased risk. Researchers believe biological factors, such as nutrient deficiency in the second pregnancy, may be a factor.

A recent study indicates if a woman takes folic acid before pregnancy or early in pregnancy, she may reduce her child's risk of autism. Experts don't know how much folic acid is needed to help prevent autism. If this is a concern of yours, don't go overboard and take a lot of folic acid. Discuss it with your healthcare provider, and follow his or her advice.

Exercise for Week 17

• • • • • • •

Sit on the floor with your legs out straight in front of you. Lift your arms straight out in front of you to shoulder height. "Walk" forward on your buttocks for 6 paces, then return to the starting position by "walking" backward. Repeat 7 times forward and backward. *Strengthens abdominal muscles and lower-back muscles.*

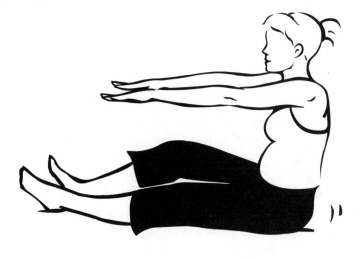

• • • • • • •

Week 18

Age of Fetus—16 Weeks

How Big Is Your Baby?

Baby's crown-to-rump length is 5 to 5½ inches (12.5 to 14cm) by this week. Weight of the fetus is about 5¼ ounces (150g).

How Big Are You?

If you put your fingers sideways and measure, your uterus is about two finger-widths (1 inch) below your bellybutton. It's the size of a cantaloupe or a little larger.

Total weight gain to this point should be 10 to 13 pounds (4.5 to 5.8kg), but this can vary. If you've gained more weight than this, talk to your healthcare provider. You may need to see a nutritionist. You still have more than half of your pregnancy ahead of you, and you'll definitely gain more weight.

How Your Baby Is Growing and Developing

Baby continues to develop, but the rapid growth rate slows. As you can see in the illustration on page 184, your baby has a human appearance now.

Blood from your baby flows to the placenta through the umbilical cord. In the placenta, oxygen and nutrients are carried from your blood to fetal blood. At birth, baby must go rapidly from depending on you for oxygen to depending on its own heart and lungs. The foramen ovale closes at birth, and blood goes to the right ventricle and the lungs for oxygenation. It is truly a miraculous conversion.

Changes in You

Does Your Back Ache?

Between 50 and 80% of all pregnant women have back and hip pain at some time. Pain usually occurs during the third trimester as your tummy grows larger. However, pain may begin early in pregnancy and last until well after delivery (up to 5 or 6 months).

It's more common to have mild backache than severe problems. You may need to be careful getting out of bed or getting up from a sitting position. In extreme cases, some women find it difficult to walk.

The hormone *relaxin* may play a part. It's responsible for relaxing joints that allow your pelvis to expand to deliver baby. When joints relax, it may lead to

Dad Tip
. . . .

You may be surprised how tired your pregnant partner seems. Doing anything may take a lot of effort on her part, especially if she works outside your home. You can help out by offering to run errands. Take her dry cleaning in, and pick it up when it's ready. Stop by the bank for her. Take her car to a car wash. Return her library books or rented DVDs.

pain in the lower back and legs. Other factors include your weight gain (another good reason to control weight), larger breasts and a bigger tummy, which can cause a shift in posture. Check with your healthcare provider if back pain is a problem for you.

Lumbar-spine pain (LSP) is an aching feeling that spreads throughout the center lower back. It often begins in the first or second trimester. If you've had lower-back pain before pregnancy, you may experience this discomfort during pregnancy. A prenatal yoga class may offer relief. Staying off your feet is also a good remedy.

Actions You Can Take to Relieve Back Pain. There are some things you can do to prevent or lessen back pain. Don't gain too much weight or gain weight too quickly. Stay active; swimming, walking and nonimpact aerobics may be beneficial. Stretching gently may also help. Practice good posture.

Try to get off your feet and lie on your side for 30 minutes each day. Lie on your side when you nap or sleep. If you have other children, nap when they do.

With lower-back pain, use an ice pack for up to 30 minutes three or four times a day. If pain lasts, switch to a heating pad,

sticking with the same regimen. It's OK to take acetaminophen for a short time for back pain.

Prenatal massage may help relieve pain. Ask your healthcare provider if he or she can suggest some qualified massage therapists. A lower-back brace or pregnancy-support garment may be recommended.

If pain becomes constant or severe, talk to your healthcare provider. Discomfort may also indicate more serious problems.

Inflammatory Bowel Disease (IBD)
Inflammatory bowel disease (IBD) describes two medical problems—ulcerative colitis and Crohn's disease. IBD affects about 2 million Americans. (IBD is not the same as IBS—irritable bowel syndrome. See Week 30 for a discussion of IBS.)

With *ulcerative colitis,* the inner lining of the intestine gets swollen, and ulcers develop. It may be most severe in the rectal area and cause frequent diarrhea. The problem seems to run in families, but IBD can be caused by other factors, including environment and diet.

A third of all women with ulcerative colitis relapse during pregnancy, usually

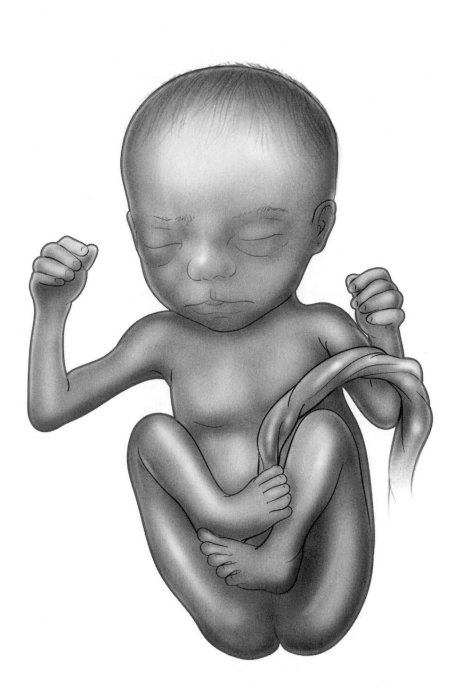

By this week, baby is about
5 inches (12.5cm) from crown to rump.
It looks much more human now.

Avodart and Propecia

• • • • • • • • • • •

You may have heard on TV or read in magazines that pregnant women shouldn't handle certain medications, especially Avodart and Propecia. Should you take these warnings seriously? Can you harm your growing baby by just touching them? You shouldn't handle either of these pills during pregnancy because of possible problems if pills are crushed or broken, then handled. Medication could be absorbed into your body and cause problems for your baby. If contact is accidentally made, wash the area immediately with soap and water.

during the first trimester. Flare-ups occur most often during the first trimester and immediately after birth.

Crohn's disease is a chronic illness in which the intestine or bowel becomes inflamed and scarred. It often affects the part of the small intestine called the *ileum* but can occur in any part of the large or small intestine, stomach, esophagus and even the mouth. Symptoms include chronic diarrhea, rectal bleeding, weight loss, fever, abdominal pain and/ or tenderness and a feeling of fullness in the lower-right abdomen.

If you have active Crohn's disease, getting pregnant may be more difficult. During pregnancy, a flare-up may occur, most often in the third trimester, but flare-ups are often mild and respond to treatment.

IBD and Pregnancy. Most women who have IBD have a normal pregnancy and give birth to a healthy baby. If you didn't talk to your healthcare provider before you got pregnant, contact your healthcare provider as soon as you confirm pregnancy.

If your IBD is in remission when you get pregnant, it may stay in remission during pregnancy. This happens with about 65% of all pregnant women. If your disease is active, it will probably remain active throughout pregnancy.

Women who have severe IBD have a higher risk of problems. You may lose fluid and nutrients, which can lead to fever, fatigue, weight loss and malnutrition. You may be seen more often during pregnancy, and you may have more tests during pregnancy. Experts believe it's safe to have various tests during pregnancy, but avoid X-rays and CT scans. Ask your pregnancy healthcare provider about an MRI if one is recommended.

You may be prescribed anti-inflammatory drugs and/or immunosuppressive agents to treat IBD. Sulfasalazine, mesalamine, balsalazide and olsalazine don't hurt the baby. Infliximab (Remicade) and adalimumab (Humira) may be necessary during pregnancy and breastfeeding. Avoid methotrexate during pregnancy.

If symptoms don't respond to medication, surgery may be necessary. If needed during pregnancy, it should be performed during the second trimester.

The type of delivery you have depends on the condition of the tissues around the vagina and anus. A Cesarean may be recommended if you develop a fistula or to reduce your risk of developing fistulas.

How Your Actions Affect Your Baby's Development

Can Pregnant Women Receive Salt Therapy?

Salt therapy is also known as *halotherapy*. Proponents of this drug-free, noninvasive treatment claim salt treatments help ease various health problems related to asthma, allergies, bronchitis, sinusitis, snoring, sleep apnea and other respiratory illnesses. They believe exposure to salt heals respiratory tissues, and the ionized salt particles also help boost the immune system.

With salt therapy, you don't consume salt. Instead, you breathe it in; the amount of salt entering your respiratory system is very low. A machine on the outside of the salt-therapy room produces dry saline aerosol, which is blown into the room through an opening in the wall. In addition, the walls of the salt-therapy room are covered with mineral salt. Salt entering the lungs is believed to kill bacteria, reduce inflammation and help loosen mucus.

Halotherapy is becoming more popular all over the country, and pregnant women want to know if it's safe for them. Because salt therapy is a completely drug-free treatment, it can be an alternative medicine choice for women who do not want to take over-the-counter or prescribed medication for various respiratory problems. Pregnant women who have engaged in salt therapy often find relief for their congestion and other respiratory problems.

If you tried salt therapy before pregnancy, talk to your healthcare provider about continuing its use. There are no known negative effects on pregnant women with the use of salt therapy, but it's something you should discuss at a prenatal appointment.

Exercise in the Second Trimester

Pregnant women can usually participate safely in many exercise activities throughout pregnancy. Listen to your body. It will tell you when it's time to slow down.

Many activities are safe for a woman with a normal pregnancy. Swimming can be good for you. The support and buoyancy of the water can be relaxing. If you swim, swim throughout pregnancy. Exercising in the shallow end of a swimming pool can also be beneficial. Just don't overdo it.

Walking is great during pregnancy. Two miles of walking at a good pace is adequate. As pregnancy progresses, you may need to decrease your speed and distance. Walking is an exercise you can begin at just about any time during pregnancy. If you jog, check with your healthcare provider. You may need to change to walking.

A stationary bike can give you a good workout. If you're comfortable riding a regular bicycle and have safe places to ride, you can enjoy this activity with your partner or family. Your balance changes as your body changes, so take care; getting on and off a bicycle may be more difficult. If you participate in spinning,

> ## *Tip for Week 18*
> · · · · · · · · · · ·
> During exercise, your oxygen demands increase. Your body is heavier, and your balance may change. You may also tire more easily. Keep these points in mind as you adjust your fitness program.

talk with your healthcare provider about continuing during pregnancy.

If you're interested in participating in other sports activities, talk about it at a prenatal appointment. Some activities will be OK; others will not be.

Your Nutrition

You need about 30mg of iron a day to meet the increased needs of pregnancy. Baby draws on your iron stores to create its own stores for its first few months of life. This helps protect baby from iron deficiency if you breastfeed.

Your prenatal vitamin contains about 60mg of iron, which should be enough for you. If you must take iron supplements, take your iron pill with a glass of orange juice or grapefruit juice to increase the iron absorption. Avoid drinking milk, coffee or tea with your iron supplement; they prevent the body from absorbing the mineral.

If you feel tired, have trouble concentrating, suffer from headaches, dizziness or indigestion, or if you get sick easily, you may have iron deficiency. An easy way to check is to examine the inside of your lower eyelid. If you're getting enough iron, it should be dark pink. Your nail beds should also be pink.

Your body absorbs only 10 to 15% of the iron you consume. You need to eat iron-rich foods on a regular basis to maintain those stores. Foods rich in iron include chicken, red meat, organ meats (liver, heart, kidneys), egg yolks, dark chocolate, dried fruit, spinach, kale and tofu. Combining a vitamin-C food and an iron-rich food ensures better iron absorption. A spinach salad with orange sections is a good example.

If you eat a well-balanced diet and take your prenatal vitamin every day, you may not need additional iron. Discuss it with your healthcare provider if you're concerned.

· ·

Gaining more than the recommended weight can make pregnancy and delivery harder on you. And extra pounds may be hard to lose afterward, so keep watching what you eat. Choose food for the nutrition it provides you and your growing baby.

· ·

You Should Also Know

Chronic Fatigue Syndrome (CFS)
Chronic fatigue syndrome (CFS) is a condition in which a person experiences long periods of severe fatigue not directly caused by another condition. Resting doesn't relieve symptoms. CFS affects about 1 million Americans; 80% are women. Research suggests about 65% of all people diagnosed with the problem also have symptoms of

fibromyalgia. (For more on fibromyalgia, see Week 21.)

Many women with chronic fatigue syndrome have had successful pregnancies and healthy babies. Symptoms improve in some pregnant women. Improvement usually occurs after the first trimester and may be due to pregnancy hormones.

If you have CFS and are pregnant, you will probably need extra rest during pregnancy. Some women need bed rest. Within weeks of delivery, about half of all new mothers relapse or feel worse than before pregnancy. This may be caused by the demands of taking care of a newborn along with the loss of pregnancy hormones. We don't know if women with CFS pass the condition to their babies during pregnancy or breastfeeding.

Talk to your healthcare provider about any over-the-counter or prescription medicine you take. Some medicine may need to be stopped or dosages reduced. Folic acid has been shown to be beneficial before and during pregnancy.

Bladder Infections

A urinary-tract infection (UTI) is the most common problem involving your bladder or kidneys experienced during pregnancy. Other names for urinary-tract infections are *bladder infections* and *cystitis*. Symptoms include the feeling of urgency to urinate, frequent urination and painful urination, particularly at the end of urinating. A severe UTI may cause blood in the urine.

Your healthcare provider may do a urinalysis and urine culture at your first prenatal visit. He or she may check your urine for infection at other times during pregnancy and when bothersome symptoms arise.

Help avoid infection by not holding your urine. Empty your bladder as soon as you feel the need. It also helps to empty the bladder after having intercourse. Drink plenty of fluid; cranberry juice may help. Don't take cranberry supplements without first checking with your healthcare provider.

If you have a UTI during pregnancy, call your healthcare provider. Bacteria could pass through the placenta and affect baby. If left untreated, UTIs can cause other pregnancy problems.

Many antibiotics are safe to treat a UTI infection, but some may not be safe during pregnancy. Your healthcare provider can advise you. Take the full course of any antibiotic prescribed for you. It may be harmful to baby if you don't treat the problem!

. . . .

If UTIs are a problem, try eating less poultry and pork. These foods may contain an antibiotic-resistant form of E. coli.

. . . .

Other Kidney Problems. A more serious problem resulting from a bladder infection is *pyelonephritis*, which occurs in 1 to 2% of all pregnant women. Symptoms include frequent urination, a burning sensation during urination, the feeling you need to urinate and nothing will come out, high fever, chills and back pain.

Pyelonephritis may require hospitalization and treatment with intravenous antibiotics. If you have pyelonephritis

Keep Your Urinary Tract Healthy

• • • • • • • • • • • •

- Don't hold your urine—go when you feel the urge.
- Drink at least 100 ounces of fluid every day to flush bacteria from the urinary tract; include cranberry juice.
- Urinate immediately after sexual intercourse.
- Don't wear tight underwear or slacks.
- Wipe from the front of the vagina to the back after a bowel movement.

or recurrent bladder infections during pregnancy, you may have to take antibiotics throughout pregnancy to prevent reinfection.

Another problem involving the kidneys and bladder is *kidney stones (renal calculi, nephrolithiasis)*. They occur about once in every 1500 pregnancies. Kidney stones cause severe pain in the back or lower abdomen and may cause blood in the urine.

Pain with kidney stones may be severe enough to require hospitalization. A kidney stone can usually be treated with pain medication and by drinking lots of fluids. In this way, the stone may be passed without surgical removal or lithotripsy (an ultrasound procedure).

Exercise for Week 18

• • • • • • •

Stand with your feet flat on the floor and your arms by your sides. As you lift your arms straight in front of you and over your head, lunge forward with your right leg. Step back into the starting position as you lower your arms to your sides. Repeat 7 times, then lunge with your left leg. *Tones and strengthens arms, upper back, back of legs and buttock muscles.*

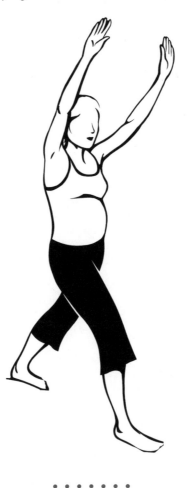

• • • • • • •

Week 19

Age of Fetus—17 Weeks

How Big Is Your Baby?

Crown-to-rump length of the growing fetus is 5¼ to 6 inches (13 to 15cm) by this week. Your baby weighs about 7 ounces (200g). It's incredible to think your baby will increase its weight more than 15 times between now and delivery!

How Big Are You?

You can feel your uterus about ½ inch (1.3cm) below your bellybutton. The illustration on page 192 gives you an idea of the relative size of you, your uterus and your growing baby. A side view really shows the changes in you!

Your total weight gain at this point should be between 8 and 14 pounds (3.6 and 6.3kg). Only about 7 ounces (200g) is baby. The placenta weighs about 6 ounces (170g); the amniotic fluid weighs another 11 ounces (320g). The uterus weighs 11 ounces (320g). Your breasts have each increased in weight by about 6½ ounces (180g). The rest of the weight you have gained is increased blood volume and other maternal stores.

How Your Baby Is Growing and Developing

Around this time, your baby begins hearing sounds from you—your beating heart, lungs filling with air, swishing blood and digesting food. "Hearing" in a fetus is really a matter of feeling vibrations in the skull that are transmitted to baby's inner ear. Baby "hears" your voice as it vibrates through your bones. Research shows lower-pitched sounds are heard more clearly in utero than high-pitched ones.

Hydrocephalus

With *hydrocephalus*, fluid accumulates in baby's skull, causing enlargement of baby's head. Brain tissue is compressed by the fluid, which is a major concern. Occurring in about 1 in 2000 babies, it is responsible for about 12% of all severe birth defects. The problem is often associated with spina bifida, meningomyelocele and omphalocele.

Ultrasound is the best way to diagnose the problem. Hydrocephalus can usually be seen on ultrasound by 19 weeks of pregnancy. Occasionally it is

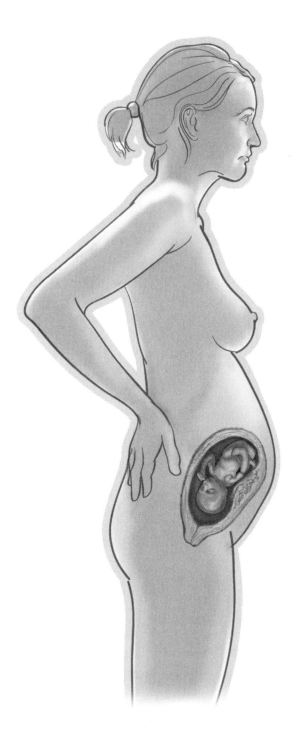

Comparative size of the uterus at 19 weeks of pregnancy
(fetal age—17 weeks). The uterus can be felt
just under the umbilicus (bellybutton).

found by routine exams and by "feeling" or measuring your uterus.

Treatment while the fetus is still in the uterus may be done in some cases. There are two ways to treat hydrocephalus inside the uterus. In one method, a needle passes through the mother's abdomen into the area of the baby's brain; some fluid is removed to relieve pressure on baby's brain. In another method, a small plastic tube is placed into the area where fluid collects in the brain. This tube is left in place to drain fluid continuously.

Hydrocephalus is a high-risk problem. These procedures are highly specialized and should be performed only by someone experienced in the latest techniques. It requires consultation with a perinatologist specializing in high-risk pregnancies.

Changes in You

Feeling Dizzy

Feeling dizzy during pregnancy is a fairly common symptom, often caused by low blood pressure (hypotension). It usually doesn't appear until the second trimester.

There are two common reasons for hypotension during pregnancy. *Supine hypotension* can be caused by the enlarging uterus putting pressure on your aorta and vena cava, and occurs when you lie down. Help ease or prevent it by not sleeping or lying on your back. *Postural hypotension* is caused by rising rapidly from a sitting, kneeling or squatting position. The problem is cured by rising slowly.

If you're anemic, you may feel dizzy. Your blood is checked routinely during pregnancy for this problem. Your healthcare provider can tell you if you have anemia.

Pregnancy also affects blood-sugar levels. High blood sugar (hyperglycemia) or low blood sugar (hypoglycemia) can make you feel dizzy or faint. Many healthcare providers routinely test pregnant women for blood-sugar problems. Avoid or improve the problem by eating a balanced diet, not skipping meals and not going a long time without eating. Carry a piece of fruit or several crackers with you for a quick boost in blood sugar when you need it.

· ·

Feeling dizzy or lightheaded? Cross your ankles and squeeze your thighs together, or squeeze a rubber ball in your hand. Both actions tense muscles; this improves blood flow to your head, which can help you stop feeling faint.

· ·

Thrombophilia

Some women experience blood clots during pregnancy; the term *thrombophilia* describes the condition. Thrombophilia encompasses a broad range of blood-clotting disorders. Inherited thrombophilias occur in up to 10% of women.

Many healthcare providers don't screen women for this problem. Ask for a test if you have a family history of the disorder. Some researchers have found inherited thrombophilias are tied to second- or third-trimester fetal loss, not first-trimester loss.

If a blood test shows you have a problem, your healthcare provider may advise aspirin and heparin during pregnancy. This treatment has been shown to be effective for some women.

Complications from thrombophilia can recur in subsequent pregnancies. Some preventive treatments include folic-acid supplementation, the use of heparin and a low-dose aspirin regimen.

How Your Actions Affect Your Baby's Development

Warning Signs during Pregnancy

Many women are nervous because they don't think they will know if something important or serious happens during pregnancy. Most pregnant women have few, if any, problems. If you're concerned, the list below includes the most important symptoms to watch for. Call your healthcare provider if you experience any of the following:

- vaginal bleeding
- severe swelling of the face or fingers
- severe abdominal pain
- loss of fluid from the vagina, usually a gush of fluid, but sometimes a trickle or continuous wetness
- a big change in baby's movement or a lack of movement

- high fever (more than 101.6F) or chills
- severe vomiting or an inability to keep food or liquid down
- blurring of vision
- painful urination
- a severe headache or one that won't go away
- an injury or accident, such as a fall or automobile accident, that causes you concern about the well-being of your baby

Later in pregnancy, if you can't feel baby moving, sit or lie down in a quiet room after eating a meal. Focus on how often the baby moves. If you don't feel at least 10 fetal movements in 2 hours, call your healthcare provider.

Be sure to talk about any concerns you have at a prenatal appointment. Don't be embarrassed to ask questions; he or she has probably heard it before. Your healthcare provider would rather know about problems while they may be easier to deal with.

You may not have a high-risk pregnancy at the beginning of your pregnancy. But if problems develop with you or baby, you may be referred to a perinatologist, an OB who cares for women with high-risk pregnancies. You may be able to return to your regular healthcare provider for your delivery. Or you may

> ## *Eat More Meals Every Day!*
> ....
> Eating frequent, small meals during the day may provide better nutrition to baby than if you eat three large meals. Though you're eating the same amount of calories, there is a difference. Studies show keeping your blood level of nutrients constant (by eating frequent, small meals) is better for baby than if you eat a large meal, then don't eat again for quite a while. Eating three larger meals means nutrient levels rise and fall during the day, which isn't as good for the growing baby. Eating small meals frequently can also help ease or avoid some pregnancy problems.

have to deliver your baby at a hospital that has specialized facilities or can administer specialized tests and/or care to you or your baby.

Your Nutrition

Herbal Use in Pregnancy
If you normally use herbs and botanicals—in the forms of teas, tinctures, pills or powders—to treat various medical and health problems, stop! Don't use any herbal remedy during pregnancy without checking first with your healthcare provider!

You may believe an herbal remedy is OK, but it could be dangerous during pregnancy. For example, if you're constipated, you may decide to use senna as a laxative. However, senna may cause a miscarriage. Or you may have used St. John's wort before pregnancy. Avoid it now—St. John's wort can interfere with various medicines. Avoid dong quai, pennyroyal, rosemary (used for digestive problems, not cooking), juniper, thuja, blue cohosh and senna during pregnancy.

Play it safe—be extremely careful with *any* substance your healthcare provider has not specifically recommended for you. Always check with him or her first before you take anything!

You Should Also Know

Allergies during Pregnancy
Allergies occur when the immune system reacts to a substance as if it's harmful. Common reactions include nasal congestion, sneezing, runny nose, and itchy eyes and inner ears. Allergies can be caused by pollen in grasses, weeds, trees and mold.

Nearly 10% of all pregnant women have seasonal allergies. They may get a little worse during pregnancy. Some fortunate women notice they get better during pregnancy, and symptoms improve.

....

If you have hay fever during early pregnancy, your baby is 6 times more likely to have hay fever.

....

If you use allergy medicine, don't assume it's safe during pregnancy. Some may not be advised, such as sudafed during the first trimester. Many are combinations of several medicines. Ask your healthcare provider about your medicine, whether prescription or non-prescription, including nasal sprays.

Medicines that are OK to use during pregnancy include antihistamines and decongestants. Ask your healthcare provider which brands are safest for you. For a nonmedicine treatment, add lime to water and drink it. Lime is a natural antihistamine and may help reduce symptoms. Ask your healthcare provider about increasing your magnesium intake—it relaxes airways and helps relieve congestion. Be sure to get enough omega-3 fatty acids because they help deal with itching and swelling.

Try to avoid anything that triggers your allergies. If dust bothers you, keep windows closed. Put a dab of petroleum jelly inside your nostrils to help catch pollen before you breathe it in. Use the air conditioner in your car and home. Don't hang clothes, towels or sheets outside to dry.

Avoid outdoor activities in the morning, when the pollen is usually at its worst. Stay inside on cloudy days—a drop in barometric pressure may result in headaches and/or sinus pressure. Be careful with pools—pollen can collect in outdoor pools. Wear a pollen-filtering mask when you're outside. Take a shower as soon as you come in from outdoors to wash away pollen.

Thoroughly clean the inside of your home. Wear a mask when you vacuum, and use a vacuum cleaner with a HEPA filter. Use a humidifier if you live in a very dry climate. Clean the filter in your home at least once a month.

Under your healthcare provider's supervision, you can continue taking allergy shots, but don't start them now.

Nasal Congestion

Congestion during pregnancy is normal in many women. It can be especially bad during allergy season when you're pregnant, so you may feel very stuffed up! Pregnancy can cause increased blood flow to mucous membranes.

Decongestants reduce nasal swelling by narrowing blood vessels in the nose. Most experts agree you can use Afrin as short-term relief to help reduce swelling. For longer relief, talk to your healthcare provider about using products, such as Nasalcrom, which are considered safe during pregnancy. You may also consider visiting a salt-therapy spa. Discuss it with your healthcare provider.

If you have a ragweed allergy, don't eat bananas, cucumbers, zucchini, melons or sunflower seeds. Avoid drinking chamomile tea. These are all in the ragweed family and may make symptoms worse.

Is Body-Hair Removal OK during Pregnancy?

Some women wax their legs and/or underarms and want to know if they can continue during pregnancy. This type of waxing is OK and shouldn't cause any problems during pregnancy. Bikini waxes are also OK while you're pregnant. Just be careful around the pubic area, and avoid Brazilian waxes. They involve putting hot wax on the tissue on either side of the vaginal opening (labia), which could be more sensitive when you're pregnant.

If you're into the "hairless-body craze," you either clip, shave, wax or depilate (remove with chemical cream) body hair in the genital area. If you wax, be aware skin irritation from hair removal may increase your risk of contracting a minor STD called *molluscum contagiosum* or *pox infection*. It may also increase your risk of developing genital warts. Signs of infection are raised white bumps in the affected area. In some cases, bumps spread up the abdomen or down the thigh. It can be spread when you scratch irritated skin. Shaving the genital area may increase the risk of occurrence.

If you stop removing hair from the genital area and let it grow out, the rash associated with the infection usually disappears in a year without treatment. There is also little evidence of scarring.

. . . .

More than 35% of all pregnant women snore. Recent studies show snoring has no damaging effect on baby's growth or development.

. . . .

Will You Be a Single Mother?

In the past years, we have seen an increase in the number of single moms. Today, over 40% of all babies in the United States are born to unmarried women. Many concerns are shared by all single moms-to-be. This discussion reflects some of the issues they have raised.

If you will be a single mother, seek support from family and friends. Mothers of young children can identify with your experiences—they've had similar ones recently. If you have friends or family members with young children, talk with them.

Raising a child alone can be both challenging and joyful. A single mother must take extra-good care of herself physically and emotionally. It's important to have a strong support system of family and/or friends. Many single moms find it easier to live and parent when they share expenses and daily activities with family or friends by living together.

Identify people you can count on for help during your pregnancy and after baby arrives. You may want to choose someone to be with you when you labor and deliver, and to be there to help afterward. A doula can be a good choice for you if you have natural childbirth. Your insurance company may even pay for a doula's services.

Childbirth classes are offered in many places for single moms. Many hospitals and birthing centers have options for single women when they give birth. Ask at your healthcare provider's office for further information.

After birth, you'll need support when you take baby home. Consider asking family members, friends and neighbors to help out. You'll probably need the most help the first month home. Some chores and errands people can do include some alone time for you, laundry, cooking, cleaning and shopping.

If you find yourself feeling apart from family and friends, make friends with other single moms for emotional and spiritual support. This can also provide

Protect Your Documents

• • • • • • • • • • •

Once you've made your will, keep the original in a safe place. If an attorney prepares yours, he or she will keep an original at the office. You might consider keeping a copy in a fireproof safety box at home. If you choose a relative to be the executor of your estate, you might also consider giving him or her a copy to have at hand.

you a support group for social inter-action and exchanging child care and other tasks.

You Need a Will. If you don't have a will, now's the time to make one. If you al-ready have a will, check it before baby's birth for changes or additions you may want to make.

Your will should name a legal guard-ian for your child in case something happens to you. Naming a guardian can be one of the most important things you do. Without a will that names a guard-ian, the courts decide who will care for your child.

After you decide on a guardian, ask that person before naming him or her in your will. Choose at least two people who could be the guardian of your child, and ask them both. If they accept, put their names in your will, and denote first and second choices.

If you want someone else to handle finances for your child, you can name a separate property guardian. This per-son's main responsibility is to take care of any financial assets you leave your child.

It's probably a good idea to have an attorney draw up your will. If you're unmarried, an attorney may be helpful

in covering all the necessary aspects so your child and/or partner will inherit your assets.

Check Your Insurance. Check your in-surance coverage before baby's birth. You must arrange where money will come from to care for your child in case of your death. You also need enough disability insurance to provide for your future and baby's future.

If something happens to you, you want to know your child will be fi-nancially taken care of until he or she is grown. This is most often provided through a life-insurance policy. You need enough life insurance to cover raising your child through college into adulthood.

Examine other types of insurance you have. Look at coverage you have now, and determine what type of cover-age you'll need after baby's arrival. It's time to make necessary changes!

When your employer provides insur-ance, check with the human resources (HR) representative for specific infor-mation about the insurance and its benefits. Don't overlook this important resource.

Check your health insurance policy to see what the time limit is for adding

> ### Dad Tip
> • • • • • • • • • • •
> You're nearly halfway through your pregnancy. Time may be passing very quickly for you both. Make an effort to spend some couple time together. When you can, take some time off from work or other obligations. Together, focus on the pregnancy and preparing for the birth of your baby. You might even suggest a babymoon to guarantee you have quality couple time together. See the discussion in Week 27.

baby to your health insurance. In some cases, a baby must be added within 30 days following birth or no coverage will be provided.

If you have an accident that requires you to take time off your job, disability insurance is good coverage to have. It pays you a predetermined amount of money while you're disabled. Most employers provide some disability insurance, but every working parent should have enough insurance to cover between 65 and 75% of his or her income.

Legal Questions. You may have many legal questions about your situation. It's important to get answers. The questions below have been posed by women who chose to be single mothers. They are legal questions that should be reviewed with an attorney in your area who specializes in family law.

- A friend who had a baby by herself told me I should consider the legal ramifications of this situation. What was she talking about?
- I've heard that in some states, if I'm unmarried, I have to get a special birth certificate. Is that true?
- I'm having my baby alone, and I'm concerned about who can make medical decisions for me and my

expected baby. Can I do anything about this concern?
- I'm not married, but I am deeply involved with my baby's father. Can my partner make medical decisions for me or our baby if I have problems during labor or after the birth?
- What are the legal rights of my baby's father if we are not married? Do my partner's parents have legal rights in regard to their grandchild (my child)?
- My baby's father and I went our separate ways before I knew I was pregnant. Do I have to tell him about the baby?
- I chose to have donor (artificial) insemination. If anything happens to me during my labor or delivery, who can make medical decisions for me? Who can make decisions for my baby?
- I got pregnant by donor insemination. What do I put on the birth certificate under "father's name"?
- Is there a way I can find out more about my sperm donor's family medical history?
- As my child grows up, she may need some sort of medical help (such as a donor kidney) from

a sibling. Will the sperm bank supply family information?

- I had donor insemination, and I'm wondering about the rights of the baby's father to be part of my child's life in the future. Should I be concerned?
- Someone joked that my child could marry its sister or brother some day and wouldn't know it because I had donor insemination. Is this possible?

If the baby's father could claim custody of your child, work out details with an attorney. Don't assume you will automatically have sole custody if the father wasn't a participant in the pregnancy and/or birth.

Exercise for Week 19

• • • • • • •

Stand with your right side about 2 feet away from the wall. Put your left foot 12 inches in front of your right foot. Bend both knees slightly. Place your right hand on the wall for support. Lift your left arm up and stretch toward the wall, bending your head. Next, encircling your head with your left arm, touch your right ear. Hold for 5 seconds. Return to standing position. Repeat 5 times, then turn and stretch for the wall with your right arm. *Stretches lower-back and side muscles.*

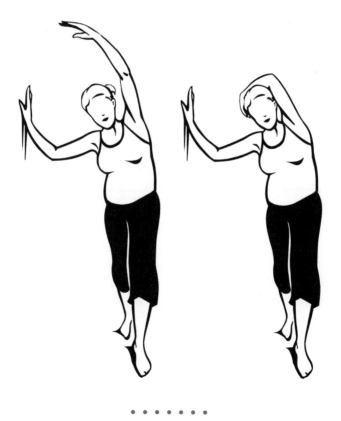

• • • • • • •

Week 20

Age of Fetus—18 Weeks

How Big Is Your Baby?

At this midpoint in your pregnancy, crown-to-rump length is 5⅔ to 6½ inches (14 to 16cm). Your baby weighs about 9 ounces (260g).

How Big Are You?

Congratulations—20 weeks marks the midpoint. You're halfway through your pregnancy! Your uterus is probably about even with your bellybutton. Your healthcare provider has been watching your growth and the enlargement of your uterus. Growth to this point may have been irregular but usually becomes more regular after the 20th week.

Measuring the Growth of Your Uterus

Measuring your uterus helps keep track of baby's growth. Your healthcare provider may use a measuring tape or his or her fingers and measure by finger breadth. He or she needs a point of reference against which to measure growth. Some healthcare providers measure from your bellybutton. Many measure from the pubic symphysis, the place where the pubic bones meet in the middle-lower part of your abdomen, 6 to 10 inches (15.2 to 25.4cm) below the bellybutton. It may be felt near your pubic hairline.

Not every healthcare provider measures the same way, not every woman is the same size and babies vary in size. Measurements differ among women and are often different for a woman from one pregnancy to another.

If you see a healthcare provider you don't normally see or if you see someone new, you may measure differently. This doesn't mean there's a problem or that someone is measuring incorrectly. It's just that everyone measures a little differently.

After this point in pregnancy, you should grow almost ½ inch (1cm) each week. If you're 8 inches (20cm) at 20 weeks, at your next visit (4 weeks later), you should measure about 10 inches (24cm).

If you measure 11¼ inches (28cm) at this point in pregnancy, an ultrasound may be recommended to see if you're carrying twins or if your due date is correct. If you only measure 6 inches (15 to 16cm), your due date could be wrong, or there may be a concern about

Tip for Week 20
. . . .

If you have an ultrasound test now, it may be possible to find out the sex of the baby, but baby must cooperate. You have to be able to see the genitals. Even if the sex looks obvious, ultrasound operators have been known to make mistakes!

intrauterine-growth restriction (IUGR) or some other problem.

Within limits, changing measurements are a sign of fetal well-being and fetal growth. If they aren't normal, it can be a warning sign. If you're concerned about your size and the growth of your pregnancy, discuss it with your healthcare provider.

How Your Baby Is Growing and Developing

Your Baby's Skin

The skin covering your baby began growing from two layers, the *epidermis*, which is on the surface, and the *dermis*, which is the deeper layer. By this point, there are four layers. One of these layers contains ridges, which are responsible for patterns on fingertips, palms and soles. They are genetically determined.

When a baby is born, its skin is covered by a white substance that looks like paste, called *vernix*. It is secreted by the glands in the skin beginning around this week. Vernix protects your growing baby's skin from amniotic fluid.

Hair appears around 12 to 14 weeks and grows from the epidermis. Hair is first seen on the baby's upper lip and eyebrow. This hair is usually shed around the time of birth and is replaced by thicker hair from new follicles.

Ultrasound Pictures

The illustration on page 204 shows an ultrasound exam (and an interpretive illustration) in a pregnant woman at about 20 weeks. An ultrasound may be easier to understand when it is actually being done. The pictures are more like motion pictures.

If you look closely at the illustration, it may make more sense to you. Read the labels, and try to visualize the baby inside the uterus. An ultrasound picture is like looking at a slice of an object. The picture you see is 2-dimensional.

Ultrasound at this time helps confirm or establish your due date. If two or more babies are present, they can usually be seen. Some fetal problems can also be seen at this time.

. . . .
Don't have one of those ultrasound "keepsakes" done at your local mall. It may be risky to you and baby because untrained technicians doing the test may not use equipment correctly.
. . . .

Percutaneous Umbilical-Cord Blood Sampling (PUBS)

Percutaneous umbilical-cord blood sampling (PUBS), also called *cordocentesis*, is a test done on the fetus inside your uterus. The test is done to detect blood disorders, infections and Rh-incompatibility.

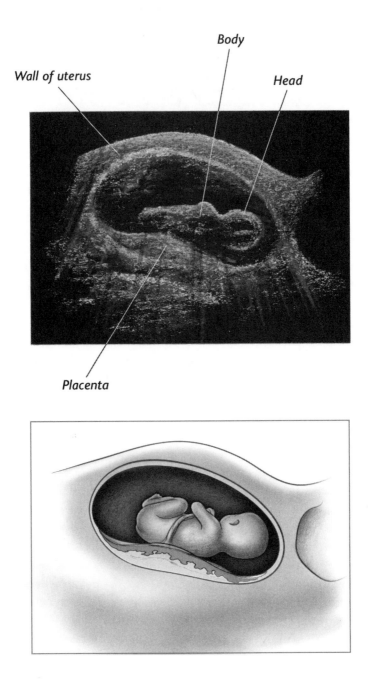

Wall of uterus

Body

Head

Placenta

Ultrasound of a baby at 20 weeks gestation
(fetal age—18 weeks). The interpretive illustration
may help you see more detail.

Dad Tip
· · · · · · · · · · ·

Around this time, your partner may have an ultrasound exam of your growing baby. You might want to be there for this fun test—it's the first time you can actually see baby move! Ask your partner to consider your schedule when making the appointment for her ultrasound.

Results are available in a few days. The test carries a slightly higher risk of miscarriage than amniocentesis.

Guided by ultrasound, a needle is inserted through the mother's abdomen into a tiny vein in the umbilical cord. A small sample of the baby's blood is removed for analysis.

PUBS results can help prevent life-threatening anemia that may develop if the mother is Rh-negative and has antibodies that are destroying baby's blood. If you're Rh-negative, you should receive RhoGAM after this procedure.

· ·

Air pollution could affect baby's birthweight. Fumes from traffic and various industries contribute to air pollution. Studies show women who live in smoggy areas often give birth to babies that weigh less than babies born in smog-free areas.

· ·

Changes in You

Stretching Abdominal Muscles

Your abdominal muscles are stretched and pushed apart as your baby grows. Muscles attached to the lower portion of your ribs run vertically down to your pelvis. They may separate in the midline. These muscles are called the *rectus muscles*; when they separate, it is a hernia called a *diastasis recti*.

You may notice the separation when you lie down and raise your head, tightening abdominal muscles. It may look like there's a bulge in the middle of your tummy. You might even feel the edge of the muscle on either side of the bulge. What you feel in the gap between the muscles is the uterus. You may feel the baby's movement more easily here. It isn't painful and doesn't harm you or baby.

If this is your first baby, you may not notice the separation. With each pregnancy, separation may be more noticeable. Exercising can strengthen these muscles, but you may still have the bulge or gap. After pregnancy, these muscles tighten and the gap closes. The separation won't be as noticeable, but it may still be present.

Rheumatoid Arthritis (RA)

Rheumatoid arthritis (RA) is an autoimmune disease that affects 1 in every 1000 pregnant women. Symptoms include joint pain, tenderness, swelling and stiffness. During pregnancy, symptoms may improve and even disappear. Nearly 75% of women with RA feel better when they're pregnant. Less pain may mean you need less medication.

Some medicines used to treat RA can be dangerous to a pregnant woman, but many are safe. Be sure to talk to your healthcare provider about medicines you take for your rheumatoid arthritis before you get pregnant.

Talk to your doctor about using over-the-counter medications during pregnancy. We have new warnings for use of acetaminophen throughout your pregnancy. See Week 7. NSAIDs should not be used in later pregnancy because they may increase the risk of heart problems in baby. Prednisone is usually acceptable, although methotrexate should never be used because it may cause miscarriage and birth defects. Enbrel is a prescription medication used to treat RA. Don't use it without checking first with your healthcare provider.

West Nile virus (WNV) is spread to humans by mosquito bites. Symptoms appear within 3 to 14 days and include fever, headache, fatigue, swollen lymph nodes, body aches and possibly a skin rash. If you're pregnant, avoid mosquito-infested areas, use screens on windows and doors, wear protective clothing and use an EPA-registered repellent. If you become ill, call your healthcare provider. There is no treatment for West Nile fever, but if your healthcare provider believes you may have contracted the illness, diagnostic testing can be done 2 to 4 weeks after onset of the illness. After baby's birth, if you have symptoms of West Nile virus, don't breastfeed.

RA may not affect your labor and delivery; however, 25% of women have a preterm birth. It may be harder to find comfortable labor positions if you have joint restrictions.

Symptoms may return a few months after baby is born. See your

rheumatologist within 4 weeks of having your baby. He or she may want you to restart medicine you stopped taking during pregnancy. If you breastfeed, discuss the choice of medications with your healthcare provider.

How Your Actions Affect Your Baby's Development

Sexual Relations

As you get larger, sexual intercourse may become difficult because of discomfort for you. With some imagination and different positions (ones in which you aren't on your back and your partner isn't directly on top of you), you can continue to enjoy sex.

If you feel emotional pressure from your partner—either his concern about the safety of intercourse or requests for frequent sexual relations—discuss it openly with him. Ask your partner to come to a prenatal visit to discuss these things with your healthcare provider.

If you're having problems with contractions, bleeding or other complications, you and your partner should talk with your healthcare provider. Together you can decide whether you should continue to have sexual relations. If your healthcare provider advises against sex, ask whether this means no intercourse or no orgasm.

Body Art

We have seen an increase in piercings and tattoos in women. An understanding of some of the problems that may occur with piercings or tattoos during pregnancy may help you understand

You May Be Sexier than You Think

. . . .

Pregnancy is sexy! We know many men think their pregnant partner is more beautiful and sexier than ever before, especially during this middle part of pregnancy. Below are reasons men have given us as to why they think their pregnant partner is sexy.

- Pregnancy hormones may increase your sexual desire. Discovering different ways to make love can be fun. Sex during pregnancy often requires some creative thinking on both your parts.
- Your pregnancy makes him walk like a man. For many men, their partner's pregnancy is a source of pride.
- You may have more cleavage (or cleavage when you've never had it before). Your curves can be sexy. Your changing figure turns him on.
- Your hair may be luxurious, nails may be long and skin glowing, smoother and softer.
- The level of commitment you feel toward each other may intensify your intimacy. Having a child together may be the ultimate act of trust.
- You're carefree because you don't have to worry about birth control.

why your healthcare provider may have concerns.

Body piercing has been around since ancient civilization and is popular again. The most common form of piercing is pierced earlobes—many women have pierced ears. This is a low-risk type of piercing your healthcare provider won't be concerned about. However, if you have any other piercings, bring them to his or her attention.

Many places on the body may be pierced, including the eyebrow, nostril, nasal septum, lips, tongue, nipples, navel, labia and clitoral hood; these piercings may cause your healthcare provider concern. With any type of piercing, there's the possibility of scar-tissue formation. Nipple piercing can damage milk ducts, which could interfere with breastfeeding. Navel jewelry must be removed; leaving it in the navel could lead to ripping or tearing.

With oral piercing, there's a chance for infection and for swallowing jewelry. If you have any oral piercings, your healthcare provider may discuss removing them before delivery. The anesthesiologist may be concerned about keeping your airway open if jewelry is not removed. Because no one can predict what labor and delivery will involve, it may be safer to remove the jewelry as you get closer to your due date.

Like body piercing, *tattoos* have been part of many cultures for thousands of years. Many people have tattoos; the most common sites are the arms, chest, back, abdomen and legs. Some problems pregnant women with tattoos can have include infection, allergic reaction, formation of scar tissue at the tattoo site, stretch marks in the area of the tattoo and removal of an unwanted tattoo.

Don't be surprised to see a change in your tattoo if it's located on a body part or in an area that can be affected by pregnancy. For example, the cute little butterfly on your abdomen may grow very large during pregnancy, and stretch marks may run through it. After pregnancy, skin may remain stretched, and the cute little butterfly droops and sags until skin returns to "normal" after pregnancy, which may not be like "normal" before pregnancy.

Tattoo removal during pregnancy is not recommended. Neither is getting a new tattoo. You don't want to increase your chances of getting an infection, which is a risk when you get a tattoo. Wait until after baby's birth to receive or to remove a tattoo.

There have been rumors that women who have tattoos on their lower backs can't have regional anesthesia, such as epidurals and spinal anesthesia. However, no studies have shown this to be true. Discuss any concerns you have about anesthesia and your tattoos with your healthcare provider.

Your Nutrition

Many women use sugar and/or artificial sweeteners before pregnancy. Are they safe during pregnancy?

Caloric sweeteners include processed and unprocessed sugars, such as granulated sugar, brown sugar, corn syrup, honey, agave nectar and raw sugar. Caloric content ranges from 16 to 22 calories per teaspoon. If you use caloric sweeteners, you're adding empty calories to your meal plan.

Artificial (noncaloric) sweeteners help a woman cut calories. Some common artificial sweeteners include aspartame, acesulfame K, sucralose, stevia and saccharin. Research indicates artificial sweeteners are probably safe to use in small amounts during pregnancy. However, avoid them if you can. Eliminate any substance you don't really need from the foods and beverages you eat and drink. Do it for the good of your baby.

You Should Also Know

Hearing Your Baby's Heartbeat

It may be possible to hear your baby's heartbeat with a stethoscope at 20 weeks. Before we had Doppler equipment to hear the heartbeat and ultrasound to see the heart beating, a stethoscope helped the listener hear baby's heartbeat. This usually occurred after quickening for most women.

The sound you hear through a stethoscope may be different from what you're used to hearing at the office. It isn't loud. If you've never listened through a stethoscope, it may be difficult to hear at first. It gets easier as baby gets larger and sounds become louder.

If you can't hear the heartbeat with a stethoscope, don't worry. It's not always easy for a healthcare provider who does this on a regular basis!

If you hear a swishing sound (baby's heartbeat), you have to differentiate it from a beating sound (mother's heartbeat). A baby's heart beats rapidly, usually 120 to 160 beats every minute. Your heartbeat or pulse rate is slower, in the range of 60 to 80 beats a minute. Ask your healthcare provider to help you distinguish the sounds.

Grandma's Remedy
· · · · · · · · · · ·

If you want to avoid using medication, try a folk remedy. If you experience foot odor, spray some antiperspirant on your feet—it helps reduce odor and may prevent skin cracking.

Could You Have Osteoporosis?

Osteoporosis is a bone disease in which bones lose density and the spaces within them grow larger, resulting in increased chance of breakage. It's typically diagnosed in older, postmenopausal women. However, it's now being diagnosed in younger women.

We believe low-calorie diets, excessive exercise and drinking lots of diet soda may be possible causes. In addition, low body weight, anemia and amenorrhea may add to the problem. Women who smoke or drink a lot of alcohol may increase that risk.

Osteoporosis at a young age can be serious. Bones may become so thin they actually break. In later years, osteoporosis may be severe.

If you believe you may have a problem, talk to your healthcare provider about it. If you do have osteoporosis, it could have an effect on you during your pregnancy.

Exercise for Week 20

• • • • • • •

Kneel on your hands and knees, with your wrists directly beneath your shoulders and your knees directly beneath your hips. Keep your back straight. Contract your tummy muscles, then extend your left leg behind you at hip height. At the same time, extend your right arm at shoulder height. Hold 5 seconds, and return to the kneeling position. Repeat on your other side. Start with 4 repetitions on each side, and gradually work up to 8. *Strengthens buttocks muscles, back muscles and leg muscles.*

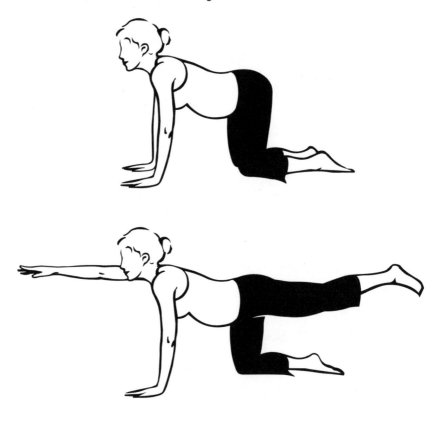

• • • • • • •

Week 21

Age of Fetus—19 Weeks

How Big Is Your Baby?

Your baby now weighs about 10½ ounces (300g); its crown-to-rump length is about 7¼ inches (18cm). It's about the size of a large banana.

How Big Are You?

When your healthcare provider measures your uterus, it's almost 8½ inches (21cm) from the pubic symphysis. Your total weight gain should be between 10 and 15 pounds (4.5 and 6.3kg). By this week, your waistline is definitely gone. Friends and relatives—and strangers—can tell you're pregnant. It would be hard to hide your condition!

How Your Baby Is Growing and Developing

Rapid growth rate of your baby has slowed. However, the baby continues to grow and to develop as different organ systems within the baby mature.

Baby's digestive system is functioning in a simple way, and baby swallows amniotic fluid. Researchers believe swallowing may help develop the digestive system. It may also condition the digestive system to function after birth. After swallowing fluid, baby absorbs much of it and passes unabsorbed matter as far as the large bowel. With ultrasound, you can see the baby swallowing.

Studies indicate full-term babies may swallow as much as 17 ounces (500ml) of amniotic fluid in a 24-hour period. It contributes a small amount to baby's caloric needs and may contribute essential nutrients to the developing baby.

Meconium

During pregnancy, you may hear the term *meconium*. It refers to undigested cells from the lining of baby's gastrointestinal tract and swallowed amniotic fluid found in baby's digestive system. It is a greenish-black to light-brown substance. It passes from baby's bowels before delivery, during labor or after birth. If meconium is present during labor, it may be an indication of fetal stress.

If baby passes meconium into amniotic fluid, baby may swallow the fluid. If it is inhaled into the lungs, baby could develop pneumonia or pneumonitis. When meconium is found at delivery,

> ## Tip for Week 21
> . . . .
>
> A good way to add calcium to your diet is to cook rice and oatmeal in skim milk instead of water.

an attempt is made to remove it from baby's mouth and throat with a small suction tube.

Changes in You

Swelling

You may notice swelling in various parts of your body, especially your lower legs and feet, particularly at the end of the day. If you're on your feet a lot, you may have less swelling if you can rest during the day.

Swelling often begins around week 24. Seventy-five percent of all pregnant women suffer from swollen fingers, ankles and feet. If your feet swell, it can help to wear pregnancy support stockings to keep blood from pooling in your feet. Ask your healthcare provider about them.

There are other things you can try to help control swelling. Prenatal massage may be good. A potassium deficiency may allow your cells to fill with water, increasing swelling, so eat plenty of raisins and bananas; both are high in potassium. Flexing your feet and ankles during the day helps keep blood circulating. You can also try standing on your tiptoes to help pump blood back to the heart. When sitting, press your toes down as if you were pushing on the gas pedal of your car to accomplish the same thing.

Blood Clots

A serious complication of pregnancy is a blood clot in the legs or groin. Symptoms include swelling of the legs accompanied by leg pain and redness or warmth over the affected area in the legs.

This problem has many names, including *venous thrombosis, thrombo-embolic disease, thrombophlebitis* and *deep-vein thrombosis*. The problem is not limited to pregnancy, but pregnancy is a time when it may be more likely to occur because blood flow slows in the legs and the blood-clotting mechanism can change.

The most probable cause during pregnancy is decreased blood flow, also called *stasis*. If you've had a previous blood clot anywhere in your body, tell your healthcare provider at the beginning of pregnancy. It's important information.

Help protect yourself by exercising, not sitting for longer than 2 hours, not smoking and not wearing tight clothing at or below your waist. Surgical stockings may help prevent the problem; heparin may be recommended in severe cases.

Superficial and Deep-Vein Thrombosis (DVT). Superficial thrombosis and deep-vein thrombosis are different conditions. *Superficial thrombosis* is a blood clot in veins close to the surface of the skin. You

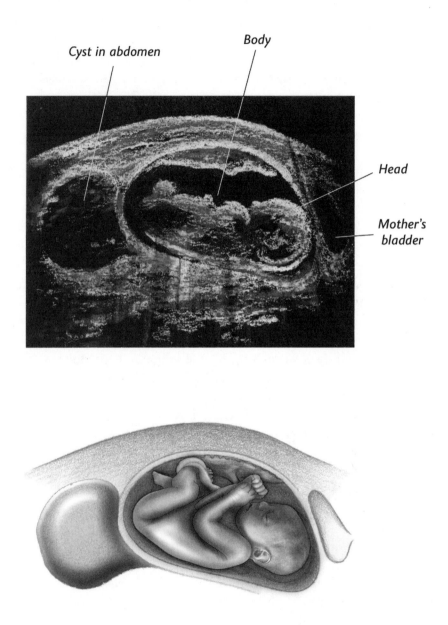

Cyst in abdomen

Body

Head

Mother's
bladder

Ultrasound may be used to detect problems. In this ultrasound of
a baby in utero, there is a cyst in the mother-to-be's abdomen.
The interpretive illustration clarifies the ultrasound image.

can see and feel these veins. This situation is treated with a mild pain reliever, elevation of the leg, support of the leg with an Ace bandage or support stockings, and occasionally heat.

Deep-vein thrombosis (DVT) occurs in a very small percentage of pregnant women. Although it's a serious complication, it can often be avoided with early treatment. If you've had a blood clot in the past, tell your healthcare provider at your first prenatal visit about any previous blood clots.

With DVT, a blood clot forms in the deeper veins in your legs. Onset can be rapid, with severe pain and swelling of the leg and thigh. Symptoms include swelling in the leg, worsening cramp or pain in one leg, discoloration of the leg, including turning red, blue or purple, and/or a feeling of warmth in the affected leg. Squeezing the calf or leg may be extremely painful, and it may be painful to walk. If you have any of these symptoms, call your healthcare provider immediately.

Ultrasound is usually used to diagnose the problem. Most major medical centers offer it.

Treating DVT. Treatment usually consists of hospitalization and anticoagulant therapy. Heparin and Lovenox (enoxaparin) are anticoagulants that can be given intravenously and are safe to use during pregnancy.

While anticoagulants are being administered, the woman must stay in bed. The leg may be elevated and heat applied. Mild pain medicine is often prescribed.

Recovery time, including hospitalization, may be 7 to 10 days. The woman will need to continue taking heparin until delivery. Following pregnancy, she will need to take an anticoagulant for up to several weeks, depending on the severity of the clot.

If a woman has a blood clot during one pregnancy, she will probably need an anticoagulant during her next pregnancies. If so, it can be given by an in-dwelling I.V. catheter or by daily injections.

One medication used to prevent or to treat deep-vein thrombosis is warfarin (Coumadin). It is not given during pregnancy because it can be harmful to the baby. Warfarin may be given to a woman after pregnancy to prevent blood clots. It may be prescribed for a few weeks or a few months, depending on the severity of the clot.

. . . .

If you eat some dark chocolate during pregnancy, baby may be happier at 6 months of age. Just don't have more than 1 ounce per day, or you might not be happier if you gain too much weight!

. . . .

How Your Actions Affect Your Baby's Development

Safety of Ultrasound

On page 213 is an illustration of an ultrasound exam, accompanied by an interpretive illustration. These show a baby inside a uterus; the mother-to-be also has a large cyst in her abdomen.

Many women wonder about the safety of ultrasound exams. Researchers have looked for potential problems for many years without finding evidence of any. Experts agree ultrasound exams don't pose any risk to you or your baby.

Ultrasound is an extremely valuable tool for diagnosing problems and answering some questions during pregnancy. If your healthcare provider recommends ultrasound, discuss it with him or her. He or she may have an important reason for doing an ultrasound exam. It could affect the well-being of your developing baby.

Craving ice can be a sign of iron-deficiency anemia; the medical term for craving ice is pagophagi. *Some experts believe your body craves ice because you have anemia—a common symptom with anemia is an inflamed tongue. The ice helps cool your tongue and makes you feel more comfortable.*

Eating Disorders—Can They Affect Pregnancy?

About 7 million women in the United States have some type of eating disorder, and eating disorders are becoming more recognized in pregnant women. Experts believe as many as 1% of all pregnant women suffer from some degree of eating disorder. The two primary eating disorders are anorexia nervosa and bulimia nervosa. Other eating disorders include restricting calories or food, and weight obsession, but those afflicted with them don't meet the anorexia or bulimia criteria.

Women with *anorexia* usually weigh less than 85% of what is normal for their age and height. They are often very fearful of becoming fat, have an unrealistic body image, purge with laxatives or by vomiting, and binge. *Bulimia* is characterized by repeated binging and purging. A bulimic binges and purges at least twice a week for a period of 3 months or more.

It's often difficult for any woman to see her body gain the weight that is normal with a pregnancy. It may be even harder for a woman with an eating disorder to see the pounds add up. It may take a lot of hard work and effort to accept these extra pounds, but you must try to do it for your good health and the good health of your baby.

Eating disorders may worsen during pregnancy. However, some women find their eating disorder gets better during this time. For some, pregnancy is the first time they can let go of their obsession about their bodies.

An eating disorder affects you and your baby! Problems associated with an eating disorder during pregnancy include:

- a weight gain that is too low or a low-birthweight baby
- miscarriage and an increased chance of fetal death
- intrauterine-growth restriction (IUGR)
- premature birth
- high blood pressure and electrolyte problems in the mother-to-be
- depression during and after pregnancy
- birth defects
- decreased blood volume

Your body is designed to provide your baby with the nutrition it needs, even if it has to take it from your body stores. You need to eat healthfully for you and baby.

Sometimes visualizing what baby looks like at a particular time can help you. Look at our illustrations of baby and read how baby is developing. Use this information to imagine how big your baby is and what it looks like at a certain time.

An eating disorder may disrupt the way nutrients are delivered to baby. More frequent prenatal visits and monitoring during pregnancy may be recommended so your healthcare provider can keep close tabs on how baby is growing. Antidepressants may also be used to help treat the problem. An eating disorder can also increase the risk of postpartum depression.

Talk to your healthcare provider about your problem as soon as possible. It's serious and can be harmful to you and your baby.

"Pregorexia." A newly recognized trend in eating disorders is called *pregorexia*. This eating disorder is not a recognized medical diagnosis, and the term is not an actual medical term. But healthcare professionals who care for pregnant women are recognizing the problem more often. Some researchers believe pregorexia is an issue for about 30% of all pregnant women.

What is pregorexia? It is the situation in which a mom-to-be doesn't gain the recommended amount of weight during pregnancy. She keeps her weight gain at a minimum through intense dieting and exercise, and she may also binge and purge.

The problem can affect women during their first pregnancy, but it may not occur until a second, or later, pregnancy. A pregnant woman doesn't gain weight *intentionally* because she's worried about having to lose weight after baby's birth or because she is fearful of giving birth to a baby that is, in her mind, "too big." Moms-to-be can become obsessed with weight gain, and their obsession becomes pregorexia.

Pregorexia can affect the fetus. If a pregnant woman engages in extended workouts, restricts calories, binges and purges, it can affect her developing baby.

We know low-birthweight babies are at risk of experiencing problems. If you find yourself beginning to have thoughts about keeping your weight gain very low during your pregnancy, talk to your healthcare provider about it immediately!

Binge-Eating Disorder (BED). Both men and women suffer from *binge-eating disorder (BED)*. It is estimated 3½% of all women in the United States are affected. What is BED? The disorder is identified when a person exhibits three or more of the symptoms described below.

- Eating a large quantity of food when you're not hungry.
- Eating a large quantity of food in a 2-hour period.
- Eating more rapidly than normal.
- Eating until you feel very uncomfortable.
- Eating alone because you don't want other people to see how much you eat.
- Feeling guilty, angry, ashamed or depressed after you overeat.

What Foods Do Pregnant Women Crave?

· · · · · · · · · · ·

Research indicates three common cravings among pregnant women.
- 33% crave chocolate
- 20% crave sweets of some sort
- 19% crave citrus fruits and juices

These episodes occur at least two times a week for a period of 6 months or longer. The disorder is further categorized by the fact the person overeating does not purge, such as by vomiting or using laxatives, and does not exercise excessively after overeating.

In the company of others, the person doesn't usually overeat. However, when alone, that person may buy favorite foods, binge on them, then hide the evidence of what was eaten.

If you suffer from BED, it's important to control it during pregnancy. Binging on foods could cause you to gain more weight than is healthy for you and baby. And the food you binge on may be high in calories and low in nutrition. If you're having problems with this disorder, contact the Binge Eating Disorder Association (BEDA). It's important to get it under control before pregnancy, when possible, but it is absolutely essential to control it during pregnancy.

Your Nutrition

Cravings

Some women experience food cravings during pregnancy. Food cravings have long been considered a nonspecific sign of pregnancy. We don't understand all the reasons you might crave a food while you're pregnant, but we believe hormonal and emotional changes add to the situation. Some believe cravings may indicate your body needs the nutrients a particular food contains, but research shows there is no proven connection between the foods you crave and nutrients you may need. Some believe cravings occur in pregnant women because taste buds change, as does a woman's sense of smell.

Craving a particular food can be both good and bad. If the food you crave is nutritious and healthful, eat it in moderation. Try to substitute healthy foods for unhealthy cravings. If you crave:

- something salty and crunchy, like potato chips, have some baked chips with humus, celery with peanut butter or popcorn
- something sweet and chewy, like candy, have some dried fruit, wheat crackers with some jam or jelly, or some trail mix
- ice cream, have some frozen ice milk or frozen yogurt, or try a fruit smoothie

If you crave foods that are high in fat and sugar or loaded with empty calories, take a little taste, but don't let yourself go crazy. Try eating another food instead of indulging in your craving, or replace

Pica—Nonfood Cravings

. . . .

Some women experience *pica* during pregnancy—they crave nonfood items, such as dirt, clay, laundry starch, chalk, ice, paint chips and other things. We don't know why pregnant women develop these cravings. Some experts believe it may be caused by an iron deficiency. Others think pica may be the body's attempt to get vitamins or minerals not being supplied in food the woman eats. Still others speculate pica cravings may be caused by an underlying physical or mental illness. Pica may be harmful to your baby and you. Eating nonfood items could interfere with nutrient absorption of healthy foods and result in a deficiency. If you have pica cravings, don't panic. Call your healthcare provider immediately. He or she will develop a plan to help you deal with the cravings.

high-calorie fare with low-calorie ones. If you crave the same nonnutritious treat over and over again, buy a few single-serve portions, and keep them in the freezer. Eat one at a time.

Be careful what you eat when you're tired. You may crave a snack that isn't healthy for you. Try eating a small healthy snack first, and wait for a bit. See if you really want the unhealthy food. Some cravings are emotional—you may be tired and out of sorts and crave a hot-fudge sundae. You may be craving comfort, not food.

If you have trouble with sugar cravings, try chewing sugar-free gum. Or go out for a treat you crave. If you have to go out, you may change your mind. Understand when you indulge your cravings for high-fat, sugary foods, you may actually increase your cravings for them!

Food Aversions

On the opposite side of cravings is food aversion. Some foods you have eaten without problems before pregnancy may now make you sick to your stomach. It's common. Again, we believe the hormones of pregnancy are involved. In this case, hormones affect the gastrointestinal tract, which can affect your reaction to some foods.

If you have food aversions, try to substitute foods to get the nutrients you need. For example, drink calcium-fortified juice if you can't drink milk. Meat making you ill? Try eggs, beans or nuts.

You Should Also Know

Will You Get Varicose Veins?

When the valves of veins are weakened or damaged, they can become *varicose*, which means abnormally swollen or dilated. During pregnancy, varicose veins appear as large, distended veins deep under the skin caused by blood-flow blockage in the veins. Normally, valves in the veins open and close to keep blood moving in one direction. With varicose veins, blood flows back through valves and pools in the veins. This causes them to stretch, swell and twist.

Varicose veins, also called *varicosities* or *varices*, occur to some degree in most pregnant women. There seems to be an inherited tendency to get varicose veins during pregnancy. It can worsen with increased age or by standing for a long time.

∙ ∙

You may experience spider veins, which are small groups of dilated blood vessels near the skin's surface. You see them most commonly on face and legs.

∙ ∙

Problems usually occur in the legs but may also be present in the vulva and rectum (hemorrhoids). Change in blood flow and pressure from the uterus can make problems worse and cause discomfort. In most instances, varicose veins become more noticeable and more painful as pregnancy progresses and may get worse as you gain more weight (especially if you stand a lot).

Symptoms vary. For some, the main symptom is a blemish or purple-blue spot on the legs with little or no discomfort, except maybe in the evening. Other women have painful bulging veins that ache or feel heavy. They may also burn, throb and swell, and look purple or blue and appear twisted, enlarged and raised above the skin. Varicose veins may also cause itching.

There are many things you can do to help deal with varicose veins. Wear medical support hose; many types are available. Ask your healthcare provider about them. Wear clothing that doesn't restrict circulation at the knee or groin. Spend as little time on your feet as you can. Lie on your side or elevate your legs when possible. This enables veins to drain more easily. Wear flat shoes when you can. Don't cross your legs; it cuts off circulation and can make problems worse.

Not sitting for long periods can help. Watch your pregnancy weight gain and eat lots of fiber. A low-salt diet may also help with varicose veins. Don't wear tight pants.

Drink citrus juice or eat citrus fruit; the vitamin C helps keep capillary and vein walls strong. Consider eating spinach, broccoli and asparagus; these foods may help lessen the severity of varicose veins and are high in vitamin K, which may help relieve symptoms.

Exercise regularly to help improve blood flow through the veins. High-impact exercise, such as step aerobics or jogging, can damage veins. Low-impact exercises, such as biking, prenatal yoga or using an elliptical trainer, may be a better choice.

Following pregnancy, swelling in the veins should go down, but varicose veins probably won't completely disappear. After-pregnancy treatment methods include laser treatment, injection and surgery.

Vaginitis

The term *vaginitis* covers a lot of conditions that cause annoying vaginal symptoms, such as itching, burning, irritation and abnormal discharge. The most common causes of vaginitis are bacterial vaginosis, vulvovaginal candidiasis and trichomoniasis. Bacterial vaginosis is the

---

Dad Tip

• • • • • • • • • • •

It's not too early to start thinking about baby names. Sometimes partners have very different ideas about names for their child. There are many books available to help you. Nearly 50% of all Americans are named after a family member. Do you plan to honor a close friend or relative by using their name? Will you use a family name? What problems could arise if you choose a peculiar, difficult-to-say or hard-to-spell name? Find out what a name means—it could help you make a decision. What do the initials spell out? What nicknames go with the name? Start thinking about it now, even if you decide you won't pick a name until after you meet your baby.

---

most common of the conditions and is discussed below.

Bacterial Vaginosis (BV). It's estimated that more than 15% of pregnant women have bacterial vaginosis (BV) during pregnancy. It is the most common vaginal infection in women of childbearing age. Some experts believe it may be caused by douching and sexual intercourse. It is also more common in women who have an IUD.

BV is caused by an imbalance or overgrowth of several types of bacteria that exist in the vagina. It may be difficult to diagnose BV because bacteria can also be found in healthy individuals. Nearly half of the women infected have no symptoms. For those who do, they may experience symptoms similar to those of a yeast infection, including itching, a vaginal odor that is "fishy," painful urination and a gray-white discharge.

Your healthcare provider can detect the problem by testing vaginal discharge for BV-causing bacteria. Antibiotics are used to treat the problem. Seven days of metronidazole (Flagyl) is the treatment of choice. If left untreated, BV can cause

problems. If you have BV, be sure it is treated.

Fibromyalgia

Fibromyalgia affects nearly 5 million American women every year. It causes muscles all over the body to ache, burn and twitch. If you suffer from it, you probably ache all over. You may also feel tingling in fingers and toes. Severe fatigue, headaches, sleep problems, abdominal pain and gastrointestinal problems may also be present. Some sufferers experience anxiety and depression.

The problem usually begins during early adulthood or middle age and causes chronic pain and other symptoms. Symptoms can come and go throughout a person's life. Although fibromyalgia is believed to be genetic, it may lie dormant until triggered by a trauma, such as childbirth.

Fibromyalgia can be hard to diagnose, and a person may suffer for a long time before finding help. It is more common when a person also suffers from irritable bowel syndrome, celiac disease or lactose intolerance.

We don't know a lot about fibromyalgia during pregnancy. We do know fibromyalgia won't harm your baby. Pregnancy can be a time of high stress, and physical and emotional stress are known triggers for fibromyalgia.

During pregnancy, your body produces many hormones, which may affect your disease. Studies have found some women experience more severe symptoms during pregnancy. The third trimester may be the worst, and symptoms may last as long as 3 months after birth.

If you suffer from fibromyalgia, bring it up at your first prenatal visit. At this time, there is no cure, and treatment is limited. The FDA has approved the drug Lyrica to help manage pain. Antidepressants and pain suppressants may also be used to treat symptoms. Discuss the use of any of these medicines with your healthcare provider.

Exercise may offer some relief. Some types of exercise to consider include yoga, exercising in the water, Pilates and stretching. Massage therapy may also help—look for a massage therapist with experience treating fibromyalgia pain who can safely perform massage on a pregnant woman.

Exercise for Week 21

· · · · · · ·

Like Kegel exercises, you can do this exercise just about anywhere. Standing or sitting, take a deep breath. While exhaling, tighten your tummy muscles as though you were zipping up a pair of tight jeans. Repeat 6 or 8 times. *Strengthens tummy muscles.*

Do this second exercise after you've been sitting a long time, such as at your desk or in a car or on a plane, or when you have to stand for long periods. When you're forced to stand in one place for a long time, step forward slightly with one foot. Place all your weight on that foot for a few minutes. Do the same with the other foot. Alternate the leg you begin with each time. *Stretches leg muscles.*

Week 22

Age of Fetus—20 Weeks

How Big Is Your Baby?

Your baby weighs about 12¼ ounces (350g). Crown-to-rump length at this time is about 7⅔ inches (19cm).

How Big Are You?

Your uterus is about ¾ inch (2cm) above your bellybutton. Your growing tummy doesn't get in your way much; you may feel pretty good. You're still able to bend over and to sit comfortably. Walking shouldn't be an effort. Morning sickness has probably passed. It's kind of fun being pregnant now!

How Your Baby Is Growing and Developing

Your baby's body grows every day. As you can see by looking at the illustration on page 224, eyelids and eyebrows are developed. Fingernails are also visible.

Your baby's organ systems are becoming specialized for their particular functions. Consider the liver. An important function of the liver is managing bilirubin, which is produced by the breakdown of blood cells. The life span of a fetal red blood cell is shorter than that of an adult; baby makes more bilirubin than an adult.

The fetal liver has a limited capacity to remove bilirubin from the fetal bloodstream. Bilirubin passes from fetal blood through the placenta to your blood. Your liver helps get rid of it. A premature baby may have trouble processing bilirubin because its own liver is not ready to take over this function. Full-term babies can also have this problem. A newborn baby with high levels of bilirubin may exhibit *jaundice.*

Changes in You

Fetal Fibronectin (fFN)

It can be hard to determine if a woman is at risk of delivering a preterm baby because many symptoms of preterm labor are similar to various discomforts of pregnancy. A test is available to help healthcare providers make this determination.

Fetal fibronectin (fFN) is a protein found in the amniotic sac and fetal membranes. After 22 weeks of pregnancy, fFN is not normally present until around week 38. When fFN is found in cervical-vaginal secretions of a pregnant

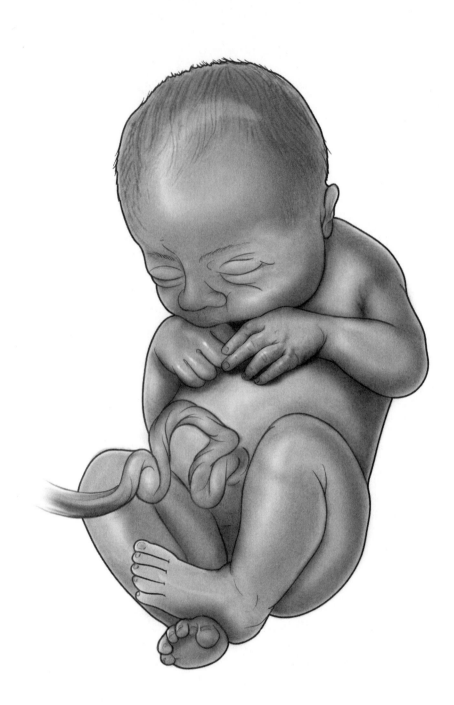

By the 22nd week of pregnancy (fetal age—20 weeks),
your baby's eyelids and eyebrows are well developed.
Fingernails now cover the fingertips.

> ## Eating Dark Chocolate
> · · · · · · · · · · ·
>
> Eating dark chocolate (at least 70% cocoa content) may help lower blood pressure and reduce the risk of anemia. Don't eat more than 3 ounces a day. Dark chocolate should replace other sweets you might want to eat.

woman after 22 weeks (before week 38), it means there is a higher risk for preterm delivery. If not found, risk of premature labor is low. fFN can rule out early delivery with 99% accuracy.

The test is similar to a Pap smear. A swab of vaginal secretions is taken from the top of the vagina, behind the cervix. It is sent to the lab, and results are available within 24 hours.

· ·

If your temperature rises above 100°F, contact your healthcare provider. A temperature above 102°F may indicate an infection is bacterial.

· ·

What Is Anemia?

Red blood cells carry oxygen throughout your body. *Anemia* is the condition in which the number of red blood cells is too low. If you suffer from anemia during pregnancy, you won't feel well, will tire easily and may experience dizziness. Treatment is important for you and your baby.

During pregnancy, the number of red blood cells increases. The amount of plasma (liquid part of the blood) also increases but at a higher rate. Your healthcare provider keeps track of these changes with a *hematocrit reading*, a measure of the percentage of the blood

that is red blood cells. This is usually done at the first prenatal visit.

Your hemoglobin level is also tested. Hemoglobin is the protein component of red blood cells. The test may be repeated once or twice during pregnancy and is done more often if you're anemic.

There is always some blood loss at delivery. If you're anemic when you go into labor, you may need a blood transfusion after your baby is born.

Follow your healthcare provider's advice about diet and supplementation if you have anemia. For a discussion of sickle-cell disease and thalassemia, two types of inherited anemia, see pages 228–230.

Iron-Deficiency Anemia. The most common type of anemia seen in pregnancy is *iron-deficiency anemia*. During pregnancy, your baby uses some of your iron stores. If you have iron-deficiency anemia, your body doesn't have enough iron to make red blood cells for you.

The goal in treating iron-deficiency anemia is to increase the amount of iron you take in. Most prenatal vitamins contain iron, but if you can't take a prenatal vitamin, you may be given 300 to 350mg of ferrous sulphate or ferrous gluconate 2 or 3 times a day. It can also be given as an injection, but it's painful and may stain the skin.

Some women develop iron-deficiency anemia during pregnancy even if they take prenatal vitamins or iron supplements. Several factors may make a woman more likely to have this condition in pregnancy, including bleeding during pregnancy, carrying multiple fetuses, previous surgery on the stomach or part of the small bowel, antacid overuse that causes a decrease in iron absorption and poor eating habits.

Side effects of iron supplementation include nausea and vomiting, with stomach upset. It may also cause constipation. If you have problems, you may need a lower dose.

To help increase your iron intake, eat more foods that are high in the mineral. Liver or spinach are good choices. Ask your healthcare provider for information on what types of foods you should include in your diet.

How Your Actions Affect Your Baby's Development

It's possible you could have diarrhea, the flu or a cold during pregnancy. These problems may raise concerns for you.

- What can I do when I feel ill?
- What medicine or treatment is OK?
- If I'm sick, should I take my prenatal vitamins?
- If I can't eat my usual diet, what should I do?

If you get sick during pregnancy, call your healthcare provider. He or she wants to know when you're feeling ill. Get his or her advice about a plan of action and recommendation as to what medicine to take to help you feel better. If any further measures are needed, your healthcare provider can recommend them.

Diarrhea during Pregnancy. If you have diarrhea, increase your fluid intake. Drink a lot of water, juice and other clear fluids, such as broth. To help you retain fluid, add 1 teaspoon of sugar to a cup of water or tea; glucose in table sugar helps the intestines absorb water instead of releasing it. A bland diet without solid food for a few days may help you feel better. If diarrhea lasts longer than 24 hours, let your healthcare provider know. Ask what medicine you can safely take for diarrhea during pregnancy.

It's OK to skip your prenatal vitamin for a few days. However, begin taking it again when your diarrhea stops. Don't take any medicine to control diarrhea without first consulting your healthcare provider. Usually a viral illness with diarrhea is a short-term problem and won't last more than a few days. You may have to stay home from work or rest in bed until you feel better.

Your Nutrition

You need to drink water during pregnancy—lots of it! Fluid helps you in many ways, and you may feel better during your pregnancy if you drink more water than you normally do.

When you don't drink water, you can become dehydrated and tire more easily. When you're dehydrated, it may reduce the amount of nutrients baby receives from you. Dehydration may also increase your risk of problems.

Grandma's Remedy

· · · · · · · · · ·

If you want to avoid using medication, try a folk remedy. If you have allergies, try some honey made by bees in your area. It contains very tiny amounts of the pollen that causes your sneezes and sniffles. Eating very small amounts of it can work like allergy shots and help you tolerate a pollen. Start with ¼ teaspoon a day, and slowly increase to 2 teaspoons a day.

Guidelines suggest you should drink 101 ounces (3 liters) of fluid—that's nearly 13 8-ounce glasses—a day during pregnancy. Water should account for at least 50 ounces of this intake. Water in food can make up another 20 ounces. The other 30+ ounces should come from milk, juice and other beverages. Sip water and other fluids throughout the day. If you decrease your consumption later in the day, you may save yourself some trips to the bathroom at night.

Don't drink a lot of caffeinated beverages. Tea, coffee and cola may contain sodium and caffeine, which act as diuretics. They essentially increase your water needs.

Some common problems women experience during pregnancy may be eased by drinking water. Headaches, uterine cramping and bladder infections may be less of a problem when you drink lots of water.

Check your urine to see if you're drinking enough. If it's light yellow to clear, you're getting enough fluid. Dark-yellow urine is a sign to increase your fluid intake. Don't wait until you get thirsty to drink something. By the time you get thirsty, you've already lost at least 1% of your body's fluids.

Fitness waters may benefit you if you're very active. Ask your healthcare provider for more information.

Your Drinking Water

The United States has one of the safest water supplies in the world, and most of the country has high-quality drinking water. Often tap water contains minerals that have been removed from bottled water. Some areas do have problems with drinking water. If water in your area doesn't rate well, use a filter to get rid of contaminants and pollutants. You may also want to use a filter if you live in an older home with lead pipes.

Chlorine is often added to drinking water to disinfect it, which may not be good for you. Check with your local water company if you're concerned.

Do not rely on bottled water as safer than tap water. One study showed nearly 35% of over 100 brands of bottled water were contaminated with chemicals or bacteria. Tap water must meet certain minimum standards if it is supplied by a municipal water company, so you know it's safe to drink. In addition, some bottled water contains sugar, caffeine and/or herbs.

You might want to check to see how much fluoride is in your drinking water.

Dad Tip
· · · · · · · · · · ·

When you ride together in the car with your partner, ask if you can help her in any way. You may offer to assist her getting in and out of the car. Ask if she needs help adjusting her seat belt or the car seat. Try to make riding and driving as easy and accessible as possible for her. You may propose trading vehicles (if you have more than one) if it's more comfortable for her to drive the other car.

Research shows we may be getting *too much* fluoride today, which can cause spotting or streaking in a child's teeth. Check with your local water company if you're concerned.

You Should Also Know

Appendicitis

Appendicitis can happen at any time, even during pregnancy. Acute appendicitis is the most common condition requiring surgery during pregnancy.

Pregnancy can make diagnosis difficult because some symptoms can be typical in a normal pregnancy, such as nausea and vomiting. Pain in the lower abdomen on the right side may be credited to round-ligament pain or a urinary-tract infection. Diagnosis may be difficult because as the uterus grows, the appendix moves upward and outward, so tenderness and pain are located in a different place than normal. See the illustration on opposite page.

Treatment of appendicitis is immediate surgery. This can be major abdominal surgery, with a 3- or 4-inch incision; it requires a few days in the hospital. Laparoscopy, with smaller incisions, is used in some situations, but laparoscopy may be harder to do during pregnancy because of the large uterus.

Rupture of a pregnant woman's appendix occurs up to 3 times more often because acute appendicitis is not diagnosed soon enough. Most physicians believe it's better to operate and remove a "normal" appendix than to risk infection of the abdominal cavity if an infected appendix bursts. Antibiotics are administered; many are safe to use during pregnancy.

Sickle-Cell Disease

Sickle-cell disease is the most common hemoglobin disorder in the United States. About 8% of Black/African Americans carry the sickle-hemoglobin gene. However, it is also found in people of Arabic, Greek, Maltese, Italian, Sardinian, Turkish, Indian, Caribbean, Latin American and Middle-Eastern descent. In the United States, most cases of sickle-cell disease occur among Black/African Americans and Latino/Hispanics. About one in every 500 Black/African Americans has sickle-cell disease.

Sickle-cell disease is inherited. Abnormal hemoglobin causes red blood cells to become stiff. Because they are stiffer, these red blood cells can get stuck in tiny blood vessels and cut off the blood supply to nearby tissues. This causes a great deal of pain and may damage organs. These abnormal red blood cells die and break down more quickly

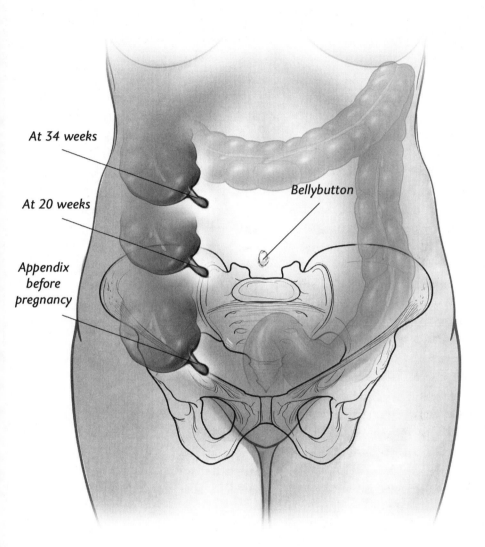

At 34 weeks

At 20 weeks

Appendix
before
pregnancy

Bellybutton

Location of the appendix at various times during pregnancy.

> ### Tip for Week 22
> • • • • • • • • • • •
>
> You need extra fluids (water is best) throughout pregnancy to help your body keep up with the increase in your blood volume. You'll know you're drinking enough fluid when your urine looks almost like clear water.

than normal red blood cells, which results in anemia.

A person who inherits the sickle-cell gene from one parent and the normal type of that gene from the other parent is said to have *sickle-cell trait*. When two people with sickle-cell trait have a child, there is a one-in-four chance the child will have the disorder. If only one parent has the trait, there is a 50–50 chance of each child having the trait, but none of the children will have sickle-cell disease.

Sickle-cell disease can also affect biracial children. To what degree depends on the ethnic group of each parent and his or her genetic makeup. A union of a Caucasian and a Black/African American will not result in a child with sickle-cell disease because Caucasians do not carry the sickle-cell gene. However, the union of a Black/African American and a person of Mediterranean or Latino/Hispanic descent could result in a child with sickle-cell disease if both parents carry the sickle-cell gene. If both parents are biracial, they could pass the disease to their children if each parent carries the gene.

Pregnancy and Sickle-Cell Disease. A woman with sickle-cell disease can have a safe pregnancy. During pregnancy, the disease may become more severe, and pain episodes may be more frequent. You will need early prenatal care and careful monitoring throughout pregnancy.

In the past, there was no effective treatment, other than blood transfusions, to prevent a pain crisis. The medication hydroxyurea was found to reduce the number of pain episodes by about 50% in some severely affected adults. We do not recommend hydroxyurea for pregnant women. However, researchers continue to study new drug treatments to help reduce complications of the disease.

A blood test can reveal whether you or your partner carry the sickle-cell trait. There also are prenatal tests to find out if baby will have the disease or carry the trait. Most children with sickle-cell disease are now identified through newborn screening tests.

Your healthcare provider will pay close attention to your sickle-cell disease during pregnancy. Work with your healthcare team to stay as healthy as possible.

Thalassemia

Thalassemia, also called *Cooley's anemia*, is not just one disease. It includes a number of different forms of anemia. The thalassemia trait is found all over the world but is most common in people from the Middle East, Greece, Italy, Georgia (the country, not the state), Armenia, Viet Nam, Laos, Thailand, Singapore, the Philippines, Cambodia, Malaysia, Burma, Indonesia, China, East

Take Precautions with All Foreign Viruses!

Recently, the Zika (or Zike) virus has received a lot of attention in the news. Zika is a rare tropical disease found in Latin America, the Caribbean, South America and some African countries. The viral infection is spread by mosquitoes/mosquito bites. Most people infected with Zika don't get sick. Those who do get the Zika virus and fall ill usually have mild symptoms—fever, rash, joint pain and red eyes lasting about a week. There is no specific vaccine or medicine to treat it. Insect repellent and clothing covering the body can help protect against mosquito bites.

The concern is that if a pregnant woman becomes infected with the virus, it can cause birth defects in some fetuses. A birth defect caused by the Zika virus is microcephaly, which causes a newborn's head to be smaller than normal because the brain does not develop properly. The exact mechanism between the Zika virus and microcephaly is being studied

It is important to be aware of various types of infections when you travel outside the United States. We suggest you always check with the Centers for Disease Control (CDC) and/or the U.S. Department of State before making travel plans. Ask if it's safe for you to travel to a specific area. Check to see if there are any illnesses in the area you will be visiting that you might be exposed to. Ask if there are any known negative effects on a fetus if you become infected.

When you return, take good care of yourself. If you experience any adverse symptoms, contact your doctor immediately.

India, Africa and Azerbaijan. It affects about 100,000 babies each year.

There are two main forms of the disease—alpha thalassemia and beta thalassemia. The type depends on which part of the hemoglobin lacks red blood cells. Most people have a mild form of the disease.

A carrier has one thalassemia gene. Most carriers lead completely normal, healthy lives. When two carriers have a child, there is a one-in-four chance their child will have the disease.

Various tests can determine whether a person has thalassemia or is a carrier. Chorionic villus sampling (CVS) and amniocentesis can detect thalassemia in a fetus. Early diagnosis is important so treatment can begin at birth to prevent complications.

Women with the thalassemia trait may be more likely to develop anemia during pregnancy. Healthcare providers may treat this with folic-acid supplementation.

Most children born with thalassemia appear healthy at birth, but during the first or second year of life they develop problems. They grow slowly and often develop jaundice.

Treatment of thalassemia includes frequent blood transfusions and antibiotics, which can prevent many complications. However, repeated blood transfusions may lead to a buildup of iron in the body. A drug called an *iron chelator* may be given to help rid the body of excess iron.

Exercise for Week 22

· · · · · · ·

Lie on your left side on the sofa, with your left knee bent. Bend your left arm, and place it under your head. Lower your right foot to the floor while keeping your leg straight. Hold for 10 seconds, then lift the straightened leg to a 45° angle; hold for 5 seconds. Do 5 complete repetitions with each leg. *Helps ease sciatica; strengthens hips and upper buttocks muscles.*

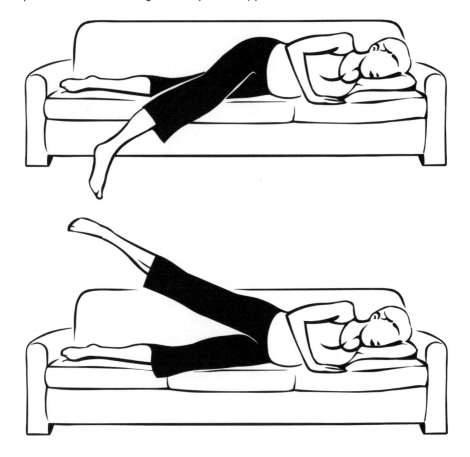

· · · · · · ·

Week 23

Age of Fetus—21 Weeks

How Big Is Your Baby?

By this week, baby weighs almost 1 pound (455g)! Its crown-to-rump length is 8 inches (20cm). Your baby is about the size of a small doll.

How Big Are You?

Your uterus extends about 1½ inches (3.75cm) above your bellybutton or about 9¼ inches (23cm) from the pubic symphysis. Your total weight gain should be between 12 and 15 pounds (5.5 and 6.8kg).

How Your Baby Is Growing and Developing

Baby's body is getting plumper but skin is still wrinkled; see the illustration on page 234. Lanugo hair on the body occasionally turns darker at this time. The baby's face and body begin to assume more of the appearance of an infant at birth.

Your baby's pancreas is important in insulin production, which is necessary for the body to break down and to use sugar. When the fetus is exposed to high blood-sugar levels from the mother-to-be, its pancreas responds by increasing the blood-insulin level. Insulin has been identified in a fetal pancreas as early as 9 weeks of pregnancy and in fetal blood as early as 12 weeks.

Blood-insulin levels are generally high in babies born to diabetic mothers. This is one reason your healthcare provider may monitor you for development of gestational diabetes.

Twin-to-Twin Transfusion Syndrome (TTTS)

Twin-to-twin transfusion syndrome (TTTS) occurs only in identical twins who share the same placenta. It does not occur in twins who each have a separate placenta. The syndrome is also called *chronic intertwin transfusion syndrome*. The condition can range from mild to severe and can occur at any point during pregnancy. It may also occur in other multiple pregnancies.

TTTS cannot be prevented; it's not a genetic disorder nor a hereditary condition. We believe it occurs in 5 to 10% of all identical-twin pregnancies.

In TTTS, twins also share some of the same blood circulation, allowing transfusion of blood from one twin to the other (thus the name). One twin

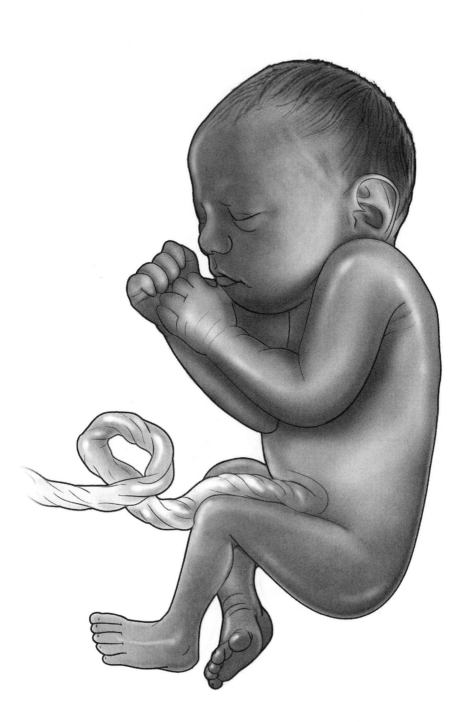

By the 23rd week of pregnancy
(fetal age—21 weeks), your baby's eyelids
and eyebrows are well developed.

> ## Dad Tip
> . . . .
> Are you also having pregnancy symptoms? Studies show as many as 50% of all fathers-to-be experience physical symptoms of pregnancy when their partner is pregnant. *Couvade*, a French term meaning "to hatch," is used to describe the condition in a man. Symptoms for an expectant father may include nausea, weight gain and cravings for certain foods.

becomes small and anemic, and its body partially shuts down blood supply to many of its organs, especially the kidneys. The other twin grows large, overloaded with blood, and produces excessive amounts of urine. This twin's blood becomes thick and difficult to pump through its body, which can lead to heart failure.

Babies are often very different in size and weight. TTTS is a progressive disorder, so early treatment may prevent complications.

Symptoms of TTTS. There are symptoms of the syndrome your healthcare provider looks for if you are expecting twins. If your abdomen enlarges quite rapidly over a 2- to 3-week period, it may be caused by the buildup of amniotic fluid in the recipient twin. The result can be premature labor and/or premature rupture of membranes. If one twin is small for its gestational age or one is big for its gestational age, it may indicate TTTS. In addition, your healthcare provider may suspect TTTS if any of the following is seen during an ultrasound:

- large difference in the size of fetuses
- difference in size between the two amniotic sacs or umbilical cords

- there is only one placenta
- evidence of fluid buildup in the skin of either fetus or fluid accumulation in some part of one fetus, such as in the scalp, abdomen, lungs or heart
- indications of congestive heart failure in the recipient twin

Diagnosing and Treating TTTS. If you know you're expecting twins, watch for rapid growth of your uterus, abdominal pain, tightness or contractions, a sudden increase in body weight or swelling in the hands and legs in early pregnancy. Alert your healthcare provider to any of these signs.

The syndrome may also be detected with ultrasound examination. It's important to find out whether twins share the same placenta, preferably in the first trimester, because in the second trimester it can be harder to learn this information.

If the syndrome is mild or undetected on ultrasound, the appearance of the twins at birth may identify it. A complete blood-cell count done after birth will show anemia in one twin and excess red blood cells in the other.

If diagnosed, the Twin to Twin Transfusion Syndrome Foundation recommends weekly ultrasounds after 16 weeks until the end of the pregnancy to monitor TTTS. They recommend this be done even if the warning signs of TTTS have decreased. The most conservative treatment is to watch and to wait. The pregnancy is followed closely with frequent ultrasound examinations, with the choice of delivering the twins by Cesarean delivery if medically necessary.

The most common treatment for TTTS is *amnioreduction*, in which large volumes of amniotic fluid are drained from the sac of the larger twin. A needle is placed through the mother's abdomen, and fluid is drained. The procedure is repeated if necessary.

In another procedure, a hole punched between the two amniotic sacs can help equalize the fluid between the sacs. However, neither of these procedures stops the twin-to-twin transfusion.

If these measures don't work, a small-scope laser procedure may be done to seal off some or all of the blood vessels the twins share. Usually only one procedure is necessary during the pregnancy. This treatment is most successful if done before 26 weeks of pregnancy.

Newborns with twin-to-twin transfusion syndrome may be critically ill at birth and require treatment in a neonatal intensive care unit. The smaller twin is treated for anemia, and the larger twin is treated for excess red blood cells and jaundice.

If you would like further information, resources are available. Contact the TTTS Foundation at www.tttsfoundation.org or call their headquarters at 800-815-9211.

Do you find your mood swings are worse? Are you still crying easily? Do you wonder if you'll ever be in control again? Don't worry. These emotions are typical at this point in pregnancy. Most experts believe hormonal changes are the culprit. If you think your partner or others are suffering from your emotional outbursts, talk about it with them. Explain these feelings are common in pregnant women. Ask them to be understanding. Then relax, and try not to get upset. Feeling emotional is a normal part of being pregnant.

Changes in You

Your healthcare provider will measure you at every visit after this point, using a measuring tape or his or her fingers. As baby grows larger, your uterus will be checked to see how much it has grown since your last visit. Within limits, changing measurements are a sign of baby's well-being and growth.

You will also be weighed and your blood pressure checked at each visit. Your healthcare provider is watching for changes in your weight gain and the size of your uterus. What's important is continual growth and change.

When shopping, pick up some healthy convenience foods, such as low-sodium canned vegetables, frozen fruits and veggies, all-natural applesauce, instant brown rice, quick-cooking oatmeal, whole-wheat tortillas and pitas, and low-fat cottage cheese and yogurt. They'll be at hand when you want them.

Loss of Fluid

Your uterus grows larger and gets heavier as pregnancy progresses. In early pregnancy, it lies directly behind the bladder. Later in pregnancy, the uterus sits on top of the bladder. As it grows, it can put a lot of pressure on your bladder. You may notice times when your underwear is damp.

You may be unsure whether you've lost urine or if you're leaking amniotic fluid. It may be difficult to tell the difference. When your membranes rupture, you usually experience a gush of fluid or a continual leaking from the vagina. If you experience this, call your healthcare provider immediately!

How Your Actions Affect Your Baby's Development

Diabetes and Pregnancy

Diabetes is one of the most common medical complications of pregnancy. It occurs in 7 to 8% of all pregnancies. It was once a very serious pregnancy problem, but today many diabetic women go through pregnancy safely. Symptoms of diabetes include more-frequent urination, blurred vision, weight loss, dizziness and increased hunger.

Diabetes is defined as a *lack of insulin in the bloodstream*. Insulin helps break down sugar and transport it to the cells. Pregnancy increases the body's resistance to insulin. If you don't have insulin, you will have high blood sugar and a high sugar content in your urine.

Type-1 diabetes causes the body to stop making insulin; *type-2* causes the body to use insulin ineffectively. The result of either type is too much sugar circulating in a woman's blood. It's important to get your diabetes under control *before* pregnancy. With the use of insulin and the development of various ways to monitor a fetus, it's uncommon to have a serious problem today.

* * *

Pregnancy is well known for its tendency to reveal women who are predisposed to diabetes. If you have trouble with high blood-sugar levels during pregnancy, you may be more likely to develop diabetes in later life.

* * *

Diabetes and Pregnancy. Diabetes can cause various problems during pregnancy. Birth defects may be more common and can occur as early as 5 to 8 weeks after the last menstrual period. Your risk for having a very large baby (macrosomia) increases and may require a Cesarean delivery.

If your diabetes is not controlled during pregnancy, baby is at greater risk. Women with poorly controlled diabetes are 3 to 4 times more likely to have a baby with heart problems or neural-tube defects.

During pregnancy, don't skip meals. Get enough exercise. Regular exercise can help keep blood-sugar levels in check and may reduce your need for medicine.

Insulin is the safest way to control diabetes during pregnancy. If you already take insulin, you may need to adjust your dosage or the timing of your dosage. You may also have to check your blood-sugar levels 4 to 8 times a day. You must balance your eating plan and your insulin at all times so your glucose levels don't climb too high. Avoid long-lasting insulin during pregnancy. It may also help if you take in more folic acid; discuss it with your healthcare provider and endocrinologist.

Some women take diabetes pills; some oral antidiabetes medications taken during pregnancy may cause problems for baby. There are safe oral medications for diabetes in pregnancy. You may have to adjust the amount of oral medication you take, or you may need to switch to insulin shots. Your healthcare provider can advise you.

Talk to your healthcare provider about getting an ultrasound of the baby's heart. A special ultrasound, called a *fetal echocardiogram*, can show if the baby has a problem. Some babies need surgery soon after they are born.

If you have type-1 diabetes, you may experience a delay in your milk coming in. You'll need to keep your breasts well stimulated to protect your milk supply.

Gestational Diabetes

Some women develop diabetes only during pregnancy, called *gestational diabetes*. It occurs when placental hormones block insulin, which normally breaks down sugar. If a pregnant woman doesn't have enough insulin, sugar builds up in the blood, which appears as diabetes. If you develop gestational diabetes, it indicates you carry a marker for diabetes. If you carry this marker, stress causes your body to metabolize sugar inefficiently.

Statistics show nearly 20% of all pregnant women are at risk of developing gestational diabetes. However, research shows only about 25% of all cases are

detected, which means nearly 75% of the cases of gestational diabetes go undiagnosed. Left untreated, gestational diabetes could lead to complications during pregnancy.

Some experts recommend screening pregnant women at risk for diabetes during the first trimester. Others recommend testing all pregnant women at 28 weeks. Tests used most often are the glucose-tolerance test (GTT) or a 1-hour glucose challenge test. New recommendations call for lower blood-sugar levels to diagnose gestational diabetes.

We believe gestational diabetes occurs for two reasons. One is the mother's body produces less insulin during pregnancy. The second is the mother's body can't use insulin effectively. Both situations result in higher blood-sugar levels.

Risk factors for developing gestational diabetes include being over 30 years old, obesity, a family history of diabetes, gestational diabetes in a previous pregnancy, previously giving birth to a baby who weighed over 9½ pounds, previously having a stillborn baby or being Black/African American, Latina/Hispanic, Asian, Native American or a Pacific Islander. In addition, if a woman was in the bottom 10th percentile of weight when she was born, she is 3 to 4 times more likely to develop gestational diabetes during pregnancy.

. . . .

Eating a diet low in fat and high in fiber may help reduce your risk of getting gestational diabetes. Increasing your intake of vitamin C may also help.

. . . .

Symptoms and Treatment for Gestational Diabetes. Good control of gestational diabetes is important. If left untreated, it can be serious for you and baby. You might experience *polyhydramnios* (excessive amounts of amniotic fluid), which can cause premature labor because the uterus becomes overdistended. Symptoms of gestational diabetes include:

- blurred vision
- tingling or numbness in hands and/or feet
- excessive thirst
- frequent urination
- sores that heal slowly
- fatigue

If your blood-sugar level is high, you may get more infections during pregnancy. You are also more likely to develop gum disease, which may raise your resistance to insulin. Treatment may help lower your risk of developing pregnancy complications.

Experts believe a woman with gestational diabetes may overfeed her fetus and cause baby to store more fat after birth. You may also have a long labor because baby is big. Sometimes a baby can't fit through the birth canal, and a Cesarean delivery is required.

Treatment for gestational diabetes includes a good nutrition plan, increased fluid intake and 30 minutes of moderate exercise every day. Your healthcare provider will probably recommend a six-meal, 2000- to 2500-calorie-per-day eating plan. If these measures don't work, medication to lower blood-sugar levels may be prescribed.

Insulin therapy is the first choice when medication is necessary. In some cases, oral medications, such as glyburide or Metformin, are used.

If gestational diabetes occurs with one pregnancy, there's about a 90% chance it will happen in future pregnancies. Your best protection is to stay within the recommended weight-gain limits your healthcare provider gives you.

After birth, nearly all women who have gestational diabetes return to normal. However, if you eat unhealthfully after pregnancy or gain weight, you could reactivate the diabetes. You also have up to a 60% chance of developing type-2 diabetes within 10 years after baby's birth and are at risk of developing *metabolic syndrome*, a collection of problems linked to heart disease. It's important to have your blood-sugar levels checked within 12 weeks after delivery and every 3 years after that.

Your Nutrition

You may need to be careful with your sodium intake during pregnancy. Taking in too much sodium may cause you to retain water, which can contribute to swelling and bloating. However, you do need some sodium every day to help deal with your increased blood volume. Aim for between 1500 and 2300mg of sodium a day.

Eat potassium-rich foods, such as raisins and bananas; potassium helps the body get rid of sodium faster. Avoid foods that contain lots of sodium or salt, such as salted nuts, potato chips, pickles, canned foods and processed foods.

Tip for Week 23

· · · · · · · · · · ·

Keeping your consumption of sodium to 2 grams (2000mg) or less a day may help you reduce fluid retention.

Read food labels. They list the amount of sodium in a serving. Some books list the sodium content of foods without labels, such as fast foods. Check them out. You'll be surprised how many milligrams of sodium a fast-food hamburger contains!

Look at the chart on page 241; it lists some common foods and their sodium content. You can see foods that contain sodium don't always taste salty. Check available information before you eat!

You Should Also Know

Sugar in Your Urine

Sugar in the urine is called *glucosuria*. It's common during pregnancy, especially in the second and third trimesters. It occurs because of changes in sugar levels and how sugar is handled in the kidneys. If extra sugar is present, you will lose it in your urine.

Many healthcare providers test every pregnant woman for diabetes, usually around the end of the second trimester. Testing is important if you have a family history of diabetes. Blood tests used to diagnose diabetes are a fasting blood-sugar test and a glucose-tolerance test (GTT).

With a fasting blood-sugar test, a normal result indicates diabetes is unlikely. An abnormal result (a high level of sugar in the blood) needs further study. Further study involves the glucose-tolerance test (GTT). At the lab, you are given a solution to drink that has a measured amount of sugar in it. It is similar to a bottle of soda pop but doesn't taste as good. After you drink the solution, blood is drawn at certain intervals, usually 30 minutes, 1 hour and 2 hours, and sometimes even 3 hours. Drawing blood at intervals reveals how your body handles sugar. If you need treatment, your healthcare provider can devise a plan for you.

Teen Pregnancy

Teen pregnancy impacts society in many ways and is defined as pregnancy in young women between the ages of 13 and 19 years of age. Young women in the 18- to 19-year-old range have the highest pregnancy rate among teens—nearly 75%. The United States continues to have the highest rates of teenage pregnancy/births in the Western world, and some ethnic groups in our country are at higher risk.

Teenage births have dropped significantly since the early 1990s. Today, about 8% of all U.S. births are to teens; 89% of teen mothers are unmarried. About 75% of all teen pregnancies are unplanned.

Pregnancy in a teenager can be difficult for many reasons. Many teens do not seek prenatal care until the second trimester. Many teenage mothers-to-be have poor eating habits, and often they don't take their prenatal vitamins. A

Sodium Content of Various Foods

· · · · · · · · · · ·

Food	Serving Size	Sodium Content (mg)
American cheese	1 slice	322
Asparagus	14½-oz. can	970
Big Mac hamburger	1 regular	963
Chicken á la king	1 cup	760
Cola	8 oz.	16
Cottage cheese	1 cup	580
Dill pickle	1 medium	928
Flounder	3 oz.	201
Gelatin, sweet	3 oz.	270
Ham, baked	3 oz.	770
Honeydew melon	½	90
Lima beans	8½ oz.	1070
Lobster	1 cup	305
Oatmeal	1 cup	523
Potato chips	20 regular	400
Salt	1 teaspoon	1938

large number of teens continue to drink alcohol, use drugs and/or smoke during pregnancy. In fact, pregnant teens have the highest smoking rate of all pregnant women.

· ·

The birth rate for women in their 30s and 40s is on the rise, while the birth rate for teens is falling.

· ·

Studies show pregnant teens are often underweight when they enter pregnancy and may not gain enough weight during pregnancy. This can lead to low-birthweight babies. Teen mothers are also more likely to give birth to premature babies. Other problems include anemia and high blood pressure. Depression during pregnancy is also higher among teens. Babies born to teen moms also have more birth defects.

Sexually transmitted diseases may be a problem for pregnant adolescents. Over 25% of all cases of STDs reported every year occur in teenagers.

A teenager who is pregnant will do herself and her baby a favor by eating a healthy diet and gaining the correct amount of weight, as determined by her healthcare provider. She should stop smoking, avoid alcohol and stay away from drugs. Getting early prenatal care and keeping all prenatal appointments is important for a successful pregnancy. A teen should address any health care problems immediately, follow her healthcare provider's advice when dealing with problems and avoid all prescription and over-the-counter medicines unless her healthcare provider tells her to take them.

Exercise for Week 23

• • • • • • •

Sit on the edge of a chair, and place both feet flat on the floor. Relax your shoulders, and curve your arms over your head. Keeping your back straight, hold in your tummy muscles while you extend one leg out in front. Using your thigh muscles only, lift your leg about 10 inches off the floor. Hold for a count of 5, then slowly lower your foot. Repeat 10 times with each leg. *Tones thigh, hips and buttocks muscles.*

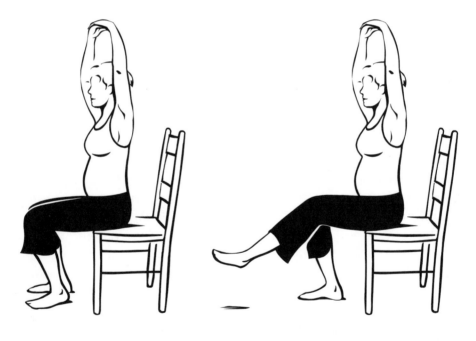

• • • • • • •

Week 24

Age of Fetus—22 Weeks

How Big Is Your Baby?

By this week, baby weighs about 1¼ pounds (540g). Its crown-to-rump length is about 8½ inches (21cm).

How Big Are You?

Your uterus is now about 1½ to 2 inches (3.8 to 5.1cm) above the bellybutton. It measures almost 10 inches (24cm) above the pubic symphysis.

How Your Baby Is Growing and Developing

Baby is filling out. Its face and body look more like that of an infant at the time of birth. Although it weighs a little over 1 pound at this point, it is still very tiny.

The baby grows in amniotic fluid inside the amniotic sac. See the illustration on page 244. Amniotic fluid has several important functions. It provides an environment in which the baby can move easily and cushions the fetus against injury. It regulates temperature. It also provides a way of assessing baby's health and maturity.

Amniotic fluid increases rapidly from an average volume of 1½ ounces (50ml) by 12 weeks of pregnancy to 12 ounces (400ml) at midpregnancy. The volume of amniotic fluid continues to increase as your due date approaches, until a maximum of about 2 pints (1 liter) of fluid is reached at 36 to 38 weeks gestation.

Makeup of amniotic fluid changes during pregnancy. During the first 20 weeks, it's similar to the fluid in your blood without blood cells, except it has a much lower protein content. As baby grows, fetal urine adds to the amount of amniotic fluid present. Amniotic fluid also contains old fetal blood cells, lanugo hair and vernix.

The fetus swallows amniotic fluid during much of pregnancy. If it can't swallow the fluid, you may develop a condition of excess amniotic fluid, called *hydramnios* or *polyhydramnios*. If the fetus swallows but doesn't urinate (for example, if the baby lacks kidneys), the volume of amniotic fluid surrounding the fetus may be very small. This is called *oligohydramnios*.

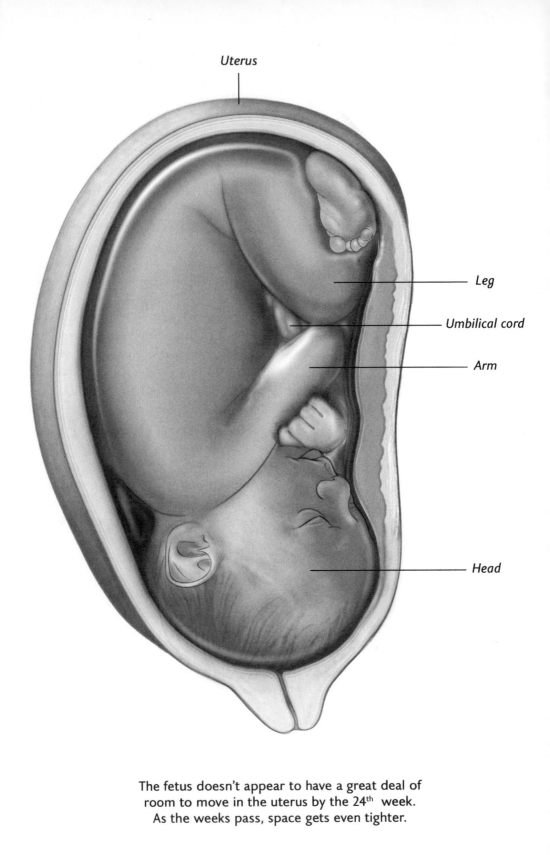

Uterus

Leg

Umbilical cord

Arm

Head

The fetus doesn't appear to have a great deal of
room to move in the uterus by the 24th week.
As the weeks pass, space gets even tighter.

Changes in You

Nasal Problems

Some women complain of stuffiness in their nose or frequent nosebleeds during pregnancy. Some experts believe these symptoms occur because of circulation changes caused by hormones during pregnancy. Mucous membranes of your nose and nasal passageways swell and bleed more easily.

A few decongestants and nasal sprays can be used during pregnancy. Some brands to consider include chlorpheniramine (Chlor-Trimeton) decongestants and oxymetazoline (Afrin, Dristan Long-Lasting) nasal sprays. Before you begin using any product, discuss it with your healthcare provider.

It may also help to use a humidifier, particularly during winter months when heating may dry out the air. Some women get relief from increasing their fluid intake and/or using a gentle lubricant in their nose, such as petroleum jelly.

. . . .

We know sounds penetrate amniotic fluid and reach your baby's developing ears inside the uterus. Ultrasounds done around this time have shown babies reacting to loud noises. If you work in a noisy place, you may want to request a quieter area. Chronic loud noise and short, intense bursts of sound may damage baby's hearing before birth. It's OK to expose your growing baby to loud noises, such as a concert, every once in a while. But if you're repeatedly exposed to noise that is so loud it forces you to shout, it may be dangerous for your growing baby.

. . . .

Depression

Depression can occur at any time during a person's life. Many things can contribute to depression, including chemical imbalances in the body, stressful life events and situations that cause anxiety and tension. If you have a history of major depression, you're at increased risk of depression occurring during pregnancy.

If you're being treated for depression when you get pregnant, it's important to continue treatment. Treating depression is as important as treating any other condition.

If you take antidepressants, don't stop unless advised by your healthcare provider to do so. Studies show up to 70% of women who stop taking antidepressants during pregnancy relapse into depression. Stopping your medication can raise stress hormones; the risks to you and your baby from depression may be greater than your risk of taking antidepressants. We know depression can be difficult to manage without drug therapy.

There may be a very small increased risk of birth defects with some medicines used to treat depression when taken during the first trimester. It may help to switch to an antidepressant that is safer during pregnancy, including fluoxetine (Prozac), citalopram and escitalopram (Lexapro). Pregnancy may affect your body's ability to use lithium. With some medications, the dose may need to be increased during the third trimester to maintain your normal mood. Talk to your healthcare provider as soon as you confirm your pregnancy.

There is some concern about the safety of Paxil during pregnancy. Research suggests using the drug in the first trimester of pregnancy may be tied to an increased risk of heart problems in baby. However, don't stop taking your antidepressant medicine without first consulting with your healthcare provider.

If you're feeling depressed, your level of vitamin D may be low. Talk about it with your healthcare provider. Other suggestions for dealing with depression include getting regular exercise and being sure you get enough B vitamins, folic acid and omega-3 fatty acids; 3.5g of omega-3 fatty acids every day has been shown to help fight depression.

Additional therapies include massage and reflexology. Another option is light therapy, similar to the type of treatment given to those who suffer from "seasonal affective disorder."

Depression during Pregnancy. Between 3 and 5% of all women experience a major depression during pregnancy. It's estimated another 15% have some degree of depression. Experts believe it's one of the most common medical problems seen in pregnant women. Depression is more common during pregnancy than after giving birth.

If left untreated, 50% of women who are depressed during pregnancy will experience postpartum depression. (For a discussion of depression after pregnancy, see Appendix B.) If you have a family history of depression, you may

be at higher risk during pregnancy. If you've been struggling with infertility or miscarriage, you may also be more prone to depression.

If you're depressed, you may not take good care of yourself. Babies born to depressed women may be smaller or born prematurely. Some women use alcohol, drugs and cigarettes in an attempt to ease their depression. You may also have trouble bonding with your baby after birth.

You may be at higher risk if you experienced mood changes when you took oral contraceptives, your mother was depressed during pregnancy, you have a history of depression, you feel sad or depressed longer than 1 week or you're not getting enough sleep and rest. If you have bipolar disorder, pregnancy can trigger a relapse, especially if you stop taking your mood-stabilizing medications.

Research shows it's better for baby if only one medicine is used during pregnancy to treat a woman's depression.

Symptoms and Treatment. It may be hard to differentiate between some normal pregnancy changes and signs of depression. Many symptoms of depression are similar to those of pregnancy, including fatigue and sleeplessness. The difference is how intense the symptoms are and how long they last. Some common symptoms of depression include:

- overpowering sadness that lasts for days, without an obvious cause

> ## *Dad Tip*
> • • • • • • • • • • •
>
> Now is a good time to explore prenatal classes in your area. Encourage your partner to find out how many classes there are, when and where to register, and the registration cost. You may be able to take classes at the hospital or birthing center where your partner plans to deliver. Try to complete the classes at least 1 month before baby is due.

- difficulty sleeping, or waking up very early
- wanting to sleep all the time or great fatigue (this can be normal early in pregnancy but usually gets better after a few weeks)
- no appetite (as distinguished from nausea and vomiting)
- lack of concentration
- thoughts of harming yourself

It can be serious if you don't get help. You may have a difficult time caring for yourself, and your risk of addictive-substance abuse, such as alcohol use and cigarette smoking, may increase. You may not be able to meet the nutritional demands of your pregnancy.

Babies born to mothers with untreated depression can have many problems. They often cry a lot, have difficulty sleeping, are fussier and are difficult to soothe.

If you have symptoms and they don't get better in a few weeks or if every day seems to be bad, seek help as soon as you recognize you might be depressed. Call your healthcare provider, or bring it up at your next prenatal visit. There are steps to take to help you feel better again. It's important to do it for yourself and your baby!

Be good to yourself during your pregnancy. Light some candles and soak in the tub. Go to your hairdresser for some pampering. Download some of your favorite music to your iPod or MP3 player. Rent a tear-jerker movie, and cry your eyes out. Buy yourself flowers. Get a pedicure, even if you can't see your feet anymore.

How Your Actions Affect Your Baby's Development

Moving during Pregnancy

Moving to a new city at any time can be stressful; when you're pregnant, it can also be challenging. How can you find a new healthcare provider? What hospital will you use?

Before you leave your old home, find a hospital in the area you're moving to that you want to use, then find a healthcare provider (who is accepting new patients) who delivers at that hospital. Do this as soon as you learn you're moving because it may take some time to get in to see the new healthcare provider for your first appointment.

A real-estate agent should be able to help in this situation. Ask about a hospital with a level-2 or level-3 nursery.

These hospitals are better able to deal with pregnancy and birth complications. Even if you don't have any problems, you'll rest easier knowing the hospital can handle an emergency.

When you've chosen the hospital, call the labor-and-delivery department and ask to speak with a supervisor. Explain your situation, and ask for recommendations for three or four obstetricians who deliver at the hospital who are accepting new patients.

When you have the names, call each office and explain your situation. Request information about fees and insurance coverage. Ask if you can get an appointment for the first week you're in town. Then make your decision about which healthcare provider you want to use and call back to confirm your appointment.

After you decide on someone, go to the healthcare provider you now see and ask for copies of your medical records. Be sure they include results of any tests you've had. Take everything with you. If the office says they'll send them to the new healthcare provider, tell them that's fine, but you must also have copies to take with you. Sending records can take a long time.

If you haven't had your alpha-fetoprotein test or a triple-screen test done and are between 15 and 19 weeks of pregnancy, ask your current healthcare provider to order them and have the results sent to you at your new address. It can take several weeks to get the results of these two tests, and it will be helpful for your new healthcare provider to

have the results when you go to see him or her. Ask your healthcare provider to write a short letter of introduction that you can give to your new healthcare provider. This is a brief summary of your pregnancy, current health and health concerns.

Your Nutrition

Many pregnant women are concerned about eating out. Some want to know if they can eat certain types of food, such as Mexican, Vietnamese, Thai or Greek food. They're concerned spicy or rich foods could be harmful to the baby. It's OK to eat out, but you might find certain foods don't agree with you.

The best types of food to eat at restaurants are those you tolerate well at home. Chicken, fish, fresh vegetables and salads are good choices. Eating foods at restaurants that feature spicy foods or unusual cuisine may cause stomach or intestinal distress. You may even notice an increase in weight from water retention after eating at a restaurant.

Avoid restaurants that serve highly salted food, food high in sodium or food loaded with calories and fat, such as gravies, fried food, junk food and rich desserts. It may be difficult to control your calorie intake at specialty restaurants.

It may be necessary to go to business lunches or to travel for your company. If so, be selective. If you can choose off the menu, look for healthy or low-fat choices. Ask about preparation—maybe a dish can be steamed instead of fried. On a business trip, take along some of

> ## Tip for Week 24
> · · · · · · · · · · ·
> Overeating and eating before going to bed at night are two major causes of heartburn. Eating five or six small, nutritious meals a day and skipping snacks before bedtime may help you feel better.

your own food. Choose healthy, nonperishable foods, such as fruits and vegetables, that don't need refrigeration.

· ·

Don't rely on a taste test to determine if food is hot enough to be safe to eat. When reheating leftovers, use a quick-reading thermometer to make sure food has reached an interior temperature of 165F. This is the temperature at which harmful bacteria are killed.

· ·

You Should Also Know

How Pregnancy Affects Your Sexual Desire

Has your sexual desire increased? Is sex the last thing on your mind? Generally, women experience one of two sex-drive patterns during pregnancy. One is a lessening of desire in the first and third trimesters, with an increase in the second trimester. The second is a gradual decrease in desire for sex as pregnancy progresses.

During the first trimester, you may experience fatigue and nausea. In the third trimester, your weight gain, enlarging abdomen, tender breasts and other issues may make you desire sex less. This is normal. Tell your partner how you feel, and try to work out a solution that pleases you both. Tenderness and understanding can help.

Pregnancy enhances the sex drive for some women. A woman may experience orgasms or multiple orgasms for the first time during pregnancy. This is due to heightened hormonal activity and increased blood flow to the pelvic area.

When to Avoid Sexual Activity

Some situations should alert you to refrain from sexual activity. If you have a history of early labor, your healthcare provider may warn against intercourse and orgasm; orgasm causes mild uterine contractions. Chemicals in semen may also stimulate contractions, so it may not be advisable for a woman's partner to ejaculate inside her.

Your healthcare provider may advise no sex if you have certain pregnancy problems. If you have a history of miscarriage, your healthcare provider may caution you against sex and orgasm. However, no data actually links the two.

Avoid some sexual practices when you're pregnant. Don't insert any object into the vagina that could cause injury or infection. Blowing air into the vagina is dangerous because it can force a potentially fatal air bubble into a woman's bloodstream. (This can occur whether or not you are pregnant.) Nipple stimulation releases oxytocin, which causes uterine contractions; discuss this practice with your healthcare provider.

An Incompetent Cervix

An *incompetent cervix* refers to painless premature dilatation (stretching) of the cervix, which usually results in delivery of a premature baby. The problem doesn't often occur before the 16th week of pregnancy. The woman doesn't realize her cervix has dilated until the baby is delivering. Diagnosis is usually made after one or more deliveries of a premature infant without any pain before delivery. Fortunately, an incompetent cervix is relatively rare.

If this is your first pregnancy, there's no way to know whether you have the problem. The cause of cervical incompetence is usually unknown. Some experts believe it occurs because of previous injury or surgery to the cervix, such as dilatation and curettage (D&C) for an abortion or miscarriage. If you've had problems in the past or have had premature deliveries and have been told you might have an incompetent cervix, share this important information with your healthcare provider.

Treatment for an incompetent cervix is usually surgical. The weak cervix is closed with a McDonald cerclage. A suture, similar to a "purse-string," is stitched around the cervix to keep it closed. The procedure is usually performed in a hospital operating room or in labor and delivery. General anesthesia or I.V. sedation is given. The procedure takes about 30 minutes; after it's over, you'll probably be monitored for a few hours before you can go home. It's normal to have a little bit of spotting or bleeding afterward.

At about 36 weeks or when you go into labor, the stitch is removed, and baby can be born normally. The suture is removed in labor and delivery without anesthesia; it takes about 5 minutes. Labor does not necessarily happen immediately after it's removed; it can occur in a few days to a few weeks.

Exercise for Week 24

• • • • • • •

Stand with your right side against the back of the sofa or a sturdy chair. Hold onto the back with your right hand. Bend your knee, and bring your left foot up behind your bottom. Grasp your foot with your left hand. Keeping your right knee slightly bent, hold for 10 seconds. Repeat for your right leg. *Strengthens quadriceps.*

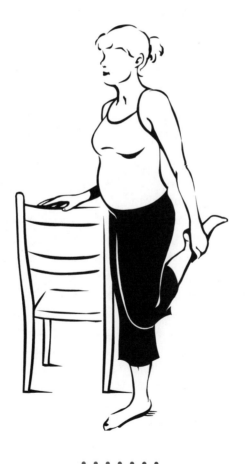

• • • • • • •

Week 25

Age of Fetus—23 Weeks

How Big Is Your Baby?

Your baby now weighs about 1½ pounds (700g), and crown-to-rump length is about 8¾ inches (22cm). These are average lengths and weights, and can vary from one baby to another and from one pregnancy to another.

How Big Are You?

Look at the illustration on page 254. Your uterus has grown to about the size of a soccer ball. When you look at a side view, you're much bigger. Your baby will have growth spurts, which may slightly affect your weight gain at certain times.

Measurement from the pubic symphysis to the top of the uterus is about 10 inches (25cm). The uterus is about halfway between your bellybutton and the lower part of your sternum (the bone between your breasts where the ribs come together). If you were seen around 20 weeks of pregnancy, you've probably grown about 1½ inches (4cm).

How Your Baby Is Growing and Developing

Survival of a Premature Baby

It may be hard to believe, but if your baby were delivered now, it would have a chance of surviving. A baby born at this time probably weighs less than 2 pounds and is extremely small. Survival can be difficult, and the baby would probably spend several months in the hospital. See the discussion of Premature Labor in Week 29.

Is Baby a Boy? A Girl?

One of the most common questions we hear is, "What is the sex of our baby?" Amniocentesis can definitely determine baby's sex. Ultrasound may predict baby's sex but is not foolproof. Some at-home tests claim to be able to determine baby's gender, but don't count on it. Some people believe a baby's heartbeat rate can indicate its sex, but there's no scientific proof of this.

A more reliable source might be a mother, mother-in-law or someone who

Tip for Week 25

· · · · · · · · · · ·

Pregnancy can be a time of communication and personal growth with your partner. Listen when he talks. Let him know he is an important source of emotional support for you.

can look at you and tell by how you're carrying the baby if it is a boy or girl. Although we make this statement with our tongues placed firmly in our cheeks, many people believe it's true. Some people claim they're never wrong about guessing or predicting the sex of a baby before birth. Again, there is no scientific basis for this method.

Your healthcare provider is more concerned about the health and well-being of you and baby. He or she will concentrate on making sure you both get through pregnancy, labor and delivery in good health.

Changes in You

Itching

Itching (pruritus gravidarum) is a common symptom during pregnancy. There are no bumps or lesions on the skin; it just itches. Nearly 20% of all pregnant women suffer from itching, often in the last weeks of pregnancy, but it can occur at any time. It may occur with each pregnancy and may also appear when you use oral contraceptives. The condition isn't harmful to you or baby.

As your uterus has grown and filled your pelvis, your skin and muscles have stretched. Itchiness may be a consequence. Lotions are OK to use to help reduce itching. Try not to scratch and

irritate your skin—that can make it worse! Ask your healthcare provider about taking antihistamines or using cooling lotions containing menthol or camphor. Often no treatment is needed.

· ·

Flavors from foods eaten by a mom-to-be pass into amniotic fluid, which may promote flavor preferences in baby before birth. By this time, baby can distinguish between sour, bitter and sweet. We know even unborn babies have a natural preference for sweet.

· ·

Stress during Pregnancy

Feeling stress is common during any woman's life. *Stress* is what you feel in situations that are difficult, dangerous or menacing. Chronic stress is stress caused by ongoing situations or problems, such as unemployment, deployment of your partner or financial problems. *Anxiety* is magnified worry and greater than justified.

· ·

Many experts believe stress in you can affect the health of your baby, so make every attempt to reduce stress in your life.

· ·

Pregnancy is stressful! Studies show pregnancy ranks #12 on a list of life's most stressful events. Normal stress probably won't hurt you or baby, but major stress may increase your risk of premature birth. Learning to manage

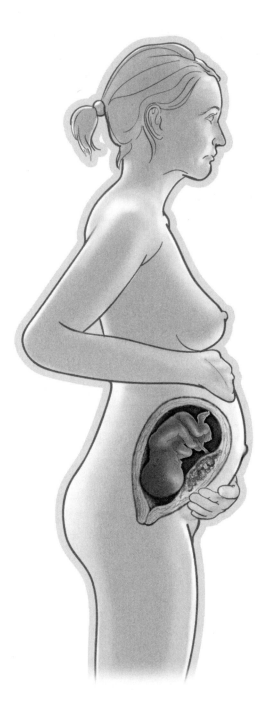

Comparative size of the uterus at 25 weeks of pregnancy
(fetal age—23 weeks). The uterus can be felt about 2 inches
(5cm) above your umbilicus (bellybutton).

Dad Tip

• • • • • • • • • •

Who knew forgetfulness could be tied to pregnancy? If you find your partner just can't remember things you ask her to do or to remember something important to you, make lists for her. Approach it with humor—you may find you get a better response.

stress can go a long way in making your life more manageable—when you're pregnant and when you're not!

During pregnancy, stress can be caused by many things. Hormone changes can cause you to react in ways that aren't normal for you, which can be stressful. Your body is changing, which stresses many women. You may have worked very hard to get and/or to maintain your figure—now that you're pregnant, there's not much you can do about it.

You may be thinking about being a good parent—the prospect can be stressful for anyone. You may not be feeling very well, which adds to the problem. You may feel stress from working or other obligations.

Relax, and take it easy! Share your concerns with your partner, or find a group of pregnant women you can talk with. Get enough sleep each night; lack of sleep can make you feel stressed. Rest during the day. Read or listen to music during a quiet period. When you feel stressed, stop and take a few slow, deep breaths to help turn off the stressed part of your nervous system.

Do something active and physical (but not too physical)—exercise can help you work off stress. Take a walk or visit the gym. Put on an exercise video

for pregnant women. Ask your partner to join you. Eat nutritiously. Having enough calories available all through the day helps you avoid "lows."

Be positive. Smiling instead of frowning can help ease stress. Think "happy thoughts." When you turn your thoughts to good things, it actually sends a chemical message to your brain that flows through your entire body and helps you relax. Do something you enjoy, and do it for you.

• •

You can go to parties while you're pregnant and still have a good time. A couple of things to remember—eat something before you go and practice portion control.

• •

How Your Actions Affect Your Baby's Development

Falling and Injuries from Falls

A fall is the most frequent cause of minor injury during pregnancy. Fortunately, a fall is usually without serious injury to the baby or mother-to-be. The uterus is well protected in the abdomen inside the pelvis. The cushion of amniotic fluid surrounding baby protects it. Your uterus and abdominal wall also offer some protection.

If you fall, contact your healthcare provider; he or she may want to examine you. You may feel reassured if you're monitored and baby's heartbeat is checked. Baby's movement after a fall can be reassuring.

Minor injuries to the abdomen are treated as though you were not pregnant, but avoid X-rays if possible. An ultrasound test may be the best choice after a fall. This is judged on an individual basis, depending on the severity of your symptoms and your injury.

Your balance and mobility change as you grow during pregnancy. Be careful during the winter when areas may be wet or icy. Many pregnant women fall on stairs; always use the handrail. Walk in well-lit areas, and try to stay on sidewalks.

. . . .

Take care when you do yard work, especially if you like to work in the garden. Sit on something that provides support. Always wear gardening gloves; rubber gloves under your gardening gloves is a great idea. And if you get a cut or puncture, contact your healthcare provider about a tetanus shot; it's safe during pregnancy.

. . . .

Slow down as you get larger; you won't be able to get around as quickly as you normally do. With the change in your balance, plus any dizziness you experience, it's important to be watchful to avoid falling.

Some signs can alert you to a problem after a fall, including bleeding, a gush of fluid from the vagina and/or severe abdominal pain. Placental abruption, when the placenta separates from the uterus, is one of the most serious problems caused by a fall.

Sometimes a bone breaks, which may require X-rays and surgery. Treatment cannot be delayed until after pregnancy; the problem must be dealt with now. If you find yourself in this situation, insist your pregnancy healthcare provider be contacted before any test is done or treatment is started.

If X-rays are required, your pelvis and abdomen must be shielded. If they can't be shielded, the need for the X-ray must be weighed against the risk it poses to baby.

Anesthesia or pain medication may be necessary with a simple break that requires setting or pinning. It is best for you and baby to avoid general anesthesia if possible. You may need pain medicine, but keep its use to a minimum.

If general anesthesia is required to repair a break, the baby should be monitored closely. Your surgeon and pregnancy healthcare provider will work together to provide the best care for you and your baby.

. . . .

When you're doing housekeeping chores, avoid oven cleaners and aerosol sprays. Be careful with chlorine bleach and ammonia; use safer products, such as vinegar and dishwashing soap. Wear rubber gloves to protect your skin.

. . . .

Your Nutrition

Pregnancy increases your need for vitamins and minerals. It's best if you can meet most of these needs through the foods you eat. However, being realistic, we know that can be hard to do. That's one reason your healthcare provider

A Balanced Meal Plan
· · · · · · · · · · ·

Below is a list of some foods to choose from each group and an appropriate serving size for each. There are many different foods to choose from.

- Breads, cereals, rice, pasta and grains, 6 to 11 servings—1 slice of bread, ½ bun, ½ English muffin, ½ small bagel, ½ cup cooked pasta, rice or hot cereal, 4 crackers, ¾ cup cold cereal
- Fruit, 2 to 4 servings—¼ cup dried fruit, ½ cup fresh, canned or cooked fruit, ¾ cup juice
- Vegetables, 3 to 5 servings—½ cup cooked vegetables, 1 cup leafy salad vegetables, ¾ cup juice
- Protein sources, 2 to 3 servings—2 to 3 ounces of cooked poultry, meat or fish, 1 cup cooked beans, ¼ cup seeds or nuts, ½ cup tofu, 2 eggs
- Dairy products, 4 servings—1 cup milk (any type), 1 cup yogurt, 1½ ounces cheese, 1½ cups of cottage cheese, 1½ cups frozen yogurt, ice milk or ice cream
- Fats, oils and sweets—limit intake of these food products; concentrate on nutritious, healthy foods

prescribes a prenatal vitamin for you—to help you meet nutritional needs.

Some women do need extra help during pregnancy; supplements are often prescribed for them. These pregnant women include teenagers (whose bodies are still growing), severely underweight women, women who ate a poor diet before conception and women who are carrying multiples. Women who smoke or drink may need supplements, as do some who have a chronic medical condition, those who take certain medications and those who have problems digesting cow's milk, wheat and other essential foods. In some cases, vegetarians may need supplements.

Your healthcare provider can discuss the situation with you. If you need more than a prenatal vitamin, he or she will advise you. Caution: never take any supplements without your healthcare provider's OK!

You Should Also Know

Thyroid Disease

The thyroid gland produces hormones to regulate metabolism and control functions in many of your body's organs. If you have a history of thyroid problems or if you take thyroid medication, discuss treatment during pregnancy with your healthcare provider.

About 2% of all pregnant women have a thyroid disorder. In fact, even if you don't have a thyroid problem before pregnancy, if there is a chance you could have a problem, it often appears during pregnancy.

Left untreated, thyroid disorders can be harmful to you and baby. Research shows women with a history of miscarriage or premature delivery, or those who have problems near delivery, may have problems with their thyroid-hormone levels. Thyroid-hormone levels may be high or low. Low levels of thyroid cause *hypothyroidism*; high levels cause *hyperthyroidism*.

Hypothyroidism is common during pregnancy. Symptoms include unusual weight gain and fatigue (both can be hard to determine during pregnancy), a hoarse voice, dry skin, dry hair and a slow pulse. If you have these symptoms, tell your healthcare provider. Left untreated, hypothyroidism can affect your baby's health. Baby may not receive adequate nutrition from you. Even with treatment, baby is at risk of being born with abnormal thyroid levels. Many babies are low birthweight.

Symptoms and Treatment. Symptoms of thyroid disease may be masked by pregnancy. Or you may notice changes during pregnancy that cause your healthcare provider to suspect the thyroid is not functioning properly. Changes can include an enlarged thyroid, changes in your pulse, redness of the palms and warm, moist palms. Because thyroid-hormone levels can change during pregnancy, your healthcare provider must be careful interpreting lab results about this hormone while you're pregnant.

The thyroid is tested primarily by blood tests (a thyroid panel), which measure the amount of thyroid hormone produced. The tests also measure thyroid-stimulating hormone (TSH). X-ray study of the thyroid (radioactive iodine scan) should not be done during pregnancy.

With hypothyroidism, thyroid replacement (thyroxin) is prescribed. It is believed to be safe during pregnancy. Your healthcare provider may check the level during pregnancy with a blood test to make sure you're receiving enough of the hormone.

If you have hyperthyroidism, treatment is the medication propyl-thiouracil. It passes through the placenta to the baby, so ask your healthcare provider to prescribe the lowest possible amount to reduce baby's risk. Blood testing during pregnancy is necessary to monitor the amount of medication needed. After delivery, it's important to test the baby and to watch for signs of thyroid problems.

Iodide is another medication used for hyperthyroidism, but it shouldn't be used during pregnancy; it can harm a developing baby. Pregnant women with hyperthyroidism should not be treated with radioactive iodine either.

. . . .

If you have acid reflux, stay away from foods that could add to the problem. Some to avoid include tomatoes, citrus fruit, and spicy and fried foods.

. . . .

Velocardiofacial Syndrome (VCFS)
Velocardiofacial syndrome (VCFS) is a genetic condition that may be hereditary. It is known by many names, including *Shprintzen syndrome, craniofacial syndrome* and *conotruncal anomaly face syndrome.* VCFS is one of the most common syndromes in humans, second only to Down syndrome in frequency.

The term *velocardiofacial* derives from three Latin words: "velum" meaning palate, "cardia" meaning heart and "facies," having to do with the face. It is

> ## Grandma's Remedy
> • • • • • • • • • • •
>
> If you want to avoid using medication, try a folk remedy. If you experience leg cramps, mix together 2 teaspoons of apple-cider vinegar and 1 teaspoon of honey in a glass of warm water, and drink it before bed.

characterized by various medical problems. Symptoms do not all occur 100% of the time. Most people with VCFS exhibit a small number of problems; many problems are relatively minor.

The exact cause of *velocardiofacial syndrome* is unknown; however, investigators have identified a chromosomal defect in people with VCFS. Most people who have been diagnosed with this syndrome are missing a small part of chromosome 22.

• •

At-home teeth whitening products are popular, and many people use them. Are they safe for pregnant women? We advise you to wait until after pregnancy to whiten your teeth. Most whitening products contain hydrogen peroxide, which can be swallowed during the whitening process. We don't have enough information about how hydrogen peroxide and other whitening agents can affect a growing baby. The substances used in tooth whiteners may also increase irritation if your gums are sensitive.

• •

Only one parent needs to have the chromosomal change to pass it along to a child. A parent with velocardiofacial syndrome has a 50/50 chance of having a child with it. However, it's estimated VCFS is inherited in only 10 to 15% of cases. Most of the time neither parent has the syndrome nor carries the defective gene.

The occurrence of congenital heart disease is most often the leading factor in diagnosis. Diagnosis is most frequently made using a genetic test called a *FISH analysis* (fluorescent in situ hybridization), which is almost 100% accurate. If the test shows chromosome 22 is not complete, the person has VCFS.

Familial Mediterranean Fever (FMF)

Familial Mediterranean Fever (FMF) occurs most often in Sephardi Jews, Armenians, Arabs and Turks. As many as one in 200 people in these populations has the disease; 20% are carriers. However, cases have occurred in other groups, particularly Ashkenazi Jews. About 50% have no family history of the disorder.

FMF is inherited and usually characterized by recurrent episodes of fever and inflammation of the abdominal membrane (peritonitis). Less frequently, pleuritis, arthritis, skin lesions and pericarditis occur.

• •

If you have regular manicures and/or pedicures, choose a salon with ventilation hoods that remove contaminated air from the area.

• •

Onset of the disease usually occurs between the ages of 5 and 15 but may also occur during infancy or much later. Attacks have no regular pattern of recurrence and usually last 24 to 72 hours. High fever is usually accompanied by pain. Abdominal pain occurs in nearly all sufferers and can vary in severity with each attack. Other symptoms include joint pain and a rash on the lower leg. Most people recover quickly and are OK until the next attack. Narcotics may be needed for pain relief.

Currently, no diagnostic test for FMF is available. The problem is diagnosed more on the basis of repeated episodes. However, researchers have identified the gene for FMF and found several different gene mutations that can cause the disease. The gene is found on chromosome 16. A protein assists in keeping inflammation under control by turning off the immune response. Without this function, an attack of FMF occurs.

Researchers continue to work to develop a blood test to diagnose FMF. With more research, it may also become easier to recognize environmental triggers that lead to attacks, which may lead to new treatments for FMF.

. . . .

If you have a burst of energy during this trimester, use it to get out of the house.

. . . .

Exercise for Week 25

• • • • • • •

Sit tall at the edge of a straight-backed side chair. Fold your arms in front of you, at shoulder height, and slowly lean forward a bit. In this position, lift your left foot off the floor, and hold for 5 seconds; be sure you are sitting erect. Lower your left leg. Do 5 times for each leg. *Stretches and strengthens abdominal muscles, thigh muscles and lower-back muscles.*

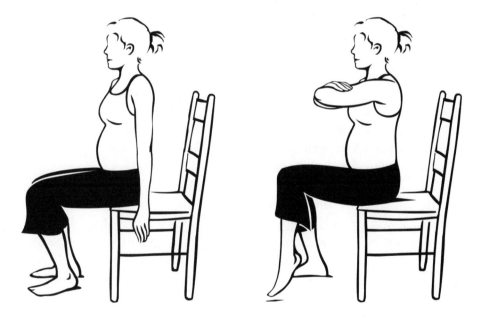

• • • • • • •

Week 26

Age of Fetus—24 Weeks

How Big Is Your Baby?

Baby now weighs almost 2 pounds (.91kg). By this week, crown-to-rump length is about 9¼ inches (23cm). See the illustration on page 264.

How Big Are You?

Your uterus is about 2½ inches (6cm) above your bellybutton or nearly 10½ inches (26cm) from your pubic symphysis. During the second half of pregnancy, you'll grow nearly ½ inch (1cm) each week. If you've been following a balanced meal plan, your total weight gain is probably between 16 and 22 pounds (7.2 to 9.9kg).

How Your Baby Is Growing and Developing

The fetus has distinct sleeping and waking cycles. You may find a pattern; at certain times of the day baby is very active, while at other times he or she is asleep. In addition, all five senses are now fully developed.

Heart Arrhythmia

By now you've heard baby's heartbeat at several visits. When listening to your baby's heartbeat, you may be startled to hear a skipped beat. An irregular heartbeat is called an *arrhythmia*. You'll hear it as regular pulsing or pounding with an occasional skipped or missed heartbeat. Arrhythmias in a fetus are not unusual and don't always indicate a problem.

If an arrhythmia is discovered before labor, you may need fetal heart-rate monitoring during labor. When an arrhythmia is detected during labor, it may be a good idea to have a pediatrician present at the delivery. He or she will make sure the baby is treated right away if a problem exists.

Changes in You

Time is passing quickly. You're approaching the end of the second trimester. You're getting bigger as your uterus, placenta and baby grow larger. Discomforts, such as back pain, pressure in

Tip for Week 26
• • • • • • • • • • •

Lying on your side (your left side is best) when you rest provides the best circulation to your baby. You may not experience as much swelling if you lie on your side.

your pelvis, leg cramps and headaches, may occur more frequently. Nearly two-thirds of pregnancy is behind you; it won't be long until baby is born.

How Your Actions Affect Your Baby's Development

Previous Weight-Loss Surgery

Before pregnancy, some women have weight-loss surgery to help them lose weight. *Bariatric surgery* is defined as surgery related to the prevention and control of obesity and related diseases. If you get pregnant after weight-loss surgery, you may have fewer risks during pregnancy than women who are morbidly obese.

Recent studies indicate women who had bariatric surgery need careful monitoring during pregnancy. Ultrasounds are a good way to monitor fetal growth. Women who have had surgery are at risk of micronutrient deficiencies, which could lead to problems for baby. Dietary supplements to help baby's growth may be prescribed. In addition, these women are more likely to give birth prematurely and have a lower-birthweight baby.

If you had lap-band surgery, it's possible to have the band adjusted so you can meet the increased nutritional needs of pregnancy. The doctor who performed the surgery can adjust the band so you and baby get the nutrition you both need.

If you had gastric-bypass surgery, studies show no particular problems associated with the procedure, especially if you waited 12 to 18 months after surgery to get pregnant. This time allows you to lose a lot of weight and restore lost nutrients. During pregnancy, you may need supplements because gastric-bypass surgery makes it harder for your body to absorb enough calcium, iron and B_{12}. Severe iron-deficiency anemia may result because you don't absorb enough of the nutrients you need.

If you've had weight-loss surgery and find out you're pregnant, call your healthcare provider immediately. Together you can plan a meal program so you and baby get the nutrients you need for a healthy pregnancy.

• •

Retin-A (tretinoin), not to be confused with Accutane (isotretinoin), is used to treat acne and to help erase fine wrinkles on the face. If you're pregnant and using Retin-A, stop using it immediately! We don't have enough data to know if Retin-A is safe to use during pregnancy. At this time, it's best to avoid using it for the sake of your baby.

• •

How to Have a Successful Labor and Delivery

It's not too early to start thinking about labor and delivery. It helps to know what makes a labor and delivery successful.

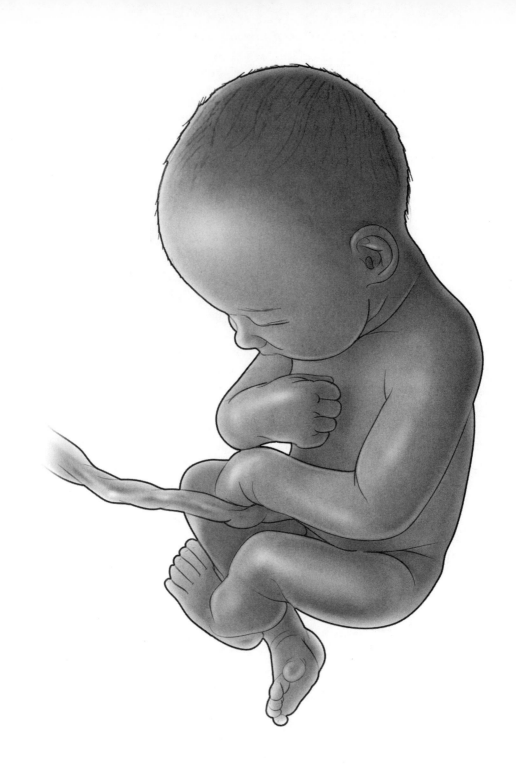

By this week, your baby weighs about 2 pounds (910g).
It is now putting on some weight and filling out.

> ## Dad Tip
> . . . .
>
> As pregnancy moves along, a lot of women start to feel unattractive. They may experience swelling in their hands and feet. They may find their hair and nails have changed. Their skin may not be normal for them. And their tummy is growing and growing! Reassure your partner that you know she's going through a lot to give your baby a healthy start in life. Take her on a date—go to dinner and a movie! Tell her she's beautiful. Take a full-view picture of her as a remembrance of how lovely she is now.

Become informed about labor and delivery. When you understand what can and will occur, you may be able to relax. Read this and our other pregnancy books, discuss questions and concerns with your healthcare provider and share information with your partner.

. . . .

Do you have a birth plan? If you do, it's important to keep an open mind and be flexible. As we've seen more times than we can count, the best-laid (birth) plans often go awry. It's crucial for you to communicate your ideas to your healthcare provider, but trust him or her to make the best decisions for you and baby during labor and delivery. After all, he or she has had a lot of experience delivering babies. And we all want the same thing—a healthy mom and a healthy baby.

. . . .

The relationships you have with your healthcare team are important. Follow medical suggestions, watch your weight, eat healthfully, take your prenatal vitamins and go to all your prenatal appointments and tests.

Being able to help make decisions about your medical care, including birth positions, pain-relief methods, feeding baby and your partner's level of participation in labor and delivery, helps you feel more in control. Discuss questions and various situations with your healthcare provider at prenatal appointments.

. . . .

You may have to rethink your expectations as to your partner's involvement in labor and delivery. Don't presume he will be an active participant just because you want him to be. Well before your due date, talk with him about how he sees his role. He may want to be completely involved, or he may want to play a smaller role. As important as it is to you, consider his feelings and expectations in this process. If he doesn't feel comfortable playing a major role and you try to force him to do it, medical personnel may have to care for you, baby and dad during labor and delivery!

. . . .

Your Nutrition

Fish Can Be Healthy during Pregnancy

Eating fish is healthy, especially during pregnancy. Pregnant women who eat fish may have longer pregnancies and give birth to babies with higher birth weights. Studies show the omega-3 fatty acids found in fish may help protect you from premature labor and other problems. Remember—the longer a

Good Fish and Shellfish Choices
• • • • • • • • • • •

Below is a list of fish that are safe to eat if you cook them thoroughly. Don't exceed a total of 12 ounces of all fish in any given week!

bass	haddock	pollack
catfish	herring	red snapper
cod	marlin	salmon
croaker	ocean perch	scrod
flounder	orange roughy	sole
freshwater perch	Pacific halibut	

The following shellfish are safe to eat if they are thoroughly cooked.

clams	lobster	scallops
crab	oysters	shrimp

In addition, fish sticks and fast-food fish sandwiches are OK to eat—they are commonly made from fish that is low in mercury.

baby stays in the uterus, the better its chances are of being strong and healthy at delivery.

Many fish are safe to eat, and you should include them in your diet. Most fish is low in fat and high in vitamin B, iron, zinc, selenium and copper. Many fish choices are excellent, healthful additions to your diet (with certain limits, as discussed below).

Omega-3 Fatty Acids. Omega-3 fatty acids are beneficial during pregnancy. They help protect your skin, reduce skin inflammation and fight depression. Fish oil is important to fetal brain development.

Anchovies, herring, mullet, mackerel (not King mackerel), salmon, sardines and trout are some fish sources of omega-3 fatty acids. Omega-3 fatty acids are also found in animal foods,

including grass-fed beef and eggs from hens fed special diets. If you're a vegetarian or you don't eat fish, add tofu, canola oil, flaxseed, soybeans, walnuts and wheat germ to your food plan. These foods contain linolenic oil, which is a type of omega-3 fatty acid.

Fish-oil capsules may be another option. If you buy fish-oil capsules, choose the filtered type because they don't contain pollutants. Take no more than 2.4g of omega-3 fatty acids a day. Fish-oil capsules may upset your stomach; if so, freeze them or take them with meals or at bedtime.

• •

Eating 12 ounces of fish every week during pregnancy may help your child enjoy better development during his or her early years.

• •

Methyl-Mercury Poisoning. Some fish are contaminated from man-made pollution. People who eat these fish are at risk of methyl-mercury poisoning.

Mercury is a naturally occurring substance and a pollution by-product. It becomes a problem when it is released into the air, then settles into the oceans and from there winds up in some types of fish, where it accumulates in their muscles. Larger fish that live longer have the highest levels of mercury because they've had the longest time to accumulate it in their system.

We know methyl mercury can pass from mother to fetus across the placenta. A fetus may be more at risk of methyl-mercury poisoning than an adult. Studies show one in five American women of childbearing age has mercury levels that are too high.

Pregnant women should limit their fish and shellfish intake to no more than *12 ounces a week*, which is two to three average servings.

There are different thoughts about pregnant women eating tuna. Canned light tuna has less mercury than albacore tuna, so eat that. Don't eat more than one 6-ounce can of any kind of tuna in a week. If you want to eat a cooked tuna steak every once in awhile, keep your total tuna intake (fresh and/or canned) to no more than 6 ounces a week. If you have questions, talk to your healthcare provider.

The amount of mercury in fish varies. Choose fish and shellfish that are lower in mercury. There is debate about eating canned tuna. Talk to your healthcare provider about it at a prenatal appointment if this is a favorite of yours. The box above contains information on canned and fresh tuna.

Some freshwater fish may also be risky to eat, such as walleye and pike. Consult local or state authorities for any advisories on eating freshwater fish. Other fish to avoid include some found in warm tropical waters; avoid the following local fish—amberjack, barracuda, bluefish, grouper, mahimahi, snapper and fresh tuna.

Some Additional Cautions about Fish. Parasites, bacteria, viruses and toxins can contaminate fish, and these can make you sick. Sushi and ceviche are fish dishes that could have viruses or parasites. Contaminated raw shellfish could cause hepatitis-A, cholera or gastroenteritis. **Avoid all raw fish during pregnancy!**

Fish can contain other environmental pollutants. Dioxin and polychlorinated biphenyls (PCBs) are found in bluefish and lake trout; avoid them. You may want to double-check tilapia. Farm-raised tilapia has low levels of omega-3 fatty acids and high levels of unhealthy omega-6 fatty acids.

We advise pregnant women not to eat sushi. However, if you're craving sushi, eat a California roll (no raw fish) or shrimp tempura. Other dishes made with cooked eel and rolls with steamed crab and veggies are OK.

If you're unsure about whether you should eat a particular fish or if you want further information, ask your healthcare provider for pamphlets about fish. Or contact the Food and Drug Administration for information.

Fish to Avoid

· · · · · · · · · · ·

The FDA recommends pregnant and breastfeeding women avoid swordfish, shark, king mackerel and tilefish. Also avoid walleye, pike, amberjack, barracuda, bluefish, grouper, mahimahi and snapper.

Home uterine monitoring helps identify women with premature labor. It combines recording uterine contractions with daily telephone contact with the healthcare provider. A recording of contractions is transmitted from a woman's home by telephone to a center where it can be evaluated. The healthcare provider may be able to view recordings at his or her office or home.

You Should Also Know

Seizures and Epilepsy

A history of seizures—before pregnancy, during a previous pregnancy or during this pregnancy—is important information you must share with your healthcare provider. (Another term for seizure is *convulsion*.) It's estimated that about 500,000 women with a seizure disorder in the United States are of childbearing age.

Seizures can occur without warning. A seizure indicates an abnormal condition related to the nervous system, particularly the brain. During a seizure, a person often loses body control. This can be serious for mom and baby.

If you have never had a problem with seizures, know that a short episode of dizziness or lightheadedness is not usually a seizure. Seizures are usually diagnosed by someone observing you and noting the symptoms previously mentioned. An electroencephalogram (EEG) may be needed to diagnose a seizure.

Epilepsy. If you have epilepsy, it's important to control your disease during pregnancy because seizures can affect you and baby in many ways. One-third of women with epilepsy will see a decrease in the number of seizures they have during pregnancy. One-third will have more seizures, and one-third will see no change at all.

During pregnancy, hormonal fluctuations can affect epilepsy. You may be at higher risk of some pregnancy problems. It's good to know more than 90% of all epileptic pregnant women give birth to healthy babies.

Medications to Control Seizures. If you take medication for seizure control or prevention, tell your healthcare provider before trying to get pregnant or at the beginning of pregnancy. Medications can be taken during pregnancy to control seizures, but some are safer than others. Ask about taking large doses of folic acid; it has proved helpful in some women.

If you have morning sickness, tell your healthcare provider about it. Nausea and vomiting can interfere with your body's ability to absorb your medications. Ask your healthcare provider to put you on the lowest dosage of one antiepileptic drug. Take your antiseizure medication exactly as it is prescribed.

Most studies show increased risk to baby when a mom-to-be takes valproate, especially in the first trimester. There's evidence baby's exposure to this medication increases the risk of autism. Talk to your healthcare provider about valproate before you become pregnant or as soon as you know you're pregnant.

Dilantin can cause birth defects in a baby. Other medications may be used during pregnancy for seizure prevention. One of the more common is phenobarbital, but there's some concern about its safety. Lamotrigine therapy alone shows no increased risk of problems in baby.

During pregnancy, kidneys may remove greater amounts of antiepileptic drugs from your system more quickly than usual. Drug levels could decrease by as much as 50%. It's important to see your neurologist every month for blood tests to check the levels in your blood. Any dosage adjustments can be made after test results are in.

You may need increased monitoring during pregnancy. If you have questions or concerns about a history of possible seizures, talk to your healthcare provider about them.

Need some help getting to sleep at night? Here are a couple of food-related treatments you might want to try. Make a piece of toast and add 1 tablespoon of peanut butter. Or have a small serving of yogurt, and add some fruit. Both of these remedies contain tryptophan, which may help you get to sleep.

Exercise for Week 26

• • • • • • •

Sit on the floor with your knees bent and your feet flat on the ground. Keep your knees about 12 inches apart. Reach underneath each thigh with your hands, then stretch back slowly until your arms are straight. Keep your feet on the floor as you return to the starting position. Repeat 8 times. *Strengthens abdominal muscles, inner thighs and pelvic floor.*

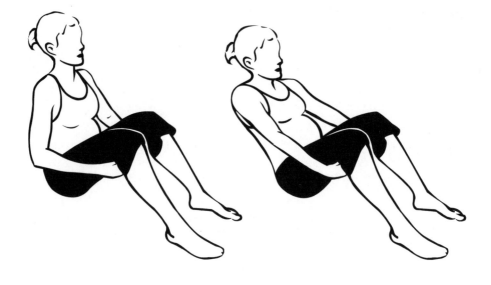

• • • • • • •

Week 27

Age of Fetus—25 Weeks

How Big Is Your Baby?

This week marks the beginning of the third trimester. We'll be adding total length of baby's body from head to toe. This will give you a better idea of how big your baby is during this last part of your pregnancy.

Your baby now weighs a little more than 2 pounds (875g), and crown-to-rump length is about 9⅔ inches (24cm) by this week. Total length is about 14⅓ inches (36cm). See the illustration on page 272.

How Big Are You?

Your uterus is about 2¾ inches (7cm) above your bellybutton. Measured from the pubic symphysis, it is more than 10½ inches (27cm) to the top of the uterus.

How Your Baby Is Growing and Developing

The retina, the part of the eye where light images come into focus at the back of the eye, is beginning to be sensitive to light. It develops layers around this time that receive light and light information and transmits them to the brain for interpretation—what we know as "sight." From here on, baby will probably be able to sense bright light. If you shine a light close to your tummy, baby may react as it senses the change in luminosity.

Baby's experiences inside the uterus impact its cognitive and sensory development.

Most people believe cataracts occur only in old age, but a *congenital cataract* can appear in a newborn baby! Instead of being transparent or clear, the lens is opaque or cloudy. This problem is usually inherited; however, it has been found in children born to mothers who had German measles (rubella) around the 6th or 7th week of pregnancy.

Another congenital eye problem is *microphthalmia*, in which the overall size of the eye is too small. It is usually the result of infections in the mom-to-be, such as cytomegalovirus (CMV) or toxoplasmosis, while baby is developing.

Changes in You

Feeling Baby Move

Feeling your baby move (quickening) is one of the more precious parts of

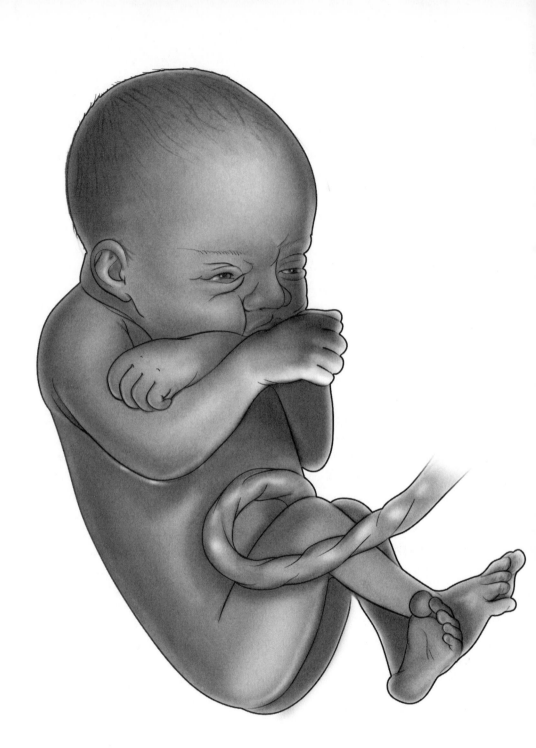

Around this time, your baby's eyelids open.
Your baby begins opening and closing its eyes
while still inside your uterus.

> ## Dad Tip
> . . . .
>
> Offer to do various jobs around the house that may be more difficult for your partner now. Cleaning the bathtub or the toilet can be a big help. Carry the laundry up and down stairs. Unload the dishwasher so you can put away heavy or awkward pieces. Add to her safety by putting away anything that belongs in a high or difficult-to-reach location.

pregnancy and can be the beginning of your bonding with baby. Many women feel they begin to connect with baby and its personality by feeling it move. Your partner can experience and enjoy baby's movements by feeling your tummy when baby is active.

Movement can vary in intensity. It can range from a faint flutter, sometimes described as a feeling of a butterfly or a gas bubble in early pregnancy, to brisk motions or even painful kicks and pressure as baby gets larger.

Women often ask how often a baby should move. They want to know if they should be concerned if the baby moves too much or doesn't move enough. This is hard to answer because your sensation can be different from that of someone else, and each baby's movement can be different. However, studies show an active baby moves at least 10 times in 2 hours. It's usually more reassuring to have a baby move frequently. But it isn't unusual for a baby to have quiet times when there is not as much activity. Many women report baby is more active at night, making it hard to sleep.

If your baby is quiet and not as active as what seems normal or what you expected, discuss it with your healthcare provider. You can always go to the office to hear baby's heartbeat if it hasn't been moving in its usual pattern. In most instances, there is nothing to worry about.

Pain Under Your Ribs When Baby Moves

Some women complain of pain under their ribs and in their lower abdomen when baby moves. This type of pain isn't an unusual problem, but it may cause enough discomfort to concern you.

Baby's movement has increased to a point where you probably feel it every day, and movements are getting stronger and harder. At the same time, your uterus is getting larger and putting more pressure on all your organs. If the pressure really is pain, don't ignore it. Discuss it with your healthcare provider. In most cases, it isn't a problem.

Discovering a Breast Lump

Discovering a breast lump is significant, during pregnancy or any other time. It's important for you to learn at an early age how to do a breast exam and to perform this on a regular basis (usually after every menstrual period). Women examining themselves find 9 out of 10 breast lumps.

Your healthcare provider will probably perform breast exams at regular intervals, usually when you have your annual Pap smear. If you have an exam every year and are lump-free, it helps assure you no lumps are present before you begin pregnancy.

It may be more difficult to feel a lump during pregnancy because of changes in your breasts. Growing breasts during pregnancy and nursing tends to hide lumps or masses in the tissue of the breast.

Continue to examine your breasts during pregnancy every 4 or 5 weeks. The first day of every month is a good time to do it. If you find a lump, you may need a mammogram or ultrasound exam. Because a mammogram is a breast X-ray, your pregnancy must be protected during the procedure, usually by shielding your abdomen with a lead apron. Pregnancy has not been shown to accelerate the course or growth of a breast lump.

Treatment during Pregnancy. Often a breast lump can be drained or aspirated. Fluid removed from the cyst is sent to the lab to see if it contains abnormal cells. If a lump or cyst can't be drained by needle, a biopsy may be necessary.

If examination of a lump signals breast cancer, treatment may begin during pregnancy. The need for radiation therapy and chemotherapy must be considered, along with the needs of the pregnancy. See also the discussion of cancer in pregnancy in Week 32.

Medicine has made great strides in treating cancer in pregnant women. Today, many women are able to receive cancer treatment and to carry their baby to full term without harm to the baby. If you have questions, ask your healthcare provider.

How Your Actions Affect Your Baby's Development

Childbirth-Education Classes

Even though it's just the beginning of the third trimester, it may be time to sign up for childbirth-education classes. If you sign up now, you may be able to finish classes before the end of your pregnancy and have time to practice what you learn. Childbirth classes are usually held for small groups of pregnant women and their partners or labor coaches. They are designed to inform you and your partner or labor coach about pregnancy, what happens at the hospital and what happens during labor and delivery.

By meeting in class on a regular basis, usually once a week for 4 to 6 weeks,

Childbirth-education classes can help parents-to-be in many ways. A class can help expecting couples:
- learn how baby develops
- alert them to warning signs of problems during pregnancy
- give tips to help identify when labor begins
- describe pain management techniques
- help practice breathing and relaxation methods
- describe what will happen during labor and delivery

> ## *Tip for Week 27*
> • • • • • • • • • • •
>
> Childbirth-education classes are not just for couples. Classes may be offered for single mothers or for pregnant women whose partners cannot come to classes. Ask at the office about classes for you.

you can learn a lot. Classes often cover a wide range of subjects, including different childbirth methods and clarification of "natural childbirth." Cesarean delivery and pain-relief methods, including epidurals, may also be discussed. The need for an episiotomy, an enema and fetal monitor are often covered. A big part of these classes is the information you need for the childbirth method you choose and the opportunity to practice it in class. These are important considerations. Discuss them with your healthcare provider, if you don't get answers in your childbirth-education classes.

Prenatal classes are not only for first-time pregnant women. If you have a new partner, if it's been a few years since you've had a baby or if you would like a review of what lies ahead, a prenatal class can help you. Childbirth classes that deal with vaginal birth after Cesarean (VBAC) may also be available. Ask at the office for information about various classes available in your area.

Classes are offered in various settings. Most hospitals that deliver babies offer classes, often taught by labor-and-delivery nurses or by a midwife. Various classes may have different degrees of involvement. This means the time commitment or depth of the subject covered is different for each type of class available.

If you have problems getting to a prenatal class because of cost or time or because you're on bed rest, it may be possible to take classes at home. Some instructors will come to you for private sessions. Or use a video.

• •

Sometimes childbirth-education instructors promote the belief there is an ideal way to give birth (vaginally). This sets many women up to believe they have failed if they end up having a Cesarean delivery. The goal in labor and delivery is a healthy mom and a healthy baby. If various procedures are used to deliver your baby safely—even if you didn't intend to employ them—rejoice that they are available to help ensure the safe delivery of your baby.

• •

Your Nutrition

Vitamin A, vitamin B and vitamin E are important vitamins you may need during pregnancy. Let's examine each vitamin and how it can help you.

Vitamin A is essential to human reproduction. Fortunately, deficiency in North America is rare. What is more concerning is the excessive use of the vitamin before conception and in early pregnancy. (This discussion concerns only the retinol forms of vitamin A, usually derived from fish oils. The beta-carotene form, of plant origin, is believed to be safe.)

The RDA (recommended dietary allowance) is 2700IU (international units) for a woman of childbearing age. The maximum dosage is 5000IU; pregnancy doesn't change these requirements. You probably get enough vitamin A from the foods you eat, so supplementation during pregnancy isn't recommended. Read food labels to keep track of your vitamin-A intake.

B vitamins help regulate the development of baby's nerves and formation of blood cells. B vitamins important in pregnancy include B_6, B_9 (folic acid/folate) and B_{12}. Vitamin B_6 helps prevent mood swings. Vitamin B_{12} helps fight depression and fatigue. If you don't take enough B_{12} during pregnancy, you could develop anemia. Taking enough vitamin B may help prevent certain birth defects.

There are many good food sources of B vitamins. Some you may enjoy include milk, eggs, tempeh, miso, collard greens and brown rice. Vitamin B_6 foods include avocado, bananas, red bell peppers, spinach, potatoes, chicken and nuts. Foods that contain vitamin B_{12} include skinless chicken breasts, lean dairy products and low-fat beef.

Vitamin E helps metabolize fats and builds muscles and red blood cells. You usually get enough vitamin E if you eat meat. Vegetarians and women who can't eat meat may have a harder time. Don't take megadoses of vitamin E; it could cause problems. Foods rich in vitamin E include olive oil, wheat germ, spinach and dried fruit. Check with your pharmacist or read the label on your prenatal vitamin to see if it supplies 100% of the recommended daily allowance.

Be cautious with every substance you take during pregnancy. If you have questions, discuss them at a prenatal visit.

You Should Also Know
Babymoons

Many expecting couples are now scheduling a *babymoon* before the end of pregnancy. A babymoon is a prebaby vacation—a trip for expectant parents to reconnect and to enjoy each other's company before baby's birth. It usually focuses on relaxing and pampering.

You can plan a weekend getaway close to home or take a trip farther afield. Some hotels and resorts now offer babymoon packages. Keep in mind it's the time you spend together that's important, whether you stay in a luxury hotel near home, find a mountain lodge to cuddle up in or relax in a condo by the sea.

A babymoon is a time to take walks, sleep in, lay by the pool, shop, eat in nice restaurants, take pictures and build memories. It's a time to enjoy each other's company before your hectic life as parents begins. Some people look forward to a babymoon so they can pamper themselves with massages and other spa treatments. Whatever you choose to do, it's a time to draw closer together.

Before You Make Plans. Discuss your plans with your healthcare provider *before* paying any deposits or buying any nonrefundable tickets. He or she may have valid reasons you shouldn't travel.

Kick Count

· · · · · · · · · · ·

Toward the end of pregnancy, you may be asked to record how often you feel baby move. This test is done at home and is called a *kick count*. It provides reassurance about baby's well-being. Your healthcare provider may use one of two common methods. The first is to count how many times baby moves in an hour. The other is to note how long it takes for baby to move 10 times. Usually you can choose when you want to do the test. After eating a meal is a good time because baby may be more active then.

If you get the OK to go, do some research. If you were thinking of going on a short cruise, check to see if the cruise line allows pregnant women to travel after a particular time in pregnancy. If you're thinking about going somewhere with activities you'd like to do, check to see if there are any restrictions on pregnant women. No matter what you plan, keep it simple and casual.

Often the best time in pregnancy to travel is during the second trimester. You're usually past morning sickness, and you haven't grown too large to enjoy moving around.

If you decide to take a babymoon, relax, share time together and enjoy the baby-free environment. It won't be long until you'll both be involved in the all-encompassing days and nights of being parents!

Lupus

Lupus is an autoimmune disorder; it is a chronic inflammatory disease that can affect more than one organ system. People with lupus have a large number of antibodies in the bloodstream that may damage organs. Affected organs include joints, skin, kidneys, muscles, lungs, the brain and the central nervous system.

The most common symptom of lupus is joint pain, which is often mistaken for arthritis. Other symptoms include lesions, fever, hypertension, rashes or skin sores.

Over 1½ million people in the United States have some form of lupus, and women have lupus much more frequently than men. Nearly 80% of cases develop in people between the ages of 15 and 45. Lupus is 2 to 3 times more common in women of color.

Lupus is diagnosed through blood tests, which look for suspect antibodies. Blood tests done for lupus are a lupus antibody test and an antinuclear antibody test.

Treating Lupus. Steroids are generally prescribed to treat lupus. The most common medicines used are prednisone, prednisolone and methylprednisolone.

Dexamethasone and betamethasone pass through the placenta and are used only when it's necessary to treat the baby as well. These medications are used in preterm labor and delivery to accelerate lung maturation.

If you use warfarin, contact your healthcare provider; warfarin should be replaced with heparin as soon as possible.

If you have high blood pressure, you may have to change medications. Don't take cyclophosphamide during the first trimester. Azathioprine and cyclosporin may be continued during pregnancy.

Lupus during Pregnancy. All lupus pregnancies should be considered high risk, although most lupus pregnancies are completely normal. "High risk" means solvable problems may occur during pregnancy and should be expected. More than 50% of all lupus pregnancies are normal, and most babies are normal, although babies may be somewhat premature.

About 35% of pregnant women with lupus have antibodies that interfere with the placenta's function. These antibodies may cause blood clots to form in the placenta that prevents it from growing and working normally. To deal with this problem, heparin therapy may be recommended.

The risk of pregnancy complications is slightly increased in a woman with lupus. It's a good idea to see your rheumatologist every month during pregnancy. If you begin to have a flare-up or other symptoms, it can be dealt with immediately.

If you had kidney damage from previous flare-ups, be on the lookout for kidney problems during pregnancy. Other common symptoms are arthritis, rashes and fatigue. Some women experience improvement in their lupus during pregnancy.

A "stress" steroid is often given to a woman with lupus during labor to protect her. After baby's birth, some experts believe steroids should be given or increased to prevent a flare-up of lupus in the mom. A woman with lupus can breastfeed; however, some medications, including prednisone, may interfere with milk production.

Exercise for Week 27

• • • • • • •

While standing in line at the grocery store, post office or anywhere else, use the time to do some "creative" exercises. These exercises help you develop and strengthen some of the muscles you'll use during labor and delivery.

- Rise up and down on your toes to work your calves.
- Spread your feet apart slightly, and do subtle side lunges to give your quadriceps a workout.
- Clench and relax your buttocks muscles.
- Do the Kegel exercise (see the exercise in Week 14) to strengthen pelvic-floor muscles.
- Tighten and hold in your tummy muscles.

You probably have to reach for things at home or at the office. When you do, make it an exercise in controlled breathing.

- Before you stretch, inhale, rise up on your toes and bring both arms up at the same time.
- When you're finished, drop slowly back on your heels.
- Exhale while slowly returning your arms to your sides.

Week 28

Age of Fetus—26 Weeks

How Big Is Your Baby?

Your baby weighs nearly 2¼ pounds (1kg). Crown-to-rump length is close to 10 inches (25cm). Total length is 14¾ inches (37cm).

How Big Are You?

Your uterus is about 3¾ inches (8cm) above your bellybutton. If you measure from the pubic symphysis, it's about 11 inches (28cm) to the top of the uterus. Your weight gain by this time should be between 17 and 24 pounds (7.7 and 10.8kg).

How Your Baby Is Growing and Developing

Until this time, the surface of baby's developing brain has appeared smooth. Around week 28, the brain begins to form characteristic grooves and indentations on the surface. The amount of brain tissue also increases.

Your baby's eyebrows and eyelashes may be present. Hair on baby's head is growing longer. The baby's body is becoming plumper and rounder because of increased fat underneath the skin. Before this time, baby had a thin appearance.

Just 11 weeks ago, baby weighed about 3½ ounces (100g). Your baby has increased its weight more than 10 times in 11 weeks! In the last 4 weeks, from the 24th week of your pregnancy to this week, weight has doubled.

Changes in You

Changing Taste Buds

Some pregnant women complain of a bad taste in their mouth; it's called *dysgeusia* and is common. It is probably caused by pregnancy hormones, which can alter taste. Some women experience a metallic or bitter taste, or they lose taste for certain foods. The good news is this condition usually disappears during the second trimester. If you have dysgeusia, try some of the following suggestions.

If sweets are too sweet, add a bit of salt to help cut sweetness in foods. Add lemon to water, drink lemonade or suck on citrus drops. Marinate fish, chicken or meat in soy sauce or citrus juice. Use plastic dinnerware; stainless steel utensils may increase a metallic taste. Brush

Nutrisystem and Jenny Craig Meal Plans
• • • • • • • • • • •

Many women have lost weight following menu plans that provide the consumer with prepackaged foods. Two of the most popular are Nutrisystem and Jenny Craig. Pregnant women want to know if they can continue to eat these foods and follow the meal plans during pregnancy. Both programs recommend a pregnant woman *not* follow their food plans because calories are too restricted. The plans do not supply enough calories for you to stay healthy and for your baby to grow and to develop during your pregnancy.

your teeth often. Gargle with baking soda and water (¼ teaspoon of baking soda in 1 cup of water), which may help neutralize pH levels.

The Placenta and Umbilical Cord

Baby is attached by the umbilical cord to the placenta. The placenta plays a critical role in baby's growth, development and survival. See the illustration on page 283. The umbilical cord contains two arteries and one vein.

• •

Studies show a baby may spend a great deal of time in utero pulling and squeezing the umbilical cord.

• •

The placenta helps move oxygen and carbon dioxide to and from baby. It's also involved in nutrition and removal of waste products from the baby. The placenta begins producing estrogen and progesterone by the 7th or 8th week of pregnancy.

Two important cell layers, the *amnion* and *chorion*, are involved in the development of the placenta and amniotic sac. Development and function of the cell layers is complicated, and their description is beyond the scope of this book. However, the amnion is the layer around the amniotic fluid in which the fetus floats.

The placenta grows at a rapid rate. At 10 weeks, it weighs about ¾ ounce (20g). At 20 weeks, it weighs almost 6 ounces (170g). In another 10 weeks, the placenta will have increased to 15 ounces (430g). At 40 weeks, it can weigh almost 1½ pounds (650g)!

Projections (villi) at the base of the placenta are firmly attached to the uterus. The villi absorb nutrients and oxygen from your blood and transport them to the baby through the umbilical vein. Baby's waste products are brought through the umbilical arteries and transferred to the maternal bloodstream to get rid of them.

At full term, a normal placenta is flat, has a cakelike appearance and is round or oval. It is about 6 to 8 inches (15 to 20cm) in diameter and ¾ to 1¼ inches (2 to 3cm) thick. The umbilical cord attached to the placenta is about 22 inches (55cm) long and is usually white. However, placentas can vary in size and shape. A large placenta (placentamegaly) may be found when a woman has syphilis or when a baby has erythroblastosis

(Rh-sensitization). A small placenta may be found with intrauterine-growth restriction (IUGR).

In multiple pregnancies, there may be more than one placenta, or there may be one placenta with more than one umbilical cord coming from it. Usually with twins, there are two amniotic sacs, with two umbilical cords running to the fetuses from one placenta.

How Your Actions Affect Your Baby's Development

Asthma in Pregnancy

Asthma is a chronic respiratory disease that causes small airways in the lungs to narrow. It is characterized by attacks of labored breathing, wheezing, shortness of breath, chest constriction and coughing. The most common causes of asthma include allergens, exercise, strong odors and cold air.

If your baby is a girl, research shows asthma attacks might worsen during pregnancy. If your baby is a boy, attacks might be better. The sex hormones produced by male fetuses are believed to have a protective effect on moms-to-be with asthma.

The problem affects about 2% of the population in the United States; one in 12 American adults is an asthma sufferer. Asthma may occur at any age, but about 50% of all asthma cases occur before age 10. Another 33% of the cases occur by age 40. About 70% of people with asthma also suffer from allergies.

Researchers believe asthma may be a genetic predisposition, and you will develop it if you are exposed to triggers. To help deal with your asthma, learn what triggers an attack, and avoid it. Measure your air flow at least once a day. Use medications to treat/control your asthma as they are prescribed.

Smog can trigger an attack and inflame the airways, causing coughing, wheezing and shortness of breath. Thunderstorms may also increase risk. Rain and lightning break pollen into very small particles, which can be more easily spread by a storm's winds.

Many asthma sufferers have heartburn; heartburn may cause asthma symptoms to worsen. Upper-respiratory infections caused by the flu may also trigger an attack.

If you have asthma and are overweight when you get pregnant, your baby is more likely to have asthma.

Pregnancy's Affect on Asthma. Asthma is the most common chronic condition in pregnancy, and all pregnant women with asthma, regardless of its severity, need to be closely monitored. About 8% of all pregnant women have asthma.

Sixty percent of women with severe asthma find control of their asthma declines during pregnancy. Only 10% of women with mild asthma experience the same effect. Some pregnant women get better during pregnancy, while others remain about the same.

Controlling asthma may help lower the risk of developing some pregnancy problems. Studies show if your asthma is under control throughout pregnancy, your pregnancy outcome can be as

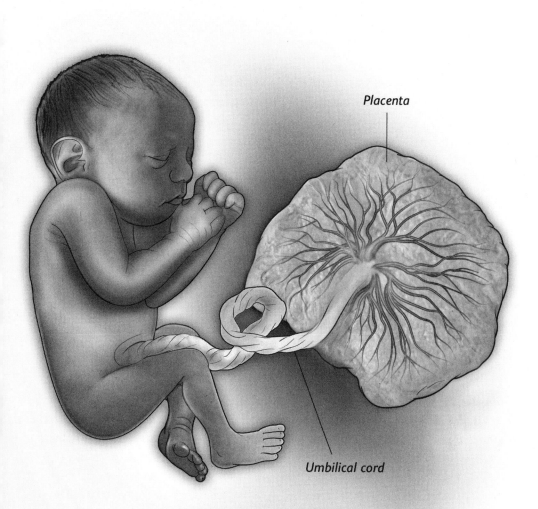

Placenta

Umbilical cord

The placenta, shown here with the fetus, carries oxygen and nutrients to the growing baby. It is an important part of pregnancy.

What Kinds of Foods Should You Eat?

You may be wondering what kinds of foods to eat and what to delete from your diet during this stage of pregnancy. Look at the chart below for some guidance.

Foods to Eat	Servings per Day
Dark green or dark yellow fruits and vegetables	1
Fruits and vegetables with vitamin C (tomatoes, citrus)	2
Other fruits and vegetables	2
Whole-grain breads and cereals	4
Dairy products, including milk	4
Protein sources (meat, poultry, eggs, fish)	2
Dried beans and peas, seeds and nuts	2
Foods to Eat in Moderation	
Caffeine	200mg
Fat	limited amounts
Sugar	limited amounts
Foods to Avoid	
Anything containing alcohol	
Food additives, when possible	

positive as a woman who doesn't have asthma. We also know asthma symptoms often improve during the last month of pregnancy due to hormonal changes.

In addition to asthma medicine you take, there are some foods you can eat to help avoid attacks. Citrus fruit, spinach, tomatoes, carrots and leafy green vegetables may reduce chances of an asthma attack. Talk to your healthcare provider about how much you should eat of any of these foods.

If your asthma is not well controlled during pregnancy, it can lead to high blood pressure in you. It may also result in a Cesarean delivery for you and low birthweight in baby. During an attack, baby may be deprived of oxygen. If you're not getting enough air, neither is baby.

It's important to have a flu shot to reduce the risk of getting severe respiratory illness, which could make asthma attacks worse. Don't smoke, and keep away from those who do smoke.

See your allergist regularly during pregnancy for a lung-function test to determine whether medication dosage needs to be adjusted. Your allergist may also suggest you monitor your breathing with a peak-flow meter to find out how open your airways are.

Asthma shouldn't be a deterrent to learning breathing techniques used in labor. Talk to your healthcare provider about it.

Treating Asthma Attacks. During pregnancy, your oxygen consumption increases by about 25%. Asthma treatment is important so baby can get the oxygen it needs to grow and to develop. The treatment plan used before pregnancy often continues to be helpful.

Research shows it's better for you to take asthma medicine during pregnancy than to risk asthma attacks and their complications. Most asthma medicine appears to be safe; however, check with your healthcare provider before using your usual prescription medication.

Asthma medication, such as terbutaline, and steroids, such as hydrocortisone or methylprednisolone, can be used during pregnancy. Aminophylline, theophylline, metaproterenol (Alupent) and albuterol (Ventolin) are also safe to use.

Studies show inhaled steroids do not seem to affect baby's growth. Inhalers work directly on the lungs, so very little medicine enters your bloodstream. However, don't use Primatene Mist during pregnancy.

If your asthma is severe, you may be given an anti-inflammatory nasal spray, such as cromolyn sodium (Nasalcrom) or an inhaled steroid, such as beclomethasone (Vanceril). Discuss the situation at one of your early prenatal visits.

Your Nutrition

If you take vitamin D, keep your intake to about 600IU/ day. Super-high levels, such as 2000IU/day, are not recommended. You can get vitamin D from various food sources, including milk, eggs, beef liver and some fish, or by supplementation, such as vitamin-D-fortified cereals. The FDA has also approved a program to allow most cheeses to be fortified with up to 20% of the daily allotment for the vitamin. Other foods are also fortified with vitamin D, such as some orange juice, yogurt and margarine. Getting enough vitamin D during pregnancy is good for baby's bones.

. . . .

Taking vitamin D may help relieve seasonal affective disorder (SAD), which can make you feel anxious, tired and sad during winter months. Ask your healthcare provider about taking vitamin D during pregnancy.

. . . .

You Should Also Know

Third-Trimester Tests

In your third trimester, you may undergo various tests to determine how you and baby are doing as labor and delivery get nearer. Below is a list of some of the common assessment tests a healthcare provider may order. Included is the week where an in-depth discussion appears for each of these tests:

- group-B streptococcus (GBS) infection test, see Week 29
- ultrasound in the third trimester, see Week 35
- home uterine monitoring, see Week 26
- kick count, see Week 27
- Bishop score, see When You're Overdue

Dad Tip
· · · · · · · · · · ·

Your partner has been feeling the baby move for a while. Around this time, you may also be able to feel it! Gently place your hand on her abdomen, and leave it there for a while. Your partner can tell you when baby is moving.

- nonstress test, see When You're Overdue
- contraction stress test, see When You're Overdue
- the biophysical profile, see When You're Overdue

Twenty-eight weeks of gestation is a time when many healthcare providers initiate or repeat certain blood tests or procedures. Testing for gestational diabetes may be done at this time.

· ·

If you are Rh-negative, you will probably receive an injection of RhoGAM at this point in pregnancy. This injection keeps you from becoming sensitized if baby's blood mixes with yours. RhoGAM protects you until delivery.

· ·

ABO Incompatibility

Blood groups are designated as types A, B, AB and O. *ABO incompatibility* is a type of blood-group difference, similar to Rh incompatibility; it can cause a disease in a newborn that destroys baby's blood cells (hemolytic disease). Type A-and-B incompatibility is the most common cause of the problem in a newborn.

The situation occurs when the mother has type O blood and her partner has type A, B or AB blood, and together they conceive a baby with type A or B blood. The mother can produce antibodies that destroy the baby's blood cells. An affected baby may have jaundice or anemia when it is born; these can both be easily treated in nearly all cases.

How Is the Baby Lying?

You may be wondering how your baby is lying inside the uterus. Is the baby head first? Is it bottom first (breech)? Is the baby lying sideways? It's difficult—usually impossible—at this point in pregnancy to tell just by feeling your abdomen. The baby changes position throughout pregnancy.

You can feel your abdomen to try to see where the head or other parts are located. In another 3 to 4 weeks, the baby's head will be harder; it will be easier at that time for your healthcare provider to determine how baby is lying.

Canavan Disease

Canavan disease, also called *Canavan sclerosis* and *Canavan-van Bogaert-Bertrand syndrome*, is a relatively common degenerative disease of the brain. Although Canavan disease may occur in any ethnic group, it's more frequent among Saudi Arabians and Ashkenazi Jews from eastern Poland, Lithuania and western Russia.

The disease is one of a group of genetic disorders called *leukodystrophies*. Canavan disease causes problems in the development of the myelin sheath, the

Tip for Week 28
· · · · · · · · · · ·

Even though delivery is several weeks away, it isn't too early to begin making plans for the trip to the hospital. This includes knowing how to reach your partner (keep all of his phone numbers with you). Also consider what you will do if he isn't near enough to take you. Who are potential drivers? How do you contact them? Make plans now!

fatty covering that acts as an insulator around nerve fibers in the brain.

There is no cure, nor is there a standard course of treatment. The disease develops in infancy, and prognosis is poor. Death usually occurs before age 4, although some children have survived into their 20s.

Canavan disease can be identified by a blood test. Both parents must be carriers of the defective gene to have an affected child. When both parents carry the Canavan gene mutation, there is a one-in-four chance with each pregnancy a child will be affected.

· ·

If you're pregnant and live in an area where bugs are a problem, it's OK to use an EPA-registered repellent. The CDC recommends repellents containing DEET or picaridin. Oil of lemon eucalyptus is another option, but it's not as long-lasting. Don't overdo it with bug sprays. Spray clothing, not your skin. Bug lights and bug candles may offer some protection. Even some plants, such as citronella plants, may help repel insects.

· ·

Is Home Birth Safe?

Home births happen. Of the 25,000 home births that occur every year in the United States, 25% (a little over 6000) are unplanned. That means the other

75% (nearly 19,000) of home births are planned. But are home births safe?

You may have heard from friends or acquaintances they had a home birth and everything went fine. Some women want to give birth at home because they feel it's "more natural." Another factor may be the high cost of labor and delivery, especially if you don't have full insurance coverage.

But research has shown giving birth at home is an extremely risky undertaking. One study showed twice as many infant deaths and serious, dangerous complications when babies are delivered at home. What can be done at home if your baby has serious problems and needs immediate medical care that can only be provided at a hospital or birthing center staffed by professionals?

There are also dangers to mom. First-time pregnant women who deliver at home have nearly triple the risk of complications after baby's birth. In addition, the chance of serious problems increases when a woman suffers from various pregnancy problems. Even carrying more than one baby increases your risk.

The American Congress of Obstetricians and Gynecologists has firmly stated that home birthing is hazardous

Grandma's Remedy

. . . .

If you want to avoid using medication, try a folk remedy. If you get a sunburn, brew up some mint tea, then cool it. Wet a small towel in the tea, and apply it to your sunburned skin. It cools the burn and may prevent peeling.

to a woman and her baby. Based on Dr. Curtis's own experiences with the aftermath of home births, we must concur. We advise any woman who is considering this option to talk to her healthcare provider about the safety and wisdom of delivering her baby at the hospital or a birthing center.

Exercise for Week 28

• • • • • • •

Sit tall in a straight-backed side chair with your knees bent, your arms relaxed at your side and your feet flat on the floor. Lift your left foot off the
floor with your leg extended. Hold for 8 seconds; be sure you are sitting
erect. Lower your left leg. Do 5 times for each leg. *Stretches hamstrings and
strengthens thigh muscles.*

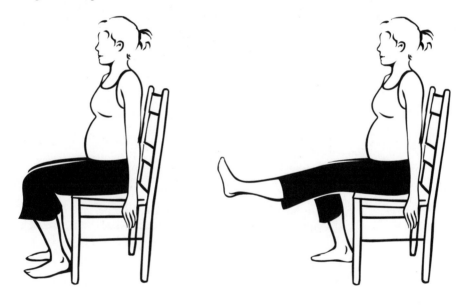

• • • • • • •

Week 29

Age of Fetus—27 Weeks

How Big Is Your Baby?

By this time, baby weighs about 2½ pounds (1.2kg). Crown-to-rump length is almost 10½ inches (26cm). Total fetal length is 15¼ inches (38cm).

How Big Are You?

Measuring from the bellybutton, your uterus is 3½ to 4 inches (7.6 to 10.2cm) above it. Your uterus is about 11½ inches (29cm) above the pubic symphysis. Your total weight gain by this week should be between 19 and 25 pounds (8.55 and 11.25kg).

How Your Baby Is Growing and Developing

Each week, we've noted the change in your baby's size. We use average weights to give you an idea of how large baby may be at a particular time. However, these are only averages; babies vary greatly in size and weight. The average baby's birthweight at full term is 7 to 7½ pounds (3.28kg to 3.4kg).

Because growth is rapid during pregnancy, infants born prematurely may be tiny. Even a few weeks less time in the uterus can have a dramatic effect on baby's size. A baby continues to grow after 36 weeks of gestation but at a slower rate.

Here are a couple of interesting facts about birthweight: Boys weigh more than girls. And the birthweight of an infant increases with the increasing number of pregnancies you have or the number of babies you deliver.

How Mature Is Your Baby?

A baby born between the 38th and 42nd weeks of pregnancy is a *term baby* or *full-term infant*. Before the 38th week, the term *preterm* can be applied to the baby. After 42 weeks of pregnancy, your baby is overdue and the term *postdate* is used.

When a baby is born before the end of pregnancy, many people use the terms *premature* and *preterm* interchangeably, but there is a difference. An infant who is 32 weeks gestational age but has mature pulmonary or lung function at the time of birth is more appropriately called a "preterm infant" than a premature infant. "Premature" best describes an infant who has immature lungs at the time of birth.

Premature Labor
and Premature Birth

Many babies born in the United States are born before their due date. Nearly 13% of all babies are premature—that's over half a million babies each year! Premature birth increases the risk of problems in a baby.

. . . .

Studies show it can be dangerous for a baby to be born even a few weeks early. Babies born before 36 weeks are more likely to develop breathing difficulties and feeding problems, and have trouble regulating body temperature. We once believed a baby's lungs were mature by 34 weeks, but we now know this isn't true. These findings may impact elective deliveries, elective Cesarean deliveries and induction of labor.

. . . .

Today, we classify premature babies into categories. The most commonly used classifications are:

- micropreemie—born before 27 weeks of pregnancy
- very premature—born between 27 and 32 weeks of pregnancy
- premature—born between 32 and 37 weeks of pregnancy
- late premature—born after 37 weeks of pregnancy

Better methods of caring for premature babies have contributed to higher survival statistics. Today, infants born as early as 25 weeks of pregnancy may survive.

The illustration on page 292 shows a premature baby with several leads attached to its body to monitor it. Many other attachments may be used, such as I.V.s, tubes and masks that provide oxygen.

It's usually best for the baby to remain in the uterus as long as possible. However, occasionally it's best for baby to be delivered early, such as when baby is not receiving adequate nutrition. Nearly 25% of preterm births are a result of pregnancy complications—baby needs to be delivered early for its health and safety.

Preterm Labor. How will you know if you are experiencing preterm labor? Signs that preterm labor may begin, or has already begun, include bleeding, a change and/or increase in vaginal discharge (watery, mucus or bloody), cramps that feel like your period or abdominal cramps, a low, dull backache, pelvic or lower-abdominal pressure, feeling as if baby is pushing down hard, ruptured membranes or contractions every 10 minutes or more often.

. . . .

Exposure to phthalates may increase your risk of delivering baby prematurely. Avoid exposure to help lessen risk. Phthalates are a group of manmade chemical compounds found in plastics, solvents, lotions, perfume, nail polish, deodorant and hairspray. Check labels to see if a product is "phthalate free" or look for the three- or four-letter acronym. If the label states any of the following, don't buy it or use it: BBP, DBP, MBP, DEHP, MEHP, DEP, MEP, DiDP, DiNP, DnHP or DnOP.

. . . .

Some actions may help stop premature labor. Stop what you're doing, and rest on your left side for 1 hour. Drink

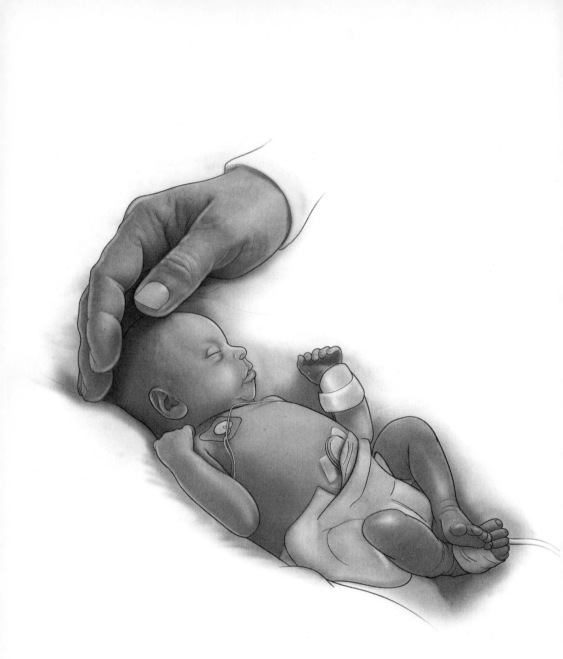

Premature baby (born at 29 weeks of pregnancy) shown with fetal monitors attached to it. Note size of adult hand in comparison.

2 to 3 glasses of water or juice. If symptoms get worse or don't go away after an hour, call your healthcare provider or go to the hospital. If symptoms go away, relax for the rest of the day. If the symptoms stop but come back, call your healthcare provider or go to the hospital.

Causes of Premature Labor and Premature Birth. In most cases, we don't know the cause of premature labor or premature birth; finding a cause may be difficult. An attempt is always made to determine what causes it so treatment may be more effective. Half of the women who go into preterm labor have no known risk factors. Your risk for preterm labor increases if you:

- had preterm labor or preterm birth in a previous pregnancy
- smoke cigarettes or use cocaine
- are carrying more than one baby
- have an abnormal cervix or uterus
- had abdominal surgery during this pregnancy
- had an infection while pregnant, such as a UTI or gum problems
- had any bleeding in the second or third trimester of this pregnancy
- are underweight
- have a mother or a grandmother who took DES (diethylstilbestrol; medication given to many pregnant women in the 1950s, 1960s and 1970s)
- have had little or no prenatal care
- are carrying a child with chromosomal disorders

Other risk factors have been identified, including giving birth at an older age, carrying a baby conceived from invitro fertilization, getting pregnant very soon after a previous birth (less than 9 months), you are Black/African American or you are under 17 or over 35. Research shows if it took you longer than 1 year to get pregnant, you may have a slightly higher chance of giving birth prematurely.

Some experts believe up to half of all premature births may be tied to infections. Iron deficiency has also been linked to an increased risk. Some researchers believe taking your prenatal vitamin every day may help cut your risk by as much as 50%!

Low HDL cholesterol and elevated homocysteine levels in a mother-to-be have been shown to be key factors associated with preterm birth. When found together, the risk of premature delivery was twice as high.

. . . .
Even if you have symptoms of premature labor, you may not deliver early.
. . . .

Tests Your Healthcare Provider May Do. One test, called *SalEst*, can help determine if a woman might go into labor early. The test measures levels of the hormone estriol in a woman's saliva. Research has shown there is often a surge in this chemical several weeks before early labor. A positive result means a woman has a 7 times greater chance of delivering her baby before the 37th week of pregnancy. Another test is fetal fibronectin (fFN). See Week 22.

There are some difficult questions to answer when premature labor begins. Is

---

Tip for Week 29
· · · · · · · · · · ·

If your healthcare provider advises bed rest, follow his or her instructions. It may be difficult for you to stop your activities and sit idly by when you have lots of things to do, but remember, it's for the good health of you and your baby!

---

it better for the infant to be inside the uterus or to be delivered? Are the dates of the pregnancy correct? Is this really labor?

Changes in You

Bed Rest

The treatment used most often for premature labor is bed rest. The term *bed rest* can cover anything from cutting back on activities to being confined to bed for 24 hours a day, getting up only to go to the bathroom or to shower. A woman is often advised to stay in bed and lie on her side. (Either side is OK.)

About 20% of all pregnant women are prescribed bed rest. However, not all experts agree on this treatment. It's OK to discuss bed rest and all of its implications with your healthcare provider if it is recommended. Ask if more tests might help or if medications are an option. Discuss getting a second opinion from a perinatologist, who deals with high-risk pregnancies.

Bed rest is often successful in stopping contractions and premature labor. If you are advised to rest in bed, it may mean you can't go to work or continue many activities. It's worth it if you can avoid premature delivery of your baby.

Bed rest is advised for other pregnancy conditions, such as pre-eclampsia,

contractions, chronic high blood pressure, incompetent cervix and placenta previa. High stress from a job or your lifestyle may also require bed rest. If serious complications arise, your healthcare provider may advise hospital treatment.

One negative aspect of bed rest is the increased risk of a blood clot in your leg, called *deep-vein thrombosis* (see Week 21 for more on deep-vein thrombosis). Other problems include muscle weakness and/or atrophy, loss of bone calcium, weight-gain issues (gaining too much or too little weight), heartburn, constipation, nausea, insomnia, depression and family tension. Discuss with your healthcare provider exercises you can do while on bed rest, such as stretching or strength training, to prevent loss of muscle tone and strength.

Lying down for quite a while can lead to you being out of shape. Take it easy getting back into the swing of things after baby is born. It can take some time to return to your normal level of activity. Don't rush into physical activities until you feel ready.

Bed-Rest Boredom Relievers. It can be pretty boring being stuck in bed. There are many things you can do to help beat bed-rest boredom. Spend the day in a room other than your bedroom. Use the living-room or family-room sofa for

Dad Tip
. . . .

After the baby is born, you may want to take time off work to help out at home and to be part of your baby's early development. The Family and Medical Leave Act was passed to help people take time off to care for family members. Ask now if it applies to you. If it does, and you plan to take time off, begin making arrangements soon.

daytime activities. Use foam mattress pads and extra pillows for comfort.

Establish a daily routine. When you get up, put on daytime clothes. Shower or bathe every day. Comb your hair, and put on lipstick. Go to bed when you normally do. Don't nap during the day; it can contribute to sleeplessness at night.

Keep a telephone close at hand, as well as reading material, the television remote control, a radio and other essentials. A laptop with Internet access can be a lifesaver; it can entertain you and keep you connected at work.

Use a cooler to keep food and drinks cold and near you. Use an insulated container for hot soup or herbal tea.

Start a journal. Our book *Your Pregnancy Journal Week by Week* is easy to use and lets you record your thoughts and feelings to share with your partner now and your child later.

Do some crafts that aren't messy, such as cross-stitch, knitting, crocheting, drawing or hand sewing. Make something for baby! Or call your favorite local charity or political organization and volunteer to make phone calls, stuff envelopes or write letters.

Use the time to plan for baby's arrival. Spend some time planning baby's room (someone else will have to carry through on it), deciding what you'll need for a layette and making a list of all the necessary items you'll need after baby comes home.

Sort! Use the time to sort through recipes, put pictures in albums, go through your coupons or make a scrapbook of information for after baby's arrival.

If you have other children at home, day care will probably be a necessity. For support, contact Sidelines (888-447-4754), a national support group that helps women with high-risk pregnancies. They can provide you with information and put you in touch with other women who have had the same experience.

How Your Actions Affect Your Baby's Development

Most of our discussion this week is devoted to the premature infant and treatment of premature labor. If you're diagnosed with premature labor and your healthcare provider prescribes bed rest and medicine to stop it, follow his or her advice!

If you have concerns about advice, discuss them. If you're told not to work or advised to reduce activities and you ignore the advice, you're taking chances with your well-being and baby's. It isn't worth taking risks. Don't be afraid to ask for a second opinion.

Your Nutrition

Potassium-rich foods, such as raisins and bananas, may help reduce your risk of premature labor. Potassium helps the body get rid of sodium faster.

We hope you've been listening to your body during pregnancy. When you feel hungry or thirsty, eat or drink something. Eating smaller, more frequent meals provides a constant supply of nutrients to your growing baby.

Keep nourishing snacks near at hand. Dried fruit and nuts are good choices when you're on the go. Know what time of day or night hunger strikes you. Be prepared.

It's OK to be different. Eat spaghetti for breakfast and cereal for lunch if that's what appeals to you. Don't force yourself to eat something that turns you off or makes you sick—there's usually an alternative. As long as you eat nourishing food and pay attention to the types of foods you eat, you help yourself and your growing baby.

You Should Also Know

Medications to Help Stop Premature Labor

Beta-adrenergic agents, also called *tocolytic agents*, may be used to suppress labor. They relax muscles and may help decrease contractions. At this time, only ritodrine (Yutopar) is approved by the FDA to treat premature labor. It is usually first given intravenously and may require a hospital stay. It may also be given as an intramuscular injection and as a pill.

When premature contractions stop, you can be switched to oral medicine, which you take every 2 to 4 hours. Ritodrine is approved for use in pregnancies over 20 weeks and under 36 weeks gestation. In some cases, medication is used without first giving an I.V. This is done most often in women with a history of premature labor or for a woman with multiple pregnancies.

Terbutaline is also used to halt premature labor. Although it has been shown to be effective, the FDA has not approved it for this use. Magnesium sulfate is used to treat pre-eclampsia, and it may also help stop premature labor. It is usually given through an I.V. and requires hospitalization. However, it is occasionally given orally, without hospitalization. You must be monitored frequently if you take magnesium sulfate.

Sedatives or narcotics may be used in early attempts to stop labor. A woman might receive an injection of morphine or meperidine (Demerol). This is not a long-term solution but may be effective in initially stopping labor.

Progesterone (17-hydroxyprogesterone) may be given to a pregnant woman if a previous baby was born prematurely. Some studies indicate a woman with a short cervix may also benefit from this treatment. Folic-acid supplementation for at least 1 year before pregnancy has been shown to decrease the occurrence of early preterm birth.

If you have premature labor, you may need to see your healthcare provider frequently. He or she will probably monitor you with ultrasound and/or nonstress tests.

Guillain-Barre syndrome (GBS)

Guillain-Barre syndrome (GBS) is an autoimmune disorder that damages nerve cells that transmit signals to your muscles. It is rare but has occurred during pregnancy. We don't know what causes GBS, but in many cases, the person had an acute infection before onset of symptoms.

Symptoms include loss of strength in the legs, numbness or tingling in the limbs, muscle weakness and a stinging sensation. Other symptoms may follow.

Eventually paralysis sets in. In most cases, a person begins to recover about 4 weeks after the onset of symptoms. Most people make a full recovery within a year.

If you experience any of these symptoms, contact your healthcare provider immediately. He or she will advise you on a course of action.

. . . .

Epstein-Barr virus (EBV) is one of the most common viruses. In the United States, as many as 95% of adults between 35 and 40 years of age have been infected. Studies of EBV during pregnancy show the virus poses little threat to baby.

. . . .

Exercise for Week 29

• • • • • • •

Kneel on the ground, sitting lightly on your heels with your feet tucked under you and your toes on the ground. Sit tall. Press your toes into the ground. Hold. Do 5 or 6 times or as often as you want. *Loosens calf and foot muscles; may help prevent leg cramps.*

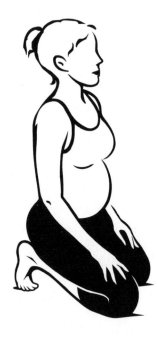

• • • • • • •

Week 30

Age of Fetus—28 Weeks

How Big Is Your Baby?

By week 30, baby weighs about 3 pounds (1.3kg). Its crown-to-rump length is a little over 10¾ inches (27cm), and total length is 15¾ inches (40cm).

How Big Are You?

It may be hard to believe you still have 10 weeks to go! You may feel like you're running out of room. Measuring from your bellybutton, your uterus is about 4 inches (10cm) above it. From the pubic symphysis, the top of your uterus measures about 12 inches (30cm).

You should be gaining about 1 pound a week. About half of this weight is concentrated in the growth of the uterus, baby, placenta and volume of amniotic fluid. Growth is mostly in your abdomen and pelvis. You may experience discomfort in your pelvis and abdomen as pregnancy progresses.

How Your Baby Is Growing and Developing

The illustration on page 300 shows a fetus and its umbilical cord. Can you see the knot in the cord? You may wonder how a knot like this can occur. We do not believe the cord grows in a knot.

A baby is usually very active during pregnancy. We believe these knots occur as baby moves around in early pregnancy. A loop forms in the umbilical cord; the baby moves through the loop, and a knot results. Your actions do not cause or prevent this kind of complication. A knot in the umbilical cord doesn't occur often.

Changes in You

Irritable Bowel Syndrome (IBS)

Irritable bowel syndrome (IBS) is a disorder of the large intestine (colon) that causes abdominal pain and abnormal bowel movements. IBS is not the same as inflammatory bowel disease (IBD). (IBD can damage the intestines and lead to more serious problems.) We don't know what causes IBS. It may be a lifelong condition, but symptoms can often be improved or relieved with treatment.

As many as 1 in 5 American adults may have symptoms of IBS. It's more common in women. Symptoms can include abdominal pain, bloating, cramping, constipation, diarrhea, gas,

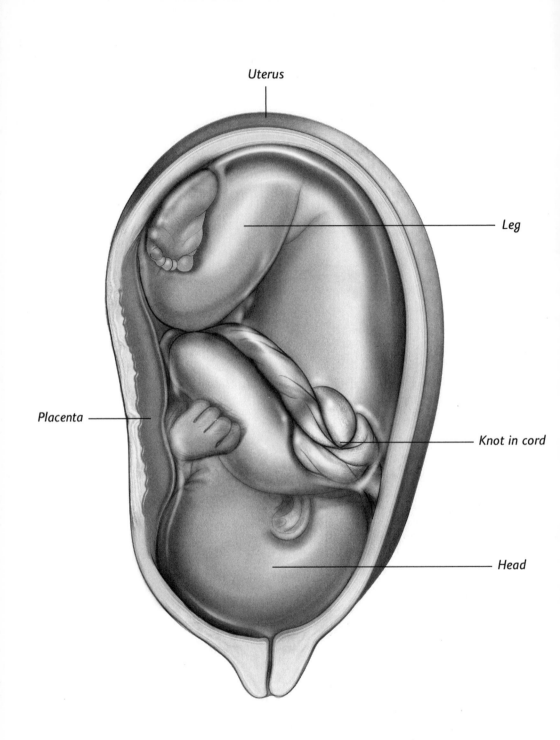

Uterus

Leg

Placenta

Knot in cord

Head

This fetus has a knot in its umbilical cord.

> ### Grandma's Remedy
> . . . .
> If you want to avoid using medication, try a folk remedy. Eat 1 teaspoon of honey before bedtime to help you sleep. Honey helps stabilize blood sugar while it increases melatonin levels and decreases stress hormones.

depression and loss of appetite. Triggers for IBS can range from gas or pressure on your intestines to certain foods, medicines and emotional stress.

IBS and Pregnancy. IBS symptoms may worsen during pregnancy, causing discomfort. The problem often is less severe during the first trimester and reappears in the second trimester. In the third trimester, symptoms may increase.

Your digestive system may slow down, causing constipation. Drink plenty of water, and eat a high-fiber diet. Do moderate, safe exercise if you have your healthcare provider's OK. Adequate rest and sleep may help. Soluble fiber supplements may reduce constipation and diarrhea.

If IBS becomes severe, you may be prescribed medication. There is no cure for the problem—the goal of treatment is to relieve symptoms. Work with your healthcare provider during pregnancy if you have IBS.

How Your Actions Affect Your Baby's Development

Bathing during Pregnancy

Many women wonder if taking a bath during pregnancy is OK. Most healthcare providers believe it's safe to bathe throughout pregnancy. They may caution you to be careful getting in or out of the bathtub. Be sure bath water is not too hot. If you think your water has broken, don't take a bath.

Women want to know how they'll know if their water breaks while they're in the tub or shower. When your water breaks, there is usually a gush of water followed by slow leakage. If your water breaks while you're bathing, you may not notice the initial gush of fluid, but you'll probably notice the leakage of fluid, which can last for quite a while.

. . . .
When you're feeling good, make some meals and freeze them. They'll be ready to go when you're too tired to cook.
. . . .

Flotation Baths and Pregnancy

Flotation baths are popular in many places in the United States. When you "take" a flotation bath, you float inside an isolation tank, which is lightless and soundproof, in salt water heated to your skin temperature. Isolation tanks are used for meditation and relaxation, and they are also used in alternative medicine. Research has concluded flotation tank sessions may provide relief for stress-related ailments and help reduce pain and swelling.

Pregnant women want to know if floating could harm their baby. Probably not. A pregnant woman may find relief in a float tank. Due to the high salt levels in the water, the flotation tank creates a zero-gravity environment. In the later stages of pregnancy, the float tank allows a woman to reduce stress on her joints when she floats in the water. It is safe to lie on your back after the 16th week of pregnancy in a float tank because you put little pressure on the blood vessels that lie beneath the uterus. The relaxed state may also help lower blood pressure and increase blood flow throughout the body.

Talk to your doctor about using a float tank during pregnancy. He or she will advise you about its safety. But if you don't want to spend the money on a flotation tank experience, go to your local pool. You'll get much of the same effect. Floating in a swimming pool will allow you to feel fairly weightless—your joints feel only 10% of your weight while you're in water. And you can do more in a pool—swim, exercise, even just walk!

Choosing Where to Give Birth

It's probably time to start considering where you want to give birth. In some situations, you may not have a choice. Or you may have several choices. Whatever birthing setup you choose, the most important considerations are the health of your baby and the welfare of you both. When you decide where to have your baby, be sure you have answers to the following questions, if you can.

- What facilities and staff are available?
- Is an anesthesiologist available 24 hours a day?
- How long does it take to respond and to perform a Cesarean delivery if necessary? (This should be 30 minutes or less.)

- Is a pediatrician available 24 hours a day?
- Is the nursery staffed at all times?
- In the event of an emergency or a premature baby that needs to be transported to a high-risk nursery, how is it done? By ambulance? Helicopter? How close is the nearest high-risk nursery, if not at this hospital?

These may seem like a lot of questions to ask, but it's good to know emergency measures can be employed in an efficient, timely manner when necessary.

There are various hospital setups available for labor and birth. With *LDRP* (labor, delivery, recovery and postpartum), the room you are admitted to at the beginning of labor is the room you labor in, deliver in, recover in and remain in for your hospital stay.

The concept of LDRP evolved because many women don't want to be moved from labor to a delivery area, then to another part of the hospital to recover. The nursery is usually close, which allows you to see your baby as often as you like and to have baby in your room for longer periods.

Another option is the *birthing room*; this generally refers to delivering baby in the same room you labor in. Even if you use a birthing room, you may have to move to another area of the hospital for recovery and the remainder of your stay.

In many places, *labor-and-delivery suites* are available; you labor in one room, then are moved to a delivery room at the time of birth. Following this, you may go to a postpartum floor, which is an area in the hospital where you will spend the remainder of your hospital stay.

Most hospitals allow you to have your baby in your room as much as you want. This is called *rooming in* or *boarding in*. Some hospitals also have a cot, couch or chair that makes into a bed so your partner can stay with you after delivery. Check availability of various facilities in the hospitals in your area.

You may think it's too early to start thinking about child care, but it's time to start thinking about it if you plan to return to work after baby's birth. Quality care is in high demand and short supply! Experts advise you to begin looking for a child-care situation at least 6 months before you need it. For some women, that may be the end of the second trimester!

Your Nutrition

Some women ask if herbal teas are safe to drink during pregnancy. Some herbal teas are probably safe to drink and include chamomile, dandelion, ginger root, lemon-balm, peppermint and nettle leaf.

You may have heard warnings about drinking peppermint tea during pregnancy. Many experts agree it's OK if you only drink one or two 6- to 8-ounce cups a day to help relieve morning sickness or upset stomach. However, it may worsen heartburn and/or GERD. Look for products that contain 100% pure peppermint leaves.

Eating small snacks during the day helps curb your hunger, stabilize your mood and meet your daily nutrient requirements.

Many "pregnancy teas" contain red-raspberry leaf. Studies show you can safely drink tea made from red-raspberry leaves during pregnancy; it may help make labor a little shorter. However, many experts advise waiting until after the first trimester to drink it because it may cause uterine contractions.

Don't overuse *any* herbal tea; a *total* of 12 to 16 ounces total a day is the maximum amount of any tea to consume. If you have questions, check with your healthcare provider.

Avoid certain herbal teas during pregnancy, including blue cohosh, black cohosh, alfalfa, yellow-dock, pennyroyal leaf, yarrow, goldenseal, feverfew, psyllium seed, mugwort, comfrey, coltsfoot, juniper, rue, tansy, cottonroot bark, large amounts of sage, senna, cascara sagrada, buckthorn, fern, slippery elm and squaw vine. We have little information on dandelion tea, stinging-nettles tea or rose hips. It may be best to avoid drinking them during pregnancy.

Benefits of Drinking Some Herbal Teas

· · · · · · · · · · ·

chamomile	aids digestion
dandelion	helps with swelling and can soothe an upset stomach
ginger root	helps with nausea and nasal congestion
nettle leaf	rich in iron, calcium and other vitamins and minerals
peppermint	relieves gas pains and calms the stomach

Avoid green tea during pregnancy. The antioxidant in green tea interferes with the body's use of folic acid. Green tea may also interfere with blood tests and can alter blood-sugar levels. In addition, it may interfere with blood clotting.

You Should Also Know

Chinese Gender Chart

One of the ways a couple can guess baby's sex is with the *Chinese gender chart.* Legend has it the calendar was found when a royal tomb was explored 700 years ago. The calendar was invented by astrologers for Chinese royalty and was used to predict the gender of royal offspring. It was kept secret until the end of the Qing Dynasty in 1911. In the 100+ years since its release, it has been widely used by Chinese people.

There's no proof it works, but couples tell us it's a fun way to try to guess if baby will be a boy or a girl. All you need are the *lunar month* the baby was conceived and the mom-to-be's *lunar age* at the time of conception.

The Chinese use a lunar calendar, which is different from a Western Gregorian calendar. If you use a Western calendar for your calculations, it'll throw off the accuracy of the Chinese gender chart.

Because the formula is complicated and based on the Chinese calendar, we suggest you go online and find a website to help your figure this all out. It can be fun to do this together as a couple during your pregnancy.

· ·

During your third trimester, you may discover your nesting instinct—the overwhelming urge to clean and get organized. Experts believe it may be caused by an increase in oxytocin.

· ·

MRSA

Methicillin-resistant Staphylococcus aureus (MRSA; sounds like MERSA) is a bacteria that causes difficult-to-treat infections. The Staphylococcus aureus bacteria, also called *staph*, are resistant to, or develop resistance to, many antibiotics. Bacteria have adapted or changed so antibiotics that were once effective no longer work. Antibiotics that *do* work against MRSA include vancomycin, doxycycline and TMP-SMZ (trimethoprim/sulfamethoxazole).

A very common location of MRSA is the nose or nostrils. Other possible sites are open wounds, I.V. catheters and the urinary tract. MRSA is passed from person to person, usually through poor hygiene practices.

Take care of cuts and scratches. MRSA can start as inflamed skin that

Tip for Week 30
. . . .

Good posture can help relieve lower-back stress and eliminate some back discomfort. Maintaining good posture may take some effort, but it's worth it if it relieves pain.

develops small red bumps like pimples. This can be accompanied by a fever or a rash. The area may be red and hot to the touch. MRSA can spread through the bloodstream. When this happens, it can cause sepsis or septic shock.

Washing your hands frequently works well in preventing MRSA. Don't share towels, soap or other personal items. If you have a cut or abrasion, keep it clean, dry and covered. If you develop any pimples or boils, keep the area tightly covered, and call your healthcare provider immediately.

Pregnant women may be at greater risk for MRSA because of decreased immunity. If either you or your partner work in a hospital, healthcare facility, school or anyplace where you have a lot of contact with people, you could be at risk. Discuss any of your concerns with your healthcare provider.

Evidence does not indicate MRSA during pregnancy causes increased risk of problems. It's very unlikely you will pass MRSA to baby during delivery. In addition, it's safe to breastfeed if you have MRSA.

Group-B Streptococcus Infection (GBS)
Group-B streptococcus (GBS) is a type of bacteria found in up to 40% of all pregnant women. A GBS infection rarely causes problems in adults but can cause life-threatening infections in newborns.

It is possible to have GBS in your system and not be sick or have any symptoms. It is recommended all women be screened for GBS between 35 and 37 weeks of pregnancy. If tests show you have the bacteria but no symptoms, you are colonized. If you're colonized, you can pass GBS to your baby.

The battle to eradicate GBS is a true medical success story. Before the 1990s, 7500 newborns contracted the infection each year; 30% of those babies died. Today, only about 1600 cases are reported each year. Much of the success has been the result of healthcare providers following the CDC guidelines. They include cultures for GBS colonization and use of antibiotics for all carriers and any woman who has given birth to an infant with proven GBS infection.

The CDC, the American Congress of Obstetricians and Gynecologists (ACOG) and the American Academy of Pediatrics (AAP) have developed recommendations to help prevent infection in newborns. They recommend all women with risk factors be treated for GBS.

Exercise for Week 30

· · · · · · ·

Sit tall on a straight-backed side chair. Hold a towel above your head, with your hands shoulder-width apart. Slowly twist from your waist to the left side as far as is comfortable for you. Return to the center, then twist to the right. Do 8 times. *Stretches spine, and strengthens shoulders and upper-back muscles.*

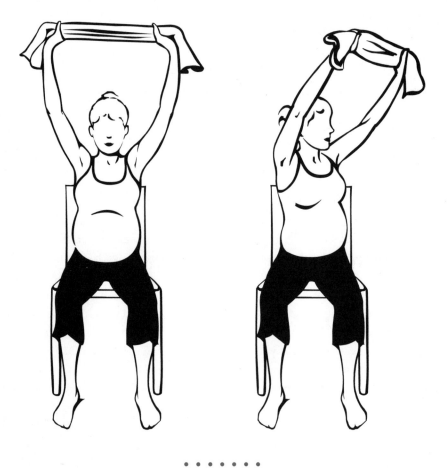

· · · · · · ·

Week 31

Age of Fetus—29 Weeks

How Big Is Your Baby?

Your baby weighs about 3⅓ pounds (1.5kg), and crown-to-rump length is 11¾ inches (28cm). Its total length is nearly 16 inches (41cm).

How Big Are You?

There is now a little more than 12 inches (31cm) from the pubic symphysis to the top of the uterus. From your bellybutton, the uterus is almost 4½ inches (11cm). Your total pregnancy weight gain should be between 21 and 27 pounds (9.45 and 12.15kg). As you can see in the illustration on page 309, your uterus now fills a large part of your abdomen.

How Your Baby Is Growing and Developing

Your healthcare provider measures you at each visit to see how your uterus and baby are growing. A problem is usually found by measuring the uterus over a period of time and finding little or no change. If you measured 10¾ inches (27cm) at 27 weeks gestation and at 31 weeks you measure only 11 inches (28cm), there might be concern about IUGR, and tests may be ordered.

Intrauterine-growth restriction (IUGR) indicates a fetus is small for its gestational age. Weight is below the 10th percentile (in the lowest 10%) for the baby's gestational age. This means 9 out of 10 babies of normal growth are larger.

When dates are correct and the pregnancy is as far along as expected and weight falls below the 10th percentile, it's cause for concern. Growth-restricted babies can have many problems.

Various conditions can raise the risk of IUGR. We know a woman who has delivered a growth-restricted baby may be more likely to do so again. Anything that results in baby receiving less nutrition can be a factor. Lifestyle choices can cause IUGR, such as smoking, alcohol use and drug use.

If you don't gain enough weight, baby may have restricted growth. Eat a healthful diet during pregnancy. Don't restrict normal weight gain.

Pre-eclampsia and high blood pressure can affect baby's growth. Some infections in mom may restrict growth. Anemia may also be a cause.

> ## Dad Tip
> ● ● ● ● ● ● ● ● ● ●
> It's time to start looking for baby equipment, such as cribs, car seats and layette items. You'll need to make some of these purchases before baby's birth. Most hospitals or birthing centers won't let you take baby home without an approved car seat.

Women who live at high altitudes are more likely to have babies who weigh less. Carrying more than one baby may also cause smaller-than-normal babies.

Other reasons for a small baby, unrelated to IUGR, include a woman who is small might have a small baby. In addition, an overdue pregnancy can lead to a smaller baby. A baby with birth defects may also be smaller.

Detecting IUGR is one important reason to keep all prenatal appointments. Measuring helps your healthcare provider determine whether your pregnancy is growing and baby is getting bigger. Ultrasound can diagnose or confirm IUGR and may also be used to assure baby is healthy and no malformations exist that must be dealt with at birth.

When IUGR is diagnosed, bed rest is one treatment. Resting on your side allows baby to receive the best blood flow; better blood flow is the best chance to improve growth. If maternal disease causes IUGR, you must be treated to improve your health.

An infant with IUGR is at risk of dying before delivery. Infants with IUGR may not tolerate labor well, and baby may need to be delivered before it is full term. Baby may be safer outside the uterus than inside it.

Changes in You

Too Much Saliva

Some women experience an increase in saliva during pregnancy; hormones are the culprit. Too much saliva is called *ptyalism*; it occurs as estrogen levels increase. The condition often runs in families. Morning sickness may also contribute to the problem.

Often when you feel queasy, you don't swallow as much as you normally do, which results in buildup of saliva. To treat the condition, drink plenty of fluid to increase swallowing. Sucking on hard candies may also offer relief.

● ●
Pineapple contains bromelain, an enzyme that helps ease swelling, inflammation and bruising. Consider adding some to your meal plan.
● ●

Swelling in Your Legs and Feet during Pregnancy

Your body produces as much as 50% more blood and body fluids during pregnancy. Some of this extra fluid leaks into body tissues. When your growing uterus pushes on pelvic veins, blood flow in the lower part of your body is partially blocked. This pushes fluid into your legs and feet, causing swelling.

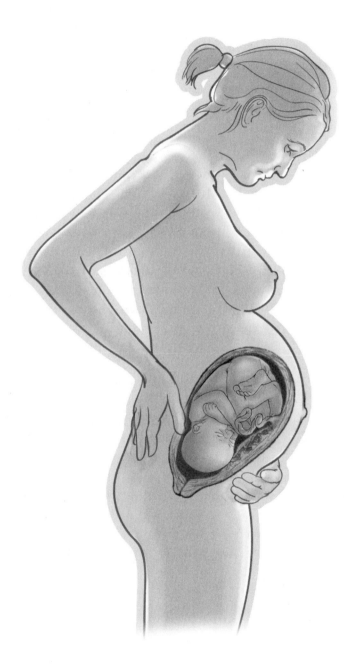

Comparative size of the uterus at 31 weeks of pregnancy
(fetal age—29 weeks). The uterus can be felt about 4½ inches
(11cm) above the bellybutton.

If you take your shoes off and leave them off for a while, you may not be able to put them back on. You may also notice wearing tight knee stockings or socks leaves an indentation in your legs. This is related to swelling. Avoid tight, restrictive clothing.

The way you sit can also affect your circulation. Crossing your legs at the knee or ankle restricts blood flow to your legs, so don't cross your legs.

How Your Actions Affect Your Baby's Development

We've already described the importance of lying on your side when resting or sleeping in Week 15. Now's the time it will pay off. You may notice you begin to retain water if you don't lie on your side.

Visiting Your Healthcare Provider

It's important to go to all prenatal appointments. It may seem not much happens at these visits, especially when everything is normal and going well. But the information collected tells your healthcare provider a lot about your condition and baby's.

Your healthcare provider is looking for signs of problems such as changes in your blood pressure or weight or inadequate growth of the baby. If problems aren't found early, they may have serious consequences for you and baby.

Childbirth Methods

It's time to start thinking about how you want to deliver your baby. Many of the methods used need a lot of time and practice to prepare you and your partner or labor coach to use them.

Some women decide they are going to labor and deliver with natural childbirth. What does this mean? The description and/or definition of natural childbirth varies. Many people equate natural childbirth with a drug-free labor and delivery. Others equate natural childbirth with the use of mild or local pain medications. Most agree natural childbirth is birth with as few artificial procedures as possible. However, a woman who chooses natural childbirth usually needs some advance instruction to prepare for it.

Childbirth Philosophies and Methods. There are various philosophies of natural childbirth. Three of the most well-known are Lamaze, the Bradley Method and Grantly Dick-Read.

Lamaze is the oldest childbirth-preparation technique. Through training, it conditions women to replace unproductive laboring efforts with fruitful ones and emphasizes relaxation and breathing as ways to relax during labor and delivery.

The *Bradley Method* embraces a basic belief in the ability of all women to give birth naturally. Classes teach many types of relaxation and inward focus. Emphasis is put on deep abdominal breathing to make labor more comfortable. Bradley includes a woman's partner; classes teach expectant parents how to stay healthy and keep their risk of complications low through good nutrition, exercise and lifestyle choices. Classes begin when pregnancy is confirmed and continue until after birth.

The *Grantly Dick-Read* method tries to break the fear-tension-pain cycle of labor and delivery through relaxation techniques. The classes were the first to include fathers in the birth experience.

Other childbirth methods are also taught. Marie Mongan, a hypnotherapist, used the work of Dr. Grantly Dick-Read to develop *hypnobirthing*. She believes if you're not afraid, pain is reduced or eliminated, so anesthetics during labor are unnecessary.

Physical therapist Cathy Daub is the founder of *Birth Works Childbirth Education*. The goal of Birth Works is to help women have more trust and faith in their ability to give birth and build self-confidence. Classes may be taken any time during pregnancy, even before you become pregnant.

Birthing from Within was developed by midwife Pam England, who believes birth is a rite of passage, not a medical event. Classes center on self-discovery. Pain-coping measures are intended to be integrated into daily life, not just used for labor.

ICEA, *ALACE* and *CAPPA* are three associations that share a similar philosophy. They believe in helping women trust their bodies and gain the knowledge necessary for making informed decisions about childbirth. Each group teaches the stages of labor and coping techniques for each stage. Class series vary in length.

Should You Consider Natural Childbirth? Natural childbirth isn't for every woman. If you arrive at the hospital dilated 1cm, with strong contractions and in pain, natural childbirth may be hard for you. In this situation, an epidural might be appropriate.

However, if you are dilated 4 or 5cm and contractions are OK, natural childbirth might be a reasonable choice. It's impossible to know what will happen ahead of time, but it helps to be aware of, and ready for, everything.

Keep an open mind during the unpredictable process of labor and delivery. Don't feel guilty or disappointed if you can't do all the things you planned. You may need an epidural. Or the birth may not be accomplished without an episiotomy. You should never feel guilty or feel you've failed if you need a Cesarean, an epidural or an episiotomy.

Beware of instructors in childbirth-education classes who tell you labor is free of pain, no one really needs a Cesarean delivery, I.V.s are unnecessary or an episiotomy is foolish. This can create unrealistic expectations for you.

The goal in labor and delivery is a healthy baby and a healthy mom. If this means you end up with a C-section, it's OK. Be grateful a Cesarean delivery can be done safely. Babies who would not have survived birth in the past can now be delivered safely. This is a wonderful accomplishment!

Your Nutrition

Salmonella bacteria can cause a lot of problems for you. Salmonella bacteria has many sources—there are over 1400 different strains! They're found in raw eggs and raw poultry. The bacteria is destroyed when a food is cooked, but

Tip for Week 31
· · · · · · · · · · · ·

Wearing rings and watches may cause circulation problems. Sometimes a ring becomes so tight on a pregnant woman's finger that the ring must be cut off by a jeweler. You might not want to wear rings if swelling occurs. Some pregnant women purchase inexpensive rings in larger sizes to wear during pregnancy. Or you could put your rings on a pretty chain and wear them around your neck or on a bracelet.

it's wise to take additional precautions. Keep in mind the following measures to stay safe.

Clean your counters, utensils, dishes and pans with hot water and soap or a disinfecting agent when you clean up. Cook with copper-alloy pots and pans. The oxidation of the copper produces a substance that kills salmonella.

Cook poultry thoroughly. Don't eat products made with raw eggs, such as Caesar salad, hollandaise sauce, homemade eggnog or homemade ice cream. Don't taste cake batter, cookie dough or anything else that contains raw eggs before it's cooked.

When you eat eggs, be sure they're cooked thoroughly. Boil eggs for at least 7 minutes. Poach eggs for 5 minutes. Fry them on each side for 3 minutes—cook them so the yolk and white are firm. Don't eat "sunny-side up" eggs.

You Should Also Know

*Carpal Tunnel Syndrome
during Pregnancy*

If you have carpal tunnel syndrome, you have pain in the hand and wrist that can also extend into the forearm and shoulder. It's caused when the median nerve in the wrist is squeezed by swelling in the wrist and arm area. Symptoms can be numbness, tingling or burning of the inner half of one or both hands. At the same time, fingers feel numb and useless. More than half of the time, both hands are involved.

Up to 25% of all pregnant women experience mild symptoms; treatment is usually unnecessary. The full syndrome, in which treatment may be needed, is less frequent; it occurs in only 1 to 2% of pregnant women.

Treatment depends on symptoms. Splints are often used during sleep and rest to keep the wrist straight. Symptoms usually disappear after delivery. Occurrence of carpal tunnel syndrome during pregnancy does not mean you'll suffer from it after baby's birth. In rare cases, symptoms may recur long after pregnancy, and surgery may be necessary.

Pregnancy-Induced Hypertension (PIH)
When high blood pressure occurs only during pregnancy, it is called *pregnancy-induced hypertension (PIH)* or *gestational hypertension*. The problem usually disappears after baby is born.

With PIH, the systolic pressure (the first number) increases to higher than

140mm of mercury or a rise of 30mm of mercury over your beginning blood pressure. A diastolic reading (the second number) of over 90mm or a rise of 15mm of mercury also indicates a problem. An example is a woman whose blood pressure at the beginning of pregnancy is 100/60. Later in pregnancy, it is 132/91. This signals she may be developing high blood pressure or pre-eclampsia.

We have seen articles in magazines and newspapers that incorrectly equate high blood pressure with pre-eclampsia. They are not the same problem. High blood pressure is one common *sign* of pre-eclampsia, but it must be accompanied by other serious symptoms for you to be diagnosed with pre-eclampsia. See below. Follow your healthcare provider's advice about taking care of high blood pressure, but don't panic.

Your healthcare provider will check your blood pressure at every prenatal appointment. That's one of the reasons to keep all your prenatal appointments.

What Is Pre-eclampsia?

Pre-eclampsia describes a group of symptoms that occur only during pregnancy or shortly after delivery. Pre-eclampsia seems to be on the rise; the condition affects 1 in 20 pregnancies and accounts for over 15% of all maternal deaths during pregnancy.

. . . .

A father-to-be's age may play a role in pre-eclampsia. One study showed the problem is 80% higher among women whose partners are 45 years or older.

. . . .

No one knows what causes pre-eclampsia. It occurs most often during a woman's first pregnancy. Women over 35 years old having their first baby are more likely to develop high blood pressure and pre-eclampsia. Some experts believe stress may be a contributing factor.

Pre-eclampsia occurs more often in women who have had chronic high blood pressure and pre-eclampsia in a previous pregnancy. Checking your blood pressure and weight at every prenatal visit can alert your healthcare provider to a developing problem.

Pre-eclampsia problems are characterized by a collection of symptoms. The first four are the most common:

- **swelling (edema)**
- **protein in the urine (proteinuria)**
- **high blood pressure (hypertension)**
- **a change in reflexes (hyperreflexia)**
- swelling and pain in a foot may worsen
- rapid weight gain, such as 10 to 12 pounds in 5 days
- flulike aches and pain, without a runny nose or sore throat
- headaches
- vision changes or problems
- elevated level of uric acid
- pain under the ribs on the right side
- seeing spots

Report symptoms to your healthcare provider immediately, particularly if you've had blood-pressure problems during pregnancy!

Most pregnant women have some swelling during pregnancy. Swelling in the legs and/or hands *does not* mean you have pre-eclampsia.

. . . .

Some researchers believe if a woman has pre-eclampsia, her blood vessels may never have dilated properly from the beginning of pregnancy.

. . . .

Pre-eclampsia increases water retention, which can increase your weight. If you notice an unusual, rapid weight gain, contact your healthcare provider.

Risk factors for developing pre-eclampsia include a history of high blood pressure before pregnancy, kidney disease, blood-clotting disorders, some autoimmune disorders, being under 20 years old, delaying childbirth until after age 35, overweight or obesity, multiple fetuses, having diabetes or kidney disease, or being Black/African American.

To reduce risk, take a multivitamin regularly before getting pregnant. Eat high-fiber foods during the first trimester, and eat garlic. Five servings a week of dark chocolate may also be helpful.

There are ways to help lower your risk of developing pre-eclampsia. Get regular exercise. Take care of your teeth so you don't get gum disease. Take folic acid. Controlling asthma during pregnancy may also help lower your risk.

Treating Pre-eclampsia. Pre-eclampsia can progress to *eclampsia*—seizures or convulsions in a woman with pre-eclampsia. The goal in treating pre-eclampsia is to avoid eclampsia and seizures.

Some experts believe low-dose-aspirin therapy may help prevent pre-eclampsia. The crucial time to begin taking it is around 12 weeks of pregnancy. Talk to your healthcare provider about it if you had pre-eclampsia with a previous pregnancy.

Treatment begins with bed rest at home, which provides the greatest blood flow to the uterus. Lie on your side, not your back. Drink lots of water. Avoid salt, salty foods and foods that contain sodium, which may make you retain fluid. If a woman with pre-eclampsia has a systolic blood-pressure reading of 155 to 160mm, she should be treated with antihypertensive therapy to help prevent a stroke.

If you can't rest in bed or if symptoms don't improve, you may be admitted to the hospital and/or your baby may need to be delivered. A baby is delivered for its well-being and to avoid seizures in you.

During labor, pre-eclampsia may be treated with magnesium sulfate. It is given by I.V. to prevent seizures during and after delivery.

If you think you've had a seizure, call your healthcare provider immediately! Diagnosis may be difficult. If possible, someone who saw the possible seizure should describe it to your healthcare provider. Eclampsia is treated with medications similar to those prescribed for seizure disorders.

Exercise for Week 31

· · · · · · ·

Sit up straight in a chair or on the floor. Lace your fingers together behind your head; keep your elbows apart. Inhale and push your hands, with your fingers still together, toward the ceiling. Exhale and return your hands to the position behind your head. Repeat 5 times. *Tones arms and shoulder muscles.*

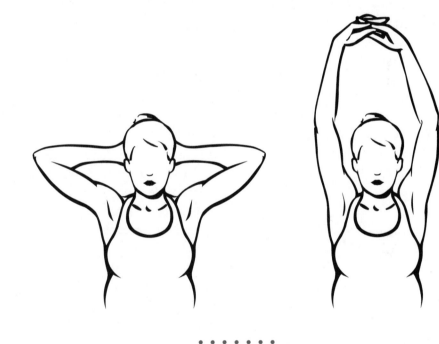

· · · · · · ·

Week 32

Age of Fetus—30 Weeks

How Big Is Your Baby?

By this week, baby weighs almost 3¾ pounds (1.7kg). Crown-to-rump length is over 11½ inches (29cm), and total length is nearly 16¾ inches (42cm).

How Big Are You?

Measurement to the top of the uterus from the pubic symphysis is about 12¾ inches (32cm). Measuring from the bellybutton, it now measures about 5 inches (12cm).

How Your Baby Is Growing and Developing

Twins? Triplets? More?

The rate of multiple births is going up—since 1980, the rate of twin births has increased 70%. Statistics show that close to 4% of all births in the United States are multiple births. If you're expecting more than one baby, you're not alone!

When talking about pregnancies of more than one baby, in most cases we refer to twins. The chance of a twin pregnancy is more likely than pregnancy with triplets, quadruplets or quintuplets (or even more!). However, we are seeing more triplet and higher-order births. A triplet birth is not very common; it happens about once in every 7000 deliveries. (Dr. Curtis has been fortunate to deliver two sets of triplets in his medical career.) Quadruplets are born once in every 725,000 births; quintuplets once in every 47 million births!

Being pregnant with two or more babies can affect you in many ways. Your pregnancy will be different, and the adjustments you may need to make may be more wide-ranging. These changes may be necessary for your health and the health of your babies. Work closely with your healthcare provider to make pregnancy healthy and safe.

A multiple pregnancy occurs when a single egg divides after fertilization or when more than one egg is fertilized. Twin fetuses usually result (over 65% of the time) from the fertilization of two separate eggs. These are called *fraternal twins* or *dizygotic (two zygotes) twins.*

About 35% of the time, twins come from a single egg that divides into two similar structures. Each has the potential of developing into a separate individual. These are known as *identical twins* or *monozygotic (one zygote) twins.*

> ## Dad Tip
> • • • • • • • • • •
>
> Together with your partner, make a list of important telephone numbers to keep with you. Include numbers for your work, your partner's work, the healthcare provider's office, the hospital, a back-up driver, babysitter or others. You may also want to make a list of numbers of people you want to call after baby's birth.

Either or both processes may be involved when more than two fetuses are formed. Triplets may result from fertilization of one, two or three eggs, or quadruplets may result from fertilization of one, two, three or four eggs.

A twin pregnancy resulting from fertility treatment often results in fraternal twins. In some cases of higher-number fetuses, a pregnancy resulting from fertility treatment can result in fraternal and identical twins.

The percentage of boys decreases slightly as the number of babies increases. As the number of babies a woman carries goes up, her chances of having girls increase.

Special Issues for Identical Twins. With identical twins, division of the fertilized egg occurs between the first few days and about day 8. If division of the egg occurs after 8 days, the result can be twins that are connected, called *conjoined twins*. (Conjoined twins used to be called *Siamese twins*.) These babies may share important internal organs, such as the heart, lungs or liver. Fortunately this is a rare occurrence.

Identical twins face some risks. There's a 15% chance they will develop a serious problem called *twin-to-twin transfusion syndrome*. Babies share one placenta. The problem occurs when one baby gets too much blood flow and the other too little. See the discussion in Week 23.

It may be important later in life for your children to know whether they were identical or fraternal because of health concerns. Before delivery, tell your healthcare provider you would like to have the placenta(s) examined (with a pathology exam) so you'll know whether babies were identical or fraternal if they are the same sex.

The Frequency of Multiples. Identical twins occur about once in every 250 births around the world. This rate doesn't seem to be influenced by age, race, heredity, number of pregnancies or medications taken for infertility (fertility drugs).

The incidence of fraternal twins *is* influenced by race, heredity, mom's age, the number of previous pregnancies and the use of fertility drugs and assisted-reproductive techniques. Fraternal twins occur in 1 out of every 100 pregnancies in white women compared to 1 out of every 79 pregnancies in black women. Certain areas of Africa have an incredibly high frequency of twins. In some places, twins occur once in every 20 births! Hispanic women also have a

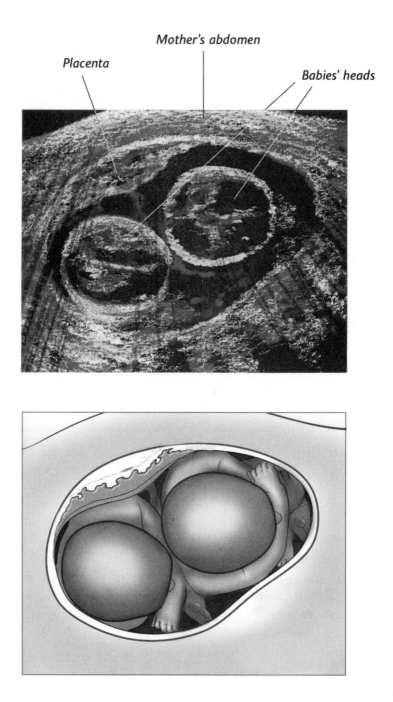

Ultrasound of twins shows two babies in the uterus.
If you look closely, you can see the two heads. The interpretive
illustration shows how the babies are lying.

slightly higher number of twin births. The occurrence of twins among Asians is less common—about 1 in every 150 births. In Japan, only 6 sets of twins are born per 1000 births, while in Nigeria that rate is over 7 times greater. In Nigeria, fraternal twins are born at a rate of 45 per 1000 births.

Heredity also plays a part. The incidence of fraternal twin births can run in families on the mother's side. In one study, the chance of a female twin giving birth to a set of twins herself was about 1 in 58 births. The study also showed if a woman is the daughter of a twin, she has a higher chance of having twins. Another study reported 1 out of 24 (4%) of twins' mothers was a twin herself.

If you've already given birth to a set of fraternal twins, your chance of having another set of twins *quadruples*! Reasons for multiple fetuses include the use of fertility drugs, in-vitro fertilization, women having babies later in life, some women having more children, being very tall or obese, recent oral contraception or taking large doses of folic acid.

Women having babies later in life accounts for nearly 35% of all multiple births. Age 30 seems to be the magic age beyond which the number of multiple births increases. Over 70% of all multiple births are to women over 30. In the United States, the highest number of multiple births occurs in women over 40; the next highest group is women between the ages of 30 and 39. Most twin births in older women are fraternal twins.

Some families are just more "blessed" than others. In one case we know of

personally, a woman had three single births. Her fourth pregnancy was twins, and her fifth pregnancy was triplets! She and her husband decided on another pregnancy; they were surprised (and probably relieved) when that pregnancy resulted in only one baby.

Discovering You're Carrying More than One Baby. Diagnosis of twins was more difficult before ultrasound was available. The illustration on page 318 shows an ultrasound of twins. You can see parts of both fetuses.

Measuring and examining you during pregnancy is important. Usually a twin pregnancy is noted during the second trimester because you're too big and growth seems too fast for one baby. Ultrasound is the best way to diagnose a multiple pregnancy.

Do Multiple Pregnancies Have More Problems? With a multiple pregnancy, the possibility of problems goes up. Possible problems include the following:

- increased risk of miscarriage and stillbirth
- birth defects
- low birthweight or growth restriction
- pre-eclampsia
- problems with the placenta or umbilical cord
- maternal anemia, bleeding or hemorrhage
- too much or too little amniotic fluid
- abnormal fetal presentations, such as breech or transverse lie
- premature labor

- difficult delivery and Cesarean delivery

Birth defects are more common among identical twins than fraternal twins. The incidence of minor problems is twice as high as it is in a single pregnancy, and major defects are also more common.

One of the biggest problems with multiple pregnancies is premature delivery. As the number of babies increases, the length of gestation and the birthweight of each baby decreases, although this is not true in every case.

The average length of pregnancy for twins is about 37 weeks. For triplets it's about 35 weeks. For every week the babies stay inside the uterus, their birthweights increase along with the maturity of organs and systems.

It's important to continue your pregnancy as long as possible; this may be achieved by bed rest. If your healthcare provider recommends bed rest, follow his or her advice. Some researchers believe use of a tocolytic agent (medication to stop labor) such as ritodrine is critical in preventing premature delivery. These medicines are used to relax the uterus to keep you from going into premature labor.

About 2% of all pregnancies are complicated by a surgical problem; the most common surgical condition is appendicitis. The second trimester is generally the safest time to perform any necessary surgery. Advantages of laparoscopic surgery include small incisions resulting in faster recovery, early return of bowel and gastrointestinal activity, smaller scars, less pain (requiring less pain medicine) and shorter hospitalization.

Weight gain is important. You may be advised to gain more than the normal 25 to 35 pounds, depending on the number of babies you carry. With twins, if you were normal weight before pregnancy, you may be advised to gain 40 to 54 pounds. With triplets, your weight gain may be between 50 and 60 pounds. If you're overweight, your healthcare provider will determine a recommended weight gain.

Follow your healthcare provider's instructions closely. Every day and every week you can keep the babies inside you are days or weeks you won't have to visit them in an intensive-care nursery while they grow, develop and finish maturing.

Delivering More than One Baby. How multiple fetuses are delivered often depends on how babies are lying in your uterus. Possible complications include abnormal presentation of one or more of the babies, the umbilical cord coming out ahead of the babies, placental abruption, fetal stress or bleeding after delivery.

Because risk is higher, safeguards are taken during labor and before delivery. These include an I.V., the presence of an anesthesiologist, the ability to perform an emergency Cesarean delivery and the availability and/or presence of pediatricians or other medical personnel to take care of the babies.

All possible combinations of fetal positions can occur. Both babies may come head first (vertex). They may come breech, meaning bottom or feet first. They may be lying sideways or oblique, meaning at an angle that is neither breech nor vertex. Or they may come in any combination of the above.

When both twins are head first, a vaginal delivery may be tried and may be accomplished safely. It may be possible for one baby to deliver vaginally, but the second one could need a Cesarean delivery if there are problems. Some healthcare providers believe delivery of multiples is more safely accomplished with a Cesarean delivery.

After delivery, healthcare providers pay close attention to bleeding in you because of the rapid change in the size of the uterus. It is overdistended with more than one baby. Medicine, usually oxytocin (Pitocin), is given by I.V. to contract the uterus to stop bleeding. Heavy blood loss could produce anemia and make a blood transfusion or long-term treatment with iron supplementation necessary.

If you're on the go and want a salad, buy a prepackaged bowl that contains dressing and toppings. It's a healthy choice on days you may be tempted to buy fast food.

Changes in You

Until this week, your visits to the healthcare provider have probably been on a monthly basis. At week 32, most healthcare providers begin seeing a pregnant woman every 2 weeks. This continues until the last month of pregnancy, then you'll probably switch to weekly visits.

By this time, you probably know your healthcare provider fairly well. Now is a good time to ask questions and to discuss concerns about labor and delivery. If there are complications or problems

later in pregnancy or at delivery, you'll be able to communicate better and know what's going on.

It may be harder to lose pregnancy weight after having twins, so stick to the weight goal your healthcare provider gives you. Carrying two babies causes more changes in your body, which may cause you to hold onto the weight you gain during pregnancy.

How Your Actions Affect Your Baby's Development

Do you wear contacts? You may want to wait until after baby is born to refill your contact-lens prescription. You may experience eye discomfort and irritation during pregnancy because of hormonal changes that change the curvature of the cornea. Hormones can also alter your vision slightly and dry your eyes. Don't use any products for dry eyes until you discuss it at a prenatal visit.

If you have problems, one solution is disposable contacts that correct for the changes. You might also try your old glasses if your contacts don't seem to work. Wait until after baby's birth to make any permanent changes. It can take up to 6 weeks for your vision to return to normal.

Your Nutrition

If you're expecting more than one baby, your nutrition and weight gain are very important during pregnancy. Food is your best source for nutrients, but take your prenatal vitamin every day. The ingredients in prenatal vitamins are

> ## Tip for Week 32
> • • • • • • • • • • •
>
> Your requirements for calories, protein, vitamins and minerals increase if you carry more than one baby. You'll need to eat about 300 calories a day more *per baby* than for a singleton pregnancy.

essential to your well-being and the well-being of your baby or babies.

Iron supplementation may be necessary. If you're anemic at the time of delivery, you might need a blood transfusion.

If you don't gain weight early in pregnancy, you have a higher chance of developing pre-eclampsia. Your babies may also be tiny.

Don't be alarmed when your healthcare provider discusses the amount of weight he or she wants you to gain. Studies show if you gain the targeted amount of weight with a multiple pregnancy, your babies are often healthier. In addition, gaining half of your weight by week 20 can help your babies, especially if they're born early.

Don't just add extra calories to your eating plan; get your calories from specific sources. Eat an extra serving of a dairy product and an extra serving of protein each day. These will provide you with the extra calcium, protein and iron necessary to meet the needs of your growing babies. Discuss the situation with your healthcare provider; he or she may suggest you see a nutritionist.

You Should Also Know

Cancer and Pregnancy

Pregnancy is a happy time for most women. Occasionally, however, serious problems can occur. Cancer in pregnancy is one serious complication that occurs rarely.

This discussion is included not to scare you but to provide you with information. It is not a pleasant subject to discuss, especially at this time. However, every woman should have this information available so you are informed if a serious problem occurs and to provide you with a resource to help you form questions for a dialogue with your healthcare provider if you wish to discuss it.

If you're now pregnant and you have had cancer in the past, tell your healthcare provider as soon as you find out you're pregnant. He or she may need to make decisions about individualized care for you during pregnancy.

Cancer during Pregnancy. Tremendous changes affect your body during pregnancy. Cancer during pregnancy is a rare occurrence and must be treated on an individual basis. Some researchers believe cancers influenced by increased hormones may increase in frequency during pregnancy. Increased blood flow may increase cancer in other parts of the body.

When cancer occurs during pregnancy, it can be very stressful. The healthcare provider must consider how to treat the cancer, but he or she is also concerned about the developing baby. How these issues are handled depends on when cancer is discovered. A woman's concerns may include the following.

- Will treatment or medications harm the baby?
- Will the malignancy affect the baby or be passed to baby?
- Will the pregnancy have to be terminated so the cancer can be treated?
- Can therapy be delayed until after delivery or after termination of the pregnancy?

Breast Cancer. Breast cancer is uncommon in women younger than 35. Fortunately, it's a rare complication of pregnancy. However, breast cancer is the most common type of cancer diagnosed during pregnancy. Of all women who have breast cancer, about 2% are pregnant at the time of diagnosis. Most evidence indicates pregnancy does not increase the rate of growth or spread of breast cancer. However, during pregnancy, it may be harder to discover breast cancer because of changes in the breasts.

Treatment of breast cancer during pregnancy varies. It may require surgery, chemotherapy and/or radiation. Recent studies indicate chemotherapy for breast cancer during pregnancy may be safe.

. . . .

Studies indicate pregnancy is safe in women with a history of breast cancer if the cancer has been successfully treated.

. . . .

A form of breast cancer you should be aware of is *inflammatory breast cancer (IBC)*. Although rare, it can occur during and after pregnancy and may be mistaken for mastitis (inflammation of the breast). Symptoms include swelling or pain in the breast, redness, nipple discharge and/or swollen lymph nodes above the collarbone or under the arm. You may feel a lump, although one is not always present.

If you experience any of these symptoms, do not panic! Nearly all of the time it will be a breast infection related to breastfeeding. However, if you're concerned, contact your healthcare provider. A biopsy is used to diagnose the problem. To learn more about IBC, visit www.ibcsupport.org.

Other Cancers. Cervical cancer is believed to occur about once in every 10,000 pregnancies. About 1% of women who have cancer of the cervix are pregnant when it's diagnosed. This cancer is curable, particularly when found and treated in its early stages.

Malignancies of the vulva, the tissue surrounding the vaginal opening, have been reported during pregnancy. It's a rare complication. Hodgkin's disease (a form of cancer) commonly affects young people. It occurs in about 1 of every 6000 pregnancies. Pregnancy does not appear to have a negative effect on the course of Hodgkin's disease.

Pregnant women who have leukemia have demonstrated an increased chance of premature labor or increased bleeding after pregnancy. Leukemia is usually treated with chemotherapy or radiation therapy.

Melanoma is a cancer derived from skin cells that produce melanin (pigment). A malignant melanoma can spread through the body. Pregnancy may cause symptoms or problems to worsen. A melanoma can spread to the placenta and baby.

Bone tumors are rare during pregnancy. However, two types of noncancerous bone tumors can affect pregnancy and delivery. These tumors, *endochondromas* and *benign exostosis*, can involve the pelvis; tumors may interfere with labor. The possibility of having a Cesarean delivery is more likely with these tumors.

Exercise for Week 32

• • • • • • •

Breath training decreases the amount of energy you need to breathe and improves the function of your respiratory muscles. Practice the different breathing exercises below for benefits in the near future (labor and delivery!).

- Breathe in through your nose, and exhale through pursed lips. Making a little whistling sound is OK. Breathe in for 4 seconds and out for 6 seconds.
- Lie back, propped on some pillows, in a comfortable position. Place your hand on your tummy while breathing. If you breathe using your diaphragm muscles, your hand will move up when you inhale and down when you exhale. If it doesn't, try using different muscles until you can do it correctly.
- Bend forward to breathe. If you bend slightly forward, you'll find it's easier to breathe. If you feel pressure as your baby gets bigger, try this technique. It may offer some relief.

Week 33

Age of Fetus—31 Weeks

How Big Is Your Baby?

Your baby weighs about 4¼ pounds (1.9kg) by this week. Its crown-to-rump length is about 12 inches (30cm), and total length is nearly 17¼ inches (44cm).

How Big Are You?

Measuring from the pubic symphysis, it's about 13¼ inches (33cm) to the top of the uterus. Measurement from your bellybutton to the top of your uterus is about 5¼ inches (13cm). Total weight gain should be between 22 and 28 pounds (9.9 and 12.6kg).

How Your Baby Is Growing and Developing

Placental Abruption

The illustration on page 328 shows placental abruption—premature separation of the placenta from the uterine wall. Normally, the placenta doesn't separate from the uterus until *after* baby is delivered. Placental abruption occurs in about 1 in every 80 pregnancies. The time of separation can vary. If it separates at the time of delivery and the infant is delivered without incident, it's not as significant as a placenta separating during pregnancy.

The cause of placental abruption is unknown. Certain conditions may increase the chance of it happening, including physical injury to the mother, a short umbilical cord, sudden change in the size of the uterus from water breaking, high blood pressure, dietary deficiency, a uterine abnormality and previous surgery on the uterus.

Studies indicate that folic-acid deficiency may play a role. Other researchers suggest smoking and alcohol use may make a woman more likely to have placental abruption.

A woman who has had placental abruption is at risk it will recur. Rate of recurrence has been estimated to be as high as 10%. This can make a subsequent pregnancy a high-risk pregnancy.

The fetus relies entirely on the placenta for its circulation. The situation is most severe when the placenta totally separates from the uterine wall. The fetus no longer receives blood from the umbilical cord, which is attached to the placenta.

Symptoms of placental abruption can vary. There may be heavy bleeding from

326

the vagina, or you may experience no bleeding at all. Vaginal bleeding occurs in about 75% of all cases. Other symptoms can include lower-back pain, tenderness of the uterus or abdomen, and contractions or tightening of the uterus.

Serious problems, such as shock, may occur with rapid loss of large quantities of blood. A large blood clot can also be a problem. Factors that clot the blood may be depleted, which can make bleeding a problem.

Ultrasound may help diagnose the problem but doesn't always provide an exact diagnosis. This is particularly true if the placenta is located at the back of the uterus where it can't be seen easily with ultrasound examination.

Can Placental Abruption Be Treated? Treatment varies based on the ability to diagnose the problem and the status of the mother and baby. With heavy bleeding, delivery of the baby may be necessary. When bleeding is not heavy, the problem may be treated more conservatively. This depends on whether the fetus is stressed or if it appears to be in immediate danger.

Placental abruption is one of the most serious problems related to the second and third trimesters of pregnancy. If you have any symptoms, call your healthcare provider immediately!

Changes in You

Fibroid Tumors

Fibroid tumors develop in the uterine wall or on the outside of the uterus. Most women with fibroids do not have problems during pregnancy, but pregnancy hormones can make fibroids grow larger.

Research shows if you have fibroids, you may have a higher chance of having problems during pregnancy. Fibroids can slightly increase the chance of miscarriage, especially if growths are large. Placental abruption may occur more readily if the placenta embeds itself over a large fibroid. Fibroids have also been known to block the opening to the cervix. Discuss the situation with your healthcare provider if you have questions.

Sleep Apnea

About 2% of all pregnant women develop sleep apnea during pregnancy, which means airways narrow and you stop breathing briefly, then resume normal breathing. This can occur up to 100 times a night, which can greatly disturb your sleep!

Lack of oxygen causes your body to release adrenaline and cortisol, which raises blood pressure and releases sugar into the bloodstream. Over time, this release of sugar into your blood may increase your risk of developing diabetes.

When it occurs during pregnancy, sleep apnea has been linked to high blood pressure, gestational diabetes, fatigue and cardiovascular problems in a mom-to-be. Some women with sleep apnea are at higher risk for developing pre-eclampsia. It can also negatively affect baby's growth and development.

Some women need a CPAP (continuous positive-airway pressure) machine to breathe more healthfully during sleep. A mask is placed over your nose and

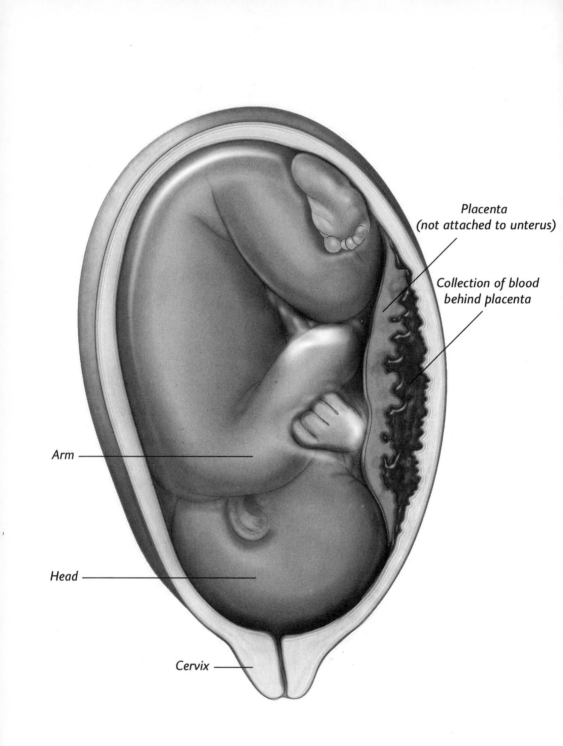

Placenta (not attached to unterus)

Collection of blood behind placenta

Arm

Head

Cervix

This illustration of placental abruption shows that the placenta has separated from the wall of the uterus.

> ## *Dad Tip*
> . . . .
>
> Is your home safe for your new baby? Things to consider when thinking about safety include pets, furniture, second-hand and third-hand smoke, window coverings or other things that could pose a danger to your little one. Start now to check for problems so you'll have time to take care of them before baby's birth.

mouth to deliver continuous air during sleep so you keep breathing. The good news is obstructive sleep apnea often disappears after baby is born.

When Your Water Breaks

Membranes around the baby that contain the amniotic fluid are called the *bag of waters*. These membranes help protect baby from infection. They usually don't break until just before labor begins, when labor begins or during labor.

Sometimes membranes break earlier in pregnancy. See the discussion below. After your water breaks, your risk of infection increases, so you need to take precautions. An infection could be harmful to your baby.

When your water breaks, there is often a gush of amniotic fluid, usually followed by leakage of small amounts of fluid. Amniotic fluid is usually clear and watery, but it may have a bloody appearance or it may be yellow or green. Women describe their water breaking as a constant wetness or water running down their leg when they stand.

Call your healthcare provider immediately when your water breaks. Tests can be done to see if your water has broken. One is a *nitrazine test*; when amniotic fluid is placed on a small strip of paper, it changes color. Another test is a *ferning test*. Amniotic fluid or fluid from the back of the vagina is taken with a swab and placed on a slide for examination under a microscope. Dried amniotic fluid looks like a fern or branches of a pine tree. Ferning may be more helpful in diagnosing ruptured membranes.

Premature Rupture of Membranes (PROM). Premature rupture of membranes (PROM) occurs when membranes rupture earlier in pregnancy. There are two categories of premature rupture. *Premature rupture of membranes (PROM)* refers to rupture of fetal membranes before the onset of labor and occurs in 8 to 12% of all pregnancies.

Preterm-premature rupture of membranes (PPROM) refers to rupture of fetal membranes *before* 37 weeks of pregnancy; it occurs in 1% of all pregnancies. The exact cause is unknown. Black/African-American women appear to have a higher incidence of PPROM than white women. Smoking is strongly correlated with PPROM. Vitamin and mineral deficiencies have also been considered causes. Uterine bleeding has been strongly tied to PPROM; infection also plays an important role in many cases. If you had PPROM with a previous pregnancy, you have a 35% chance it will occur again.

Tip for Week 33
. . . .

Don't stop eating or start skipping meals as your weight increases. You and your baby need the calories and nutrition you receive from a healthy diet.

If ruptured membranes are not detected and treated within 24 hours, infection and other serious complications may occur. A test called *Amnisure* is available to diagnose whether membranes have ruptured prematurely. The test detects a protein found in amniotic fluid. A sterile swab is inserted into the vagina, and a sample is taken. Results are available in about 10 minutes.

How Your Actions Affect Your Baby's Development

You may be gaining weight faster than at any other time during pregnancy. However, you're not putting on most of this weight—baby is! Your baby is growing and may be gaining as much as 8 ounces (½ pound) or more every week.

Heartburn may become more of a problem as baby crowds your stomach. Eating several small meals a day may make you more comfortable.

Hepatitis

Hepatitis is a serious viral infection of the liver. It's one reason all pregnant women are screened for hepatitis B at the beginning of pregnancy.

When people talk about hepatitis, it can be confusing. Six different forms of hepatitis have been identified. However, the two most common forms are hepatitis A (HAV) and hepatitis B (HBV), which we discuss here.

. . . .

We are not completely certain of the safety of the hepatitis-A vaccine. However, it's made from dead viruses, so risks may be low. Hepatitis-B vaccine is safe to receive during pregnancy but is suggested only for women who are at high risk.

. . . .

Hepatitis A (HAV). Hepatitis A (HAV) accounts for 50% of all hepatitis cases in the United States. It is transmitted by the oral-fecal path, such as drinking contaminated water, eating contaminated food or touching something contaminated with feces then touching your mouth. Fortunately, the occurrence of HAV during pregnancy is less than 1 in 1000. Symptoms include fever, malaise, anorexia, nausea, abdominal pain and jaundice.

A pregnant woman will not pass hepatitis A to her developing baby. If a pregnant woman is exposed, she may be given hepatitis immune gamma globulin to help protect her from getting the disease.

Serious complications from HAV are rare. Treatment is rest and a healthful diet. Usually a woman with hepatitis A recovers within a few months.

Hepatitis B (HBV). Hepatitis B (HBV) accounts for over 40% of all cases of hepatitis in the United States. More than 15,000 pregnant women have HBV; sexual transmission accounts for most cases. People at risk include those with a history of sexually transmitted diseases, intravenous drug use or exposure to people with HBV or to blood products that contain HBV.

During pregnancy, HBV can be passed from mother to baby. Between 10 and 20% of all babies born to moms who test positive get the disease. An infant can also get it through close contact with its mother and by breastfeeding.

HBV symptoms include nausea, flu-like symptoms, jaundice, dark urine and pain in or around the liver or upper-right abdomen. Some symptoms of HBV, such as nausea and vomiting, are common in normal pregnancies, so testing is important. Nearly half of all cases of HBV in adults have no symptoms.

If blood tests show a woman doesn't have HBV antibodies, she should be vaccinated immediately. The HBV vaccine is safe during pregnancy. She may also need to receive immune globulin.

It is now recommended that all babies be vaccinated against HBV at birth, then again at 1 week, 1 month and 6 months after birth. Ask your pediatrician about it.

Your Nutrition

Eating a well-balanced diet of fresh fruits and vegetables, dairy products, whole-grain products and protein contributes to baby's healthy development. You may be concerned about what foods to avoid. Some foods may be OK to eat when you're not pregnant but should be avoided or treated with more care now.

When possible, avoid food additives. We aren't certain how they can affect a developing baby, but if you can avoid them, do so.

. . . .
Don't eat alfalfa sprouts, radish sprouts or mung beans during pregnancy; they often have germs.
. . . .

Fresh produce can carry lots of germs; fruits and vegetables can also carry pesticides. Use soap and water to wash produce to remove any contaminants. Even if you don't eat the peel, contaminants can get on your hands if an item isn't washed. After washing, peel the fruit or vegetable if that's the way you normally eat it. If you're not going to peel it but just cut through it, rinse the skin well. If it's a root vegetable or one with grooves, like some melons, clean it with a brush, soak in a bowl of water, then rinse under running water.

Many fruits and vegetables are over 75% water, so eating them increases your fluid intake. Cook some vegetables whole to retain more vitamins. To increase your intake of some veggies, purée them and add them to sauces. For example, cook and purée carrots and add them to a spaghetti sauce.

Butternut squash is low in calories, high in beta-carotene, folate and potassium, and full of fiber and vitamin A. It may help protect you against high blood pressure and increase your immunity to illnesses. Asparagus is high in folate. Black beans are high in potassium and fiber; potassium may help control your blood pressure.

A medium artichoke is low in calories and full of folate, potassium, iron, magnesium and vitamins A, C and K. Use artichoke hearts in an omelet or casserole or top some with Parmesan cheese and bread crumbs then bake.

You Should Also Know

Whooping Cough (Pertussis)

In the last 15 years, the incidence of whooping cough, also called *pertussis*, has increased. The disease we see today is a milder form, but it still produces a nagging cough that can last a long time.

Nearly everyone has been vaccinated with the dTAP vaccine (diphtheria, pertussis and tetanus). But immunity decreases over time, leaving many people at risk. If it's been 2 years since your last tetanus/diphtheria shot, think about getting a booster.

The disease begins as a cold with a mild cough, then intense coughing begins. A person coughs until no air is left in the lungs, then takes a deep breath that produces a heaving, whooping sound. Coughing attacks may occur up to 40 times a day. Coughing may be followed by vomiting. The disease can last up to 8 weeks, and you may cough for months afterward.

If you have any symptoms of whooping cough, call your healthcare provider immediately! The faster the infection is treated, the sooner you'll feel better.

Will You Have an Episiotomy?

An *episiotomy* has been one of the most commonly performed procedures in obstetrics and has almost become routine in some places. In 2000, nearly a third of women giving birth vaginally had an episiotomy. However, many experts believe it's being used less frequently today. Many healthcare providers now let tissue between the vagina and rectum tear naturally during childbirth.

The need for an episiotomy usually becomes evident when baby's head is in the vagina. An episiotomy is necessary if a vacuum extractor or forceps will be used during the birth.

* * * * * * * *

Prenatal perineal massage started after 34 weeks of pregnancy may reduce a woman's need for an episiotomy. It may also reduce pain after childbirth. It's most helpful for first-time moms. If you're interested, discuss it with your healthcare provider.

* * * * * * * *

An episiotomy is a controlled, straight cut made from the vagina toward the rectum during delivery. It's done to help avoid tearing as baby's head passes through the birth canal. An incision may be better than a tear or rip that could go in many directions. After delivery, layers are closed with absorbable sutures that don't require removal.

Benefits of an episiotomy for a woman include less relaxation of pelvic organs with prolapse, less chance of stool and/or urine incontinence and lower likelihood of sexual dysfunction. Benefits to a baby may include more rapid delivery. However, there are disadvantages to an episiotomy. Research shows it may lead to a more-difficult recovery, sexual problems and an increased chance of incontinence.

* * * * * * * *

Some experts believe torn vaginal tissue may heal more easily than an episiotomy.

* * * * * * * *

The American Congress of Obstetricians and Gynecologists (ACOG) recommends restricted use of episiotomy, rather than routine use. Ask your healthcare provider why an episiotomy might be done and whether you will have any say in this procedure.

The description of an episiotomy includes a description of the depth of the incision. A first-degree episiotomy cuts only the skin. A second-degree episiotomy cuts the skin and underlying tissue. A third-degree episiotomy cuts the skin, underlying tissue and rectal sphincter, which is the muscle that goes around the anus. A fourth-degree episiotomy goes through the three layers and the rectal mucosa.

After baby's birth, epifoam may be prescribed. It is useful in treating the pain and itching of an episiotomy. Other medications are also safe to use, even if you breastfeed your baby. Acetaminophen with codeine or other medications may be prescribed for pain.

Exercise for Week 33

· · · · · · ·

Stand with your feet slightly apart and your knees soft, with arms by your side. Hold your tummy in. Using light weights (2 to 3 pounds each to start; if you don't have weights, use a 16-ounce can), raise your left arm to the front and your right arm to the rear; stop just below shoulder height. Don't swing your arms; control the movement. Lower your arms to the starting position. Repeat 16 times, alternating the arm to the front. *Strengthens upper body.*

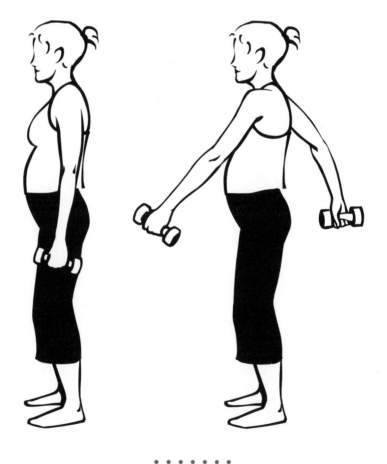

· · · · · · ·

Week 34

Age of Fetus—32 Weeks

How Big Is Your Baby?

Your baby weighs almost 4¾ pounds (2.15kg) by this week. Its crown-to-rump length is about 12¾ inches (32cm). Total length is 17¾ inches (45cm).

How Big Are You?

Measuring from your bellybutton, it's about 5½ inches (14cm) to the top of your uterus. From the pubic symphysis, it measures about 13½ inches (34cm). When your uterus grows larger at an appropriate rate, it's a sign of normal growth of baby.

. . . .

By this time, baby may turn its head in the direction of a noise.

. . . .

How Your Baby Is Growing and Developing

An ideal test to do before delivery would be able to detect fetal stress, which could indicate a problem. Ultrasound enables healthcare providers to see the baby inside the uterus, as well as to evaluate the brain, heart and other organs. Along with ultrasound, a nonstress test (NST) and a contraction stress test (CST) can indicate well-being and/or problems.

Changes in You

Stress Incontinence

During the last trimester, you may leak a little urine when you cough, sneeze, exercise or lift something. Don't panic! This is called *stress incontinence*; it's normal as your uterus grows and puts pressure on your bladder.

. . . .

One in three women experiences light bladder leakage during pregnancy.

. . . .

You can help control the problem by doing the Kegel exercise; see Week 14. Practice it now, and continue after baby arrives. It can also help you with incontinence that sometimes occurs after a baby's birth.

Bring up incontinence at a prenatal visit. It will give your healthcare provider the opportunity to rule out a urinary-tract infection, which may also cause incontinence.

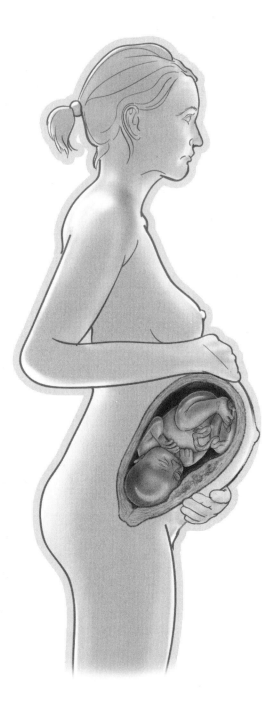

Comparative size of the uterus at 34 weeks of pregnancy
(fetal age—32 weeks). The uterus can be felt about 5½ inches
(14cm) above your bellybutton.

Physical Changes You Might Experience

A few weeks before labor begins or at the beginning of labor, you may notice a change in your abdomen. Measurement from your bellybutton or pubic symphysis to the top of the uterus may be smaller than on a previous prenatal visit. This occurs as the head of the baby enters the birth canal and is called *lightening*.

With lightening, you may have more room in your upper abdomen, giving you more room to breathe. However, you may feel more pressure in the area of your pelvis, bladder and rectum, which can make you uncomfortable. Some women have the uncomfortable feeling the baby is "falling out," which is also related to pressure baby exerts as it moves down in the birth canal.

Another feeling that may occur around this time is a "pins-and-needles" sensation. It's tingling, pressure or numbness in the pelvis or pelvic region from the pressure of the baby. It's common and shouldn't overly concern you.

The feelings described above may not be relieved until after delivery. Lying on your side may help lessen pressure on the nerves, vessels and arteries in the pelvic area. If the problem is severe, talk to your healthcare provider about it.

When you are examined, your healthcare provider may tell you your baby is "not in the pelvis" or "is high up." He or she is saying the baby has not yet come into the birth canal. If your healthcare provider says your baby is "floating" or "ballotable," it means part of the baby is felt high in the birth canal but is not fixed there. Baby may even move away from your healthcare provider's fingers when you're examined.

Don't be concerned if you don't notice the baby drop. It doesn't occur with every woman or with every pregnancy. It's common for baby to drop as labor begins or during labor.

* * *

Are you going to paint baby's room? Use nontoxic paint.

* * *

Braxton-Hicks Contractions and False Labor

Ask your healthcare provider to describe the signs of labor contractions. They are usually regular and increase in length and strength over time. You'll notice a regular rhythm to real labor contractions. Time them to know how often they occur and how long they last. When you go to the hospital may depend in part on your contractions.

Braxton-Hicks contractions are painless contractions you may be able to feel when you place your hand on your tummy. They often begin early in pregnancy and are felt at irregular intervals. They may increase in number and strength when the uterus is massaged. They are not positive signs of true labor.

False labor may occur before true labor begins. False-labor contractions can be painful and may feel like real labor to you. See the box on page 338. In most instances, they are irregular and short (less than 45 seconds). False contractions don't get longer, stronger or closer together, and they are often felt in the front of the body. With false labor, you may feel discomfort in the groin, lower abdomen or back. With true labor,

True Labor or False Labor?

Considerations	True Labor	False Labor
Contractions	Regular	Irregular
Time between contractions	Comes closer together	Does not get closer together
Contraction intensity	Increases	Doesn't change
Location of contractions	Entire abdomen	Various locations or back
Cervical change	Progressive cervical change	No cervical change
Effect of anesthetic or pain relievers	Will not stop labor	Sedation may stop or alter frequency of contractions

contractions produce pain that starts at the top of the uterus and spreads over the entire uterus, through the lower back into the pelvis. They start in the back and move to the front.

False labor seems to occur more often in women who have been pregnant before. It usually stops as quickly as it begins.

How Your Actions Affect Your Baby's Development

The end of your pregnancy begins with labor. Some women are concerned (or hope!) their actions can cause labor to begin. The old wives' tales about going for a ride over a bumpy road or taking a long walk to start labor aren't true. Going about your daily activities (unless your healthcare provider has advised bed rest) will not cause labor to start before baby is ready to be born.

Sex during late pregnancy may bring on labor. Semen contains prostaglandins that can cause contractions. Orgasm and nipple stimulation may also touch off uterine contractions.

Some parents believe baby should sleep with them in a "family bed." Many experts do not believe family bed sharing is safe. Discuss this practice with your pediatrician; safety is important.

Your Nutrition

It's a waste of time to have your cholesterol level checked during pregnancy. The level of cholesterol in your blood rises during pregnancy due to hormonal changes. Wait until after baby's birth or you stop breastfeeding to check your cholesterol.

A Vitamin-Rich Snack

When you're looking for something to snack on, you might not think of a baked potato, but it's an excellent snack! You get protein, fiber, calcium, iron, B vitamins and vitamin C when you eat one.

> ## Dad Tip
> · · · · · · · · · · ·
>
> Preregister at the hospital to save time when you finally get there for baby's birth. Ask your partner to ask at your healthcare provider's office, or ask about preregistering in your prenatal classes. If office personnel or prenatal instructors don't know, call the hospital and ask.

Bake up a few, and store them in the refrigerator. Heat one up when you're hungry. Broccoli is another food filled with vitamins. Add it to your baked potato, and top both with some plain yogurt, cottage cheese or nonfat sour cream for a delicious treat!

You Should Also Know

Getting Ready for Baby

Your baby will need many things when it comes home from the hospital. You might want to start thinking now about things baby will need so you don't get caught short if baby comes a little early.

All that baby gear you see in stores, in magazines and online looks great, doesn't it? But before you buy it all, stop and take stock of what you'll really need. Talk to friends and family members about what they absolutely had to have. You *must* have a car seat for baby to ride in when you are traveling in a vehicle. You'll also need diapers and some clothes and a place for baby to sleep. Receiving and/or swaddling blankets are pretty important. Think about these things and ask questions before investing lots of time, money and energy in acquiring things that may just gather dust.

A word of caution: be careful about buying second-hand nursery equipment or borrowing someone else's. Some items might not meet current safety standards. Before you make a purchase, check out various safety features; they help ensure baby's safety.

Car Seats. The most important piece of baby equipment you can buy is a car seat; choose one soon so you'll have it when baby is born. Once you've selected a car seat, go to your local police or fire station, and ask them to show you how to install it correctly.

Buy a new car seat—don't get a used one or borrow one from someone. You want the most up-to-date, safest car seat available. Your baby needs to ride in a car seat *every time* he rides in a car—it's the law in all 50 states.

A car seat is the best protection your baby has in case of an accident. The safest place for baby's seat is the middle of the back seat. Don't take him out of the car seat for feeding, changing or comforting while the car is moving. From the time your baby goes home from the hospital, he should ride in a car seat. One report found an average of 35 babies a year die in auto accidents on the way home from the hospital. Don't let your baby become a statistic.

There are different types of car seats available. When choosing one, be

> ## Tip for Week 34
> • • • • • • • • • • •
>
> A strip of paper, tape or a bandage can help cover a bellybutton that is sensitive or poking through your clothing.

certain it meets the safety standards of the JMPA, the CPSC and the AAP.

Pets in the Home

Nearly all pet owners consider their pets part of the family. You may have a pet that is your "baby," but now you're expecting a real baby. As soon as you learn you're pregnant, start preparing your pet for baby's arrival. An animal is sensitive to a routine, so make changes before baby is born.

If your pet has never been around an infant, he doesn't understand the changes that are going to occur when you bring baby home. Unfortunately, this can lead to behavior problems. Some things that might help include:

- find him a new sleeping area
- keep him out of your room
- let him sniff all the baby equipment you bring into the house
- play a CD of baby sounds to help desensitize him to these unusual sounds before baby comes home
- give him pet toys that don't look like baby toys and remove toys that he could confuse with baby's toys

Make any necessary changes in your pet's feeding, exercise or play schedule now. If you plan to rearrange furniture or change the functions of a room, do it early in your pregnancy to allow the animal to become familiar with the new organization.

• •

Be sure your pet is up to date on vaccinations. Have your vet check for parasites. If your pet isn't neutered, now may be the time to do it—it can help reduce aggression.

• •

An older pet may be less flexible about adding baby to the household. It may sulk, ignore you or beg for attention. Your pet may also be jealous of the time and attention you give baby. You may have to set aside some time alone with an older pet.

Some pets carry a bacteria that causes UTIs in humans. Washing hands for at least 10 seconds after patting or caring for a pet can help lower your risk. Pet foods that aren't well processed may be contaminated with salmonella. Always be sure to wash hands well after handling any pet food.

Introducing Your Dog to Baby. Pay attention to your dog's response to a baby crying. If you find your dog gets distressed, you may have to leave him with a friend or board him for a while. If you discover your dog has a tendency to bite, you may need to consider getting rid of him. You might want to consider training classes for your dog. Obedience classes can teach a dog to follow simple commands.

Introducing Your Cat to Baby. If you have a cat, you know how unpredictable she can be. It's best to keep a cat away from baby when possible; let the cat watch from a distance. If the cat slinks toward baby, it's a sign of aggression; if she shows signs of aggression, remove the cat from the area. Reward your cat for any positive actions, such as staying off furniture.

Cats usually adjust to a new baby more easily than dogs. However, cats are curious, so set up any new furniture early so kitty has a chance to check it out before baby's arrival. Don't let your cat sleep on baby furniture. Cover the crib with a mesh cover sold exclusively for this purpose. Or fill the crib with balloons—cats don't like them, especially when they pop!

Other Household Pets. Birdcages need to be cleaned every day. Wear rubber gloves; wash the gloves in bleach water and wash hands thoroughly when you're finished. Bird waste is highly toxic and may harbor bacteria. Keep birds in the cage.

Keep pocket pets, such as hamsters, mice, gerbils and guinea pigs, in their cages, away from baby. Many of these pets carry salmonella. If you have a ferret, keep it away from your baby. They have been known to attack children.

The CDC advises keeping children younger than 5 years old away from all pet reptiles. If you have a pet reptile, you may want to consider getting rid of it. They can be a source of life-threatening salmonella infections. A child can become infected from handling a reptile or by handling objects contaminated with a reptile's feces. Some cases have been reported in infants who never touched the reptiles. Researchers believe infants were infected when they were held by those who handled the reptiles!

Vasa Previa

Vasa previa is a condition in which blood vessels of the umbilical cord cross the interior opening of the cervix, lying close to it or covering it. When the cervix dilates or membranes rupture, unprotected vessels can tear or become squeezed together, which shuts off blood and oxygen to the baby. It can also occur when baby drops into position for delivery and presses on the vessels, which shuts off blood supply to baby.

Detecting the problem can be achieved with a 5-second scan with color ultrasound. The test looks at vessels lying across the cervical opening and measures the speed of the blood flow. Different rates of blood flow have distinct colors and reveal the location of the fetal blood vessels. However, this screening is not routine.

Diagnosis is difficult because there are no symptoms. Risks include placenta previa, painless bleeding, previous uterine surgery or D&C, pregnancy with multiples and in-vitro fertilization. If you have any of these risk factors, discuss having the color ultrasound with your healthcare provider.

When a woman is diagnosed with vasa previa, she may be put on bed rest the third trimester to help prevent labor.

A Cesarean delivery is done after 35 weeks of pregnancy, with a success rate of over 95%.

A "Bloody Show" and Mucus Plug

After a vaginal exam or at the beginning of early labor and early contractions, you may bleed a small amount. This is called a *bloody show*; it may occur as the cervix stretches and dilates. You should not lose a lot of blood. If it causes you concern or appears to be a large amount of blood, call your healthcare provider immediately.

Along with a bloody show, you may pass a *mucus plug*. A mucus plug creates a barrier between the vagina and uterus to protect the uterus and baby. It keeps bacteria from entering the uterus. Losing the mucus plug poses no danger to you or baby.

A mucus plug may be clear, pink, brownish or reddish in color. It may be dislodged in small pieces, or it may come out in one large piece. Losing the mucus plug can be a sign your body is preparing for labor, but it doesn't mean labor is at hand.

Timing Contractions

Most women learn in prenatal classes or from their healthcare provider how to time contractions during labor. It's important to time how long a contraction lasts and to know how often contractions occur. You can choose from two methods to do this. Ask your healthcare provider which method he or she prefers.

1. Note the time period from when a contraction starts to the time the next contraction starts. This is the most commonly used method and the most reliable.

2. Note the time period from when a contraction ends to the time the next contraction starts.

Your healthcare provider will want this information so he or she can decide when you should go to the hospital.

. . . .

You'll know it's time to head for the hospital when contractions are 4 to 5 minutes apart for at least an hour. They'll also be increasing in intensity and length, and coming closer together.

. . . .

Exercise for Week 34

· · · · · · ·

Sit on the edge of a chair. Using light weights (2 to 3 pounds each to start; if you don't have weights, use a 16-ounce can), raise your arms to shoulder level, and bend your elbows so you can point your hands toward the ceiling. Slowly bring your elbows and arms together in front of your face. Hold for 4 seconds, then slowly open to shoulder-width. Repeat 8 times; work up to 20 times. *Tightens breast muscles to help keep breasts from sagging.*

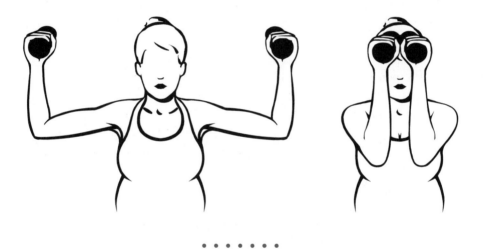

· · · · · · ·

Week 35

Age of Fetus—33 Weeks

How Big Is Your Baby?

Your baby now weighs over 5¼ pounds (2.4kg). Crown-to-rump length is about 13¼ inches (33cm), and total length is 18¼ inches (46cm).

How Big Are You?

It's about 6 inches (15cm) to the top of your uterus from your bellybutton. From the pubic symphysis, the distance is about 14 inches (35cm). By this week, your total weight gain should be between 24 and 29 pounds (10.8 and 13kg).

How Your Baby Is Growing and Changing

How Much Does Your Baby Weigh?

You've probably asked your healthcare provider several times how big your baby is or how much baby might weigh when it's born. This is one of the most frequently asked questions.

Ultrasound can be used to estimate baby's weight. Several measurements are used in a formula. Many believe ultrasound is the best way to estimate weight. However, estimates may vary as much as half a pound (225g) or more in either direction.

Even with a weight estimate, we can't tell if baby will fit through the birth canal. It's usually necessary for you to labor to see how baby fits into your pelvis and if there is room for it to pass through the birth canal.

In some women who appear to be average or better-than-average size, a 6- or 6½-pound (2.7 to 2.9kg) baby won't fit through the pelvis. Experience also shows women who are petite are sometimes able to deliver 7½-pound (3.4kg) or larger babies without much difficulty. The best test or method of assessing whether baby will deliver through your pelvis is labor.

. . . .

Baby's sucking reflex develops before birth.

. . . .

Umbilical-Cord Prolapse

With *umbilical-cord prolapse*, the umbilical cord is pushed out of the uterus when the cord passes alongside or past part of baby. Umbilical vessels are compressed, shutting off blood and oxygen to baby. It's a life-threatening emergency for baby. Fortunately, it's rare.

Tip for Week 35
• • • • • • • • • • •

Maternity bras provide extra support to your growing breasts. You may feel more comfortable wearing one during the day and at night while you sleep.

The situation may occur when there's a poor fit between the part of the baby entering the birth canal and the mother's bony pelvis. Abnormal fetal presentations, including breech, transverse lie and oblique lie, can increase the risk.

Prolapse is twice as likely to occur when a baby weighs less than 5½ pounds or when the mother-to-be has given birth at least twice before. Excessive amounts of amniotic fluid also increase the risk—when membranes rupture, the large amount of fluid released can cause the cord to pass beyond baby.

• •

Shingles occurs more often in people who are older, but it can and does occur in younger people. It can be very painful; treatment involves pain medications. A pregnant woman is at risk during the first trimester because a viral infection may affect the fetus. Around the time of delivery, the baby could contract the virus from mom. If you think you have shingles, contact your healthcare provider, who can decide on treatment for you.

• •

When the situation occurs, the healthcare provider may have to keep his or her hand inside the woman's vagina to lift the presenting part of the baby off the cord until baby can be delivered by Cesarean delivery. Lowering a woman's head or changing her position may help. Filling the woman's bladder to elevate the fetal head a little may also be done.

If steps are taken promptly to deal with the situation and deliver the baby, there is usually a good outcome.

Changes in You

Shoes and Feet

Your feet may change and/or grow during pregnancy. This can happen as your baby grows and you add pregnancy pounds. If it does (and it happens to many women!), don't panic. Give up your tie-on and strap-on shoes for slip-ons; they're much easier to get in and out of. Opt for flats—high heels and platform shoes can be dangerous. Sandals are great when they offer support. Buy a good pair.

Consider adding foot treatments to your list of "must dos"—foot massages and pedicures can help make your feet and legs feel great. A pedicure can also help you keep your toenails trimmed—a tough job when you can't even see your feet!

Emotional Changes in Late Pregnancy

As you get closer to delivery, you may become more anxious about the events to come. You may have more mood swings, or you may be more irritable. You may be concerned about insignificant or unimportant things.

While these emotions rage inside you, you'll notice you're getting bigger

Lactation Consultants

. . . .

If you want to breastfeed, it may help to consult with a lactation specialist before baby's birth. A lactation consultant is a qualified professional who can help with breastfeeding issues. Ask your healthcare provider for more information, or check at the hospital where you plan to deliver to see if they have lactation consultants on staff. For more information, see Appendix C, page 426.

and aren't able to do things you used to do. You may feel uncomfortable, and you may not be sleeping well. These things can all work together to make your emotions swing wildly from highs to lows.

Your concern about baby's health and well-being may increase during the last weeks of pregnancy. You may also fret about how well you'll tolerate labor and how you'll get through delivery. You may be concerned about whether you'll be a good mother. Emotional changes are normal; be ready for them. Talk with your partner; you may be surprised to discover he has concerns about you, the baby and his role during labor and delivery. Talking may help you understand what the other is feeling and experiencing.

Discuss emotional problems with your healthcare provider. He or she may be able to reassure you that what you're going through is normal. Take advantage of prenatal classes and information available about pregnancy and delivery.

How Your Actions Affect Your Baby's Development

Preparing for Baby's Birth

You may be feeling a little nervous about knowing when it's time to call your healthcare provider or go to the hospital. At one of your prenatal visits ask about signs to watch for. By knowing what to do, and when, you can relax a little and not worry about the beginning of labor and delivery.

During the last few weeks of pregnancy, have your suitcase packed and ready to go. See the list in Week 36 for some helpful suggestions for things you might want or need when you get to the hospital.

If possible, tour hospital facilities with your partner a few weeks before your scheduled due date. Find out where to go and what to do when you get there. Plan your route to the hospital. Have your partner drive it a few times. Plan an alternate route in case of bad weather or traffic tie-ups.

Talk with your partner about the best ways to reach him; cell phones have made it easy to stay in touch. You might have him check with you periodically.

Preregistering at the Hospital

It may save you time if you register at the hospital a few weeks before your due date. You'll be able to do this with forms you get at the office or from the hospital. It's smart to do this early because when you go to the hospital, you may be in a hurry or concerned with other things.

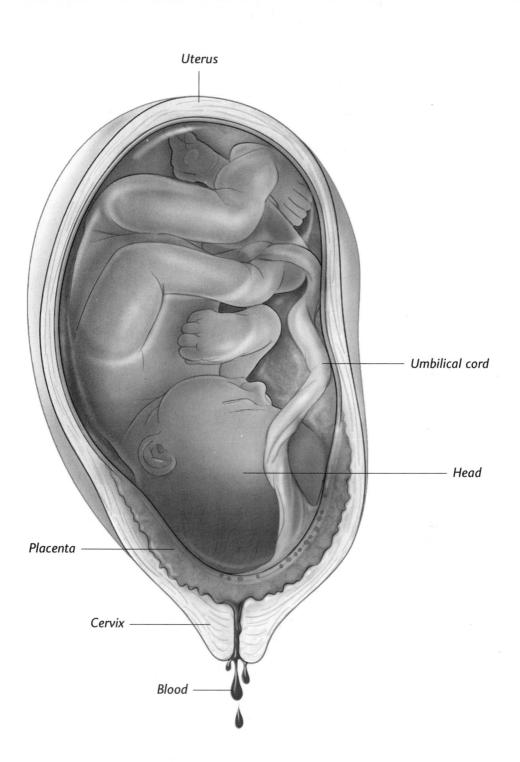

Uterus

Umbilical cord

Head

Placenta

Cervix

Blood

In this illustration of total placenta previa, note how the placenta
completely covers the cervical opening to the uterus.

> ### Dad Tip
> · · · · · · · · · · ·
> At a prenatal visit, ask the healthcare provider about your part in the delivery. There may be some things you'd like to do, such as cutting the cord or recording baby's birth. It's easier to talk about these things ahead of time. Not every new father wants an active role in the delivery. That's OK, too.

You should know certain facts that may not be included in your chart, such as your blood type and Rh-factor, the date of your last period, what your due date is and details of any past pregnancies. Write down your healthcare provider's name and your pediatrician's name.

Your healthcare provider has recorded various things that have occurred during your pregnancy. A copy of this record is usually kept in the labor-and-delivery area.

Elective Delivery

Have you heard about an elective delivery and wondered what it is? An *elective delivery* is the delivery of a baby for a non-medical reason before its due date. Some women want to deliver before they go into labor because they are uncomfortable. Other nonmedical reasons include wanting the baby born on a specific date or because baby's father will not be able to be present at the birth on the due date.

With elective delivery, there has been a trend toward earlier deliveries. This can be detrimental for baby if baby is born before he or she is fully developed. Research indicates babies are healthier if they remain in the womb until they are ready to be born. Allowing baby to be born at term may actually prevent some life-long problems.

Women should wait until at least 39 weeks of pregnancy to choose elective delivery. The difference a couple of weeks can make is dramatic. Studies indicate baby does a great deal of developing in the last 4 weeks of pregnancy. If all organs are not fully developed at birth, baby is at greater risk. For example, a baby's brain at 39 weeks weighs 1/3 more than it does at 35 weeks. Lungs and liver are also more developed. Compared to babies born at 39 weeks, studies show babies born at 37 weeks were twice as likely to have seizures, heart problems or trouble breathing.

Early elective delivery may not be good for you either. You may have harder, longer labor contractions. Early elective delivery can prolong labor because medications or procedures must be used to start labor. It can also increase the risk of having a Cesarean delivery. And higher rates of postpartum distress have been noted.

Some hospitals prohibit elective early deliveries. And some insurance companies deny payment for early deliveries performed for nonmedical reasons.

Your Nutrition

Your body continues to need lots of vitamins and minerals for baby. You'll

Nutrient Requirements during Pregnancy and Breastfeeding

· · · · · · · · · ·

Vitamins and Minerals	Pregnancy	Breastfeeding
A	800mcg	1300mcg
B$_1$ (thiamine)	1.5mg	1.6mg
B$_2$ (riboflavin)	1.6mg	1.8mg
B$_3$ (niacin)	17mg	20mg
B$_6$	2.2mg	2.2mg
B$_{12}$	2.2mcg	2.6mcg
C	70mg	95mg
Calcium	1200mg	1200mg
D	10mcg	10mcg
E	10mg	12mg
Folic acid (B$_9$)	400mcg	280mcg
Iron	30mg	15mg
Magnesium	320mg	355mg
Phosphorous	1200mg	1200mg
Zinc	15mg	19mg

need even more of them if you breast-feed! Above is a chart showing your daily vitamin-and-mineral requirements during pregnancy and breastfeeding. It's important to realize how necessary your continued good nutrition is for you and your baby.

You Should Also Know

Ultrasound in the Third Trimester

If you have an ultrasound exam in the third trimester, your healthcare provider is looking for particular information. Performed later in pregnancy, this test can:

- evaluate baby's size and growth, or check for IUGR
- determine the cause of vaginal bleeding, or vaginal or abdominal pain
- evaluate baby after an accident or injury to the mother-to-be
- monitor a high-risk pregnancy
- detect some birth defects
- monitor the growth of multiples
- measure the amount of amniotic fluid
- check whether baby is head first
- determine which delivery method to use
- find out the maturity of the placenta
- be used with amniocentesis to determine fetal lung maturity
- be used as part of a biophysical profile

What Is Placenta Previa?

With *placenta previa*, the placenta attaches to the lower part of the uterus instead of the upper wall; it lies close to the cervix or covers it. The illustration on page 347 shows placenta previa.

Placenta previa is serious because of the chance of heavy bleeding during pregnancy or during labor. There are three main types of placenta previa:

- placenta touches the cervix (low-lying placenta)
- placenta partially covers the cervix (partial placenta previa)
- placenta completely covers the cervix (total placenta previa)

The cause of placenta previa is not completely understood. Risk factors include previous Cesarean delivery, over age 30, smoking and delivery of several babies. A woman who conceives with in-vitro fertilization also has a greater chance of developing placenta previa.

The most characteristic symptom of placenta previa is painless bleeding without contractions. This doesn't usually occur until close to the end of your second trimester or later. Bleeding may occur without warning and may be extremely heavy.

Placenta previa should be considered when a woman has vaginal bleeding during the second half of pregnancy. Ultrasound is used to identify the problem because a physical exam may cause heavier bleeding. Ultrasound is accurate in the second half of pregnancy because the uterus and placenta are bigger and things are easier to see.

Your healthcare provider may advise you not to have a pelvic exam if you have placenta previa. This is important to remember if you see another healthcare provider or when you go to the hospital.

Babies are usually delivered by Cesarean delivery. The baby is delivered first, then the placenta is delivered so the uterus can contract, and bleeding can be kept to a minimum.

Exercise for Week 35

• • • • • • •

Stand with your feet apart, knees softly bent. Raise your arms so your upper arms are parallel to the floor and your hands point up into the air. Squeeze your shoulder blades together, hold for 3 seconds, then release. Do 10 times. *Improves posture, and relieves upper-back stress.*

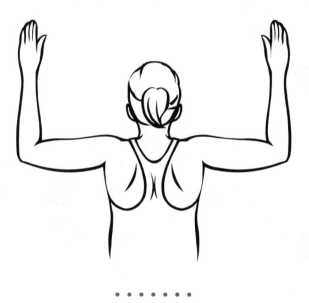

• • • • • • •

Week 36

Age of Fetus—34 Weeks

How Big Is Your Baby?

By this week, your baby weighs about 5¾ pounds (2.6kg). Its crown-to-rump length is over 13½ inches (34cm), and total length is 18⅔ inches (47cm).

How Big Are You?

From the pubic symphysis, it's about 14½ inches (36cm) to the top of the uterus. From your bellybutton, it's more than 5½ inches (14cm) to the top of the uterus.

How Your Baby Is Growing and Developing

An important part of baby's development is maturing of its lungs and respiratory system. The respiratory system is the last system to mature. Knowing how mature a baby's lungs are helps in deciding about early delivery if it must be considered. Tests can predict whether baby will be able to breathe without assistance.

Respiratory-distress syndrome (RDS), also called *hyaline membrane disease*, occurs when lungs aren't mature, and baby can't breathe on its own after birth. The baby may require a machine to breathe for it.

Several fetal-lung-maturity tests can be done before birth. Two methods for evaluating fetal-lung maturity require amniocentesis. The *L/S ratio* is done around 34 weeks of pregnancy. The test measures the ratio between lecithin and sphingomyelin, and the result indicates if baby's lungs are mature. With the *phosphatidyl glycerol (PG)* test, if phosphatidyl glycerol is present in amniotic fluid, the infant will probably not have respiratory distress at birth.

Changes in You

You have only 4 to 5 weeks until your due date. You may have gained 25 to 30 pounds (11.25 to 13.5kg), and you still have a month to go. It isn't unusual for your weight to stay the same or change very little at your weekly visits after this point.

The maximum amount of amniotic fluid surrounds baby now. In the weeks to come, your body reabsorbs some amniotic fluid, reducing the amount of room in which baby has to move. You may notice a difference in fetal movements. For some women, it feels as if baby isn't moving as much as it has been.

Restless-Leg Syndrome (RLS)

You may have restless-leg syndrome (RLS) for the first time during pregnancy; it can rob you of sleep. If you develop RLS, you feel a sensation in your legs that makes you feel as if you must move your lower limbs. Experts suggest RLS may be linked to anemia and could be caused by an iron or folic-acid deficiency.

Treatment includes increasing your iron intake and taking folic acid. Talk to your doctor before you do either. Applying a heating pad for 15 to 20 minutes may help. The good news is RLS often disappears completely after baby's birth.

What Is Labor?

It's important to understand the labor process. You'll be more informed when labor begins, and you'll know what to do. *Labor* is defined as the stretching and thinning (dilatation) of your cervix. This happens when the uterus, which is a muscle, tightens and relaxes to squeeze out the baby. The cervix must also soften and thin out (become effaced). As baby is pushed out, the cervix stretches and opens to 10cm (about 4 inches) for your baby to pass through it. (See the cervical dilation chart on page 354.)

We don't know what causes labor to begin, but there are many theories. One is hormones made by the mother and baby together trigger labor. Or the baby might produce a hormone that causes the uterus to contract.

At various times, you may feel tightening, contractions or cramps, but it isn't actually labor until there is a change in the cervix. As you can see from the discussion below, there are many aspects to labor. You'll go through them all to deliver your baby.

Every labor is different, in great part because of the level of pain you experience. Be aware that contractions can hurt.

Three Stages of Labor. There are three distinct stages of labor. In *stage one*, labor begins with uterine contractions of great enough intensity, duration and frequency to soften and dilate the cervix. The first stage ends when the cervix is fully dilated (10cm) and open enough to allow baby's head to come through it.

Stage two of labor begins when the cervix is completely dilated. This stage ends with the delivery of baby. *Stage three* begins after baby's birth and ends with delivery of the placenta and the membranes that have surrounded the fetus.

Some doctors have described a *fourth stage* of labor, referring to a time after delivery of the placenta during which the uterus contracts. Contraction of the uterus is important in controlling bleeding after delivery.

How Long Will Labor Last? The length of the first and second stages of labor can last 14 to 15 hours or more in a first pregnancy. The average length of active labor is between 6 and 12 hours. When you hear about a long labor, most of the time is spent in early labor. Contractions may start and stop, then get regular and strong.

A woman who has already had one or two children will probably have a shorter

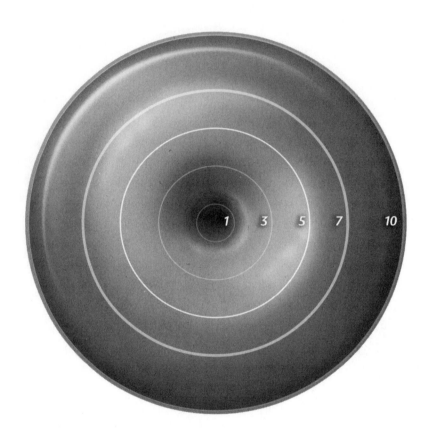

Cervical dilatation in centimeters (shown actual size).

Tip for Week 36
• • • • • • • • • •

To find a pediatrician for baby, ask for referrals. Your pregnancy doctor might be able to give you one. Or ask family, friends or people in your childbirth-education classes for names of doctors they like.

labor, but don't count on that either! The average time for labor usually decreases by a few hours for a second or third delivery.

Everyone's heard of women who barely made it to the hospital or had a 1-hour labor. For every one of those women, there are others who have labored 18, 20, 24 hours or longer. It's impossible to predict how long labor will last.

Women who listen to instrumental music (synthesizer, harp, piano, orchestra or jazz) for 3 hours during early phases of active labor experience less pain and distress. We believe the slow music helps a woman relax and distracts her from her pain.

How Your Actions Affect Your Baby's Development

Choosing Your Baby's Doctor

It's time to choose a doctor for your baby. You might choose a pediatrician, a doctor who specializes in treating children, or you might choose a family practitioner. If the doctor you are seeing during pregnancy is a family practitioner and you want him or her to care for baby, you're probably set.

It's good to meet the person who will care for baby before the birth—many pediatricians welcome it. It gives you an opportunity to discuss important matters with this new doctor.

The first visit is important, so ask your partner to go with you. You can discuss any concerns or questions about the care of your baby. Ask about the doctor's philosophy, and learn his or her schedule and "on-call" coverage.

When baby is born, baby's doctor will come to the hospital to check him or her. Selecting a pediatrician before the birth ensures your baby will see the same doctor for follow-up visits at the hospital and at the doctor's office.

Questions to Ask a Pediatrician. The questions below may help you when you talk with your pediatrician. You will probably also have other questions.

- What are your qualifications and training? Are you board certified? If not, will you be soon?
- What hospital(s) are you affiliated with? Do you have privileges at the hospital where I will deliver?
- Will you do the newborn exam? If I have a boy, will you perform the circumcision (if we want to have it done)?
- What is your availability for regular office visits and emergencies? How long is a typical office visit? Can an acutely ill child be seen the same day?

- How can we reach you in case of an emergency or after office hours?
- Who responds if you're not available? Do you have advance-practice nurses or physician assistants in your office?
- Do you return phone calls the same day? Can we contact you by email if we have routine questions? How soon do you respond?
- Are you interested in preventive, developmental and behavioral issues?
- Do you provide written instructions for well-baby and sick-baby care?
- Do you support women in their efforts to breastfeed?
- What are your fees? Do your fees comply with our insurance?
- What is the nearest (to our home) emergency room or urgent-care center you would send us to?

Analyzing Your Visit. Some issues can be resolved only by analyzing your feelings after your visit. Below are some things you and your partner might want to discuss.

- Are the doctor's philosophies and attitudes acceptable to us, such as use of medications, child-rearing practices or related religious beliefs?
- Did the doctor listen to us? Did he or she seem interested in our concerns?
- Is the office comfortable, clean and bright? Did the office staff seem cordial and easy to talk to?

By choosing someone to care for your baby before it's born, you have a chance to take part in deciding who will have that important task. If you don't, the healthcare provider who delivers your baby or hospital personnel will select someone. Another good reason for choosing someone ahead of time is if your baby has complications, you'll at least have met the person who will be treating him or her.

Your Nutrition

You may be having a harder time with your food plan than you had earlier in pregnancy. You may be bored with the food you've been eating. Baby is getting bigger, and you don't seem to have much room for food. Heartburn or indigestion may be more challenging now.

Don't give up on good nutrition! Continue to pay attention to what you eat so you can give your baby the best nutrition you can before its birth. Every day, try to eat one serving of a dark-green leafy vegetable, a serving of food or juice rich in vitamin C and one serving of a food rich in vitamin A. Many yellow foods, such as yams, carrots and cantaloupes, are good sources of vitamin A.

Keep up your fluid intake. Eat high-fiber foods for good nutrition and to help with constipation and heartburn. Keep the peel on your potatoes! They add fiber, potassium, calcium, vitamin C and vitamin B_6 to your diet. You can even mash cooked potatoes that still have the peel—they're very tasty.

You Should Also Know

How Is Your Baby Presenting?

You probably want to know at what point in your pregnancy your doctor can tell how baby is presenting for delivery. Is the baby's head down, or is the baby breech? At what point will the baby stay in the position it's in?

Usually between 32 and 34 weeks of pregnancy, you can feel baby's head in the lower abdomen below your umbilicus. Some women can feel different parts of the baby earlier than this, but baby's head may not have been hard enough until now to identify it. Baby's head has a distinct feeling; it's different from the feeling your doctor gets with a breech presentation. A breech baby has a soft, round feeling.

Beginning at 32 to 34 weeks, your doctor may feel your abdomen to determine how baby is lying inside you. This position may change many times during pregnancy.

At 34 to 36 weeks of pregnancy, baby usually gets into the position it's going to stay in. If you have a breech at 37 weeks, it's possible the baby can still turn to be head-down, but it becomes less likely the closer you get to the end of your pregnancy. (See Week 38 for further discussion.)

Packing for the Hospital

Packing for the hospital can be unnerving. You don't want to pack too early and have your suitcase staring at you. But you don't want to wait until the last minute, throw your things together and take the chance of forgetting something important.

It's a good idea to pack about 3 or 4 weeks before your due date. Pack things you'll need during labor for you and your labor coach, items you and baby will need after delivery and personal articles for your hospital stay. There are a lot of things to consider, but the list below should cover nearly all of what you might need:

- completed insurance or preregistration forms and insurance card
- 1 cotton nightgown or T-shirt, plus heavy socks, to wear during labor
- lip balm, lollipops, fruit drops or breath spray to use during labor
- books, magazines, an iPad or tablet to use during labor
- 1 or 2 nightgowns to wear after labor (bring a nursing gown if you're going to breastfeed)
- slippers with rubber soles
- 1 long robe for walking in the halls
- 2 bras (nursing bras if you breastfeed) and breast pads for leaking breasts
- 3 pairs of panties
- toiletries, including brush, comb, toothbrush, toothpaste, soap, shampoo, conditioner
- hair band or ponytail holder if you have long hair
- loose-fitting clothes for going home
- sanitary pads if the hospital doesn't supply them
- glasses (you can't wear contacts during labor)

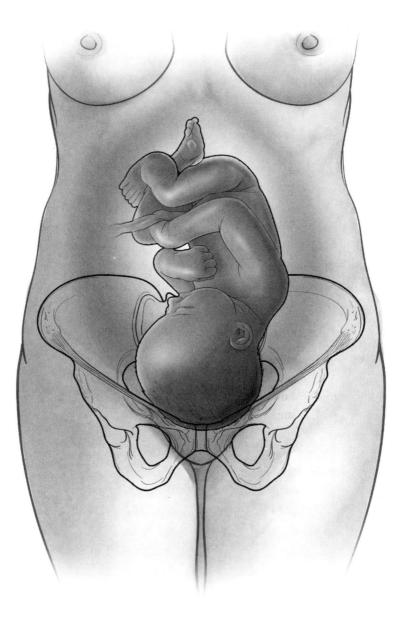

Alignment of baby with head in pelvis before delivery.
This is the preferable presentation.

You may also want to bring one or
two pieces of fruit to eat after the delivery. Don't pack them too early!

It's a good idea to include some
things in your hospital kit for your
partner or labor coach to help you both
during the birth. You might bring the
following:

- a watch with a second hand
- an item to use as a focal point
- talc or cornstarch for massaging
  you during labor
- a paint roller or tennis ball for
  giving you a low-back massage
- music downloaded on your MP3
  player, iPod or phone to listen to
- a camera
- cell-phone charger
- list of telephone numbers
- change for vending machines
- snacks for your partner or labor
  coach

The hospital will probably supply
most of what you need for baby, but you
should have a few things:

- clothes for the trip home, including an undershirt, sleeper, outer
  clothes (a hat if it's cold outside)
- a couple of baby blankets
- diapers if your hospital doesn't
  supply them

Be sure you have an approved infant
car seat for baby's first ride. Many hospitals won't let you take your baby home
without one.

What You May See in
the Delivery Room

You'll see lots of equipment when you
enter the labor and/or delivery room.
You won't recognize most of it, so below
are descriptions of equipment you may
encounter.

An *electronic vital-signs monitor* measures your heart rate and blood pressure
with a cuff to tell healthcare providers
how well you and baby are doing. *I.V.
infusion pumps* deliver fluids into your
veins if fluids are ordered.

There are various types of *birthing
beds*. In many, the bottom section can
be removed, converting the bed into a
delivery table. Some beds can also ac-
commodate alternate birthing positions.

An *epidural pump* delivers pain-relief
medication after a catheter is put in
place by an anesthesiologist. A *vacuum
extractor* helps baby through the birth
canal in some cases. An *amniohook* looks
like a crochet hook; it's used to rupture
membranes. *Suction bulbs* are used to
draw blood and mucus from baby's nose

and mouth after birth. An *infant warmer* helps stabilize baby's temperature. An *infant scale* weighs him or her.

Fetal Monitoring

A fetal monitor detects baby's heart rate and contractions; the readout is seen in the labor room, nurses' station and possibly on your healthcare provider's computer.

Every baby needs to be evaluated individually using fetal-monitor tracing and other information about your pregnancy. ACOG recommends the use of three categories to describe the results of fetal monitoring.

- *Category I*—Tracings are normal.
- *Category II*—Tracings are indeterminate; this means they aren't normal, but they aren't absolutely abnormal. They require evaluation, continued surveillance and re-evaluation. Eighty percent of all tracings fall into this category.
- *Category III*—Tracings are abnormal and require prompt evaluation. Elements used to categorize them include fetal heart rate, variability, decelerations and reaction to contractions.

Exercise for Week 36

· · · · · · ·

To help improve your posture, stand or sit on the floor, and clasp your hands behind you. Lift your arms until you feel a good stretch in your upper-chest area and upper arms. Hold for a count of 5, then lower your arms. Repeat 8 times. *Stretches arm and back muscles, and opens upper chest.*

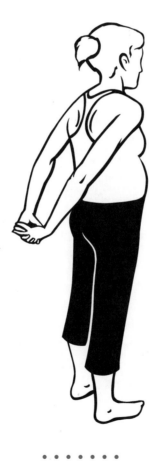

· · · · · · ·

Week 37

Age of Fetus—35 Weeks

How Big Is Your Baby?

Your baby weighs almost 6⅓ pounds (2.8kg). Crown-to-rump length is 14 inches (35cm). Its total length is around 19 inches (48cm).

How Big Are You?

Measuring from the pubic symphysis, the top of the uterus is about 14¾ inches (37cm). From the bellybutton, it is 6½ to 6¾ inches (16 to 17cm). Your total weight gain by this time should be about as high as it will go at 25 to 35 pounds (11.3 to 15.9kg).

How Your Baby Is Growing and Developing

Your baby is gaining weight, even during these last few weeks. Baby's head is usually directed down into the pelvis around this time. But in about 3% of pregnancies, the baby's bottom or legs enter the pelvis first, called a *breech presentation*; see Week 38.

. . . .

A change in pressure on your tummy, such as laying a book there, may cause baby to react by kicking vigorously.

. . . .

Changes in You

Pelvic Exam in Late Pregnancy

Your healthcare provider may do a pelvic exam to help evaluate your pregnancy. One of the first things he or she will look for is whether you're leaking amniotic fluid. If you think you are, it's important to tell your healthcare provider.

Your birth canal and cervix will be examined. The birth canal is like a tube going from the pelvic girdle through the pelvis and out the vagina. The baby travels through this tube from the uterus. During labor, the cervix usually becomes softer and thins out. Your cervix may be evaluated for its softness or firmness and the amount of thinning.

Before labor begins, the cervix is thick. When you're in active labor, the cervix thins out; when it is half-thinned, it is "50% effaced." Immediately before delivery, the cervix is "100% effaced" or completely thinned out.

The amount the cervix is open is also important. This is measured in centimeters. The cervix is fully open when the diameter of the cervical opening measures 10cm. The goal is to be a 10! Before labor begins, the cervix may be closed or open a little way, such as 1cm (nearly ½ inch).

You will be checked to see if baby's head, bottom or legs are coming first; this may be referred to as the "presenting part." The shape of your pelvic bones is also noted.

The station is then determined. Station describes the degree to which the presenting part of the baby has descended into the birth canal. If the baby's head is at a -2 station, it means the head is higher inside you than if it were at a +2 station. The 0 point is a bony landmark in the pelvis, the starting place of the birth canal.

. . . .

It may be difficult at times to tell the exact location of different parts of the baby. You may have a good idea according to where you feel kicks and punches. Ask your healthcare provider to show you on your tummy how the baby is lying. Some take a marking pen and draw on your stomach to show you how baby is lying. Leave it so you can later show your partner how baby was lying when you were seen in the office.

. . . .

Your healthcare provider may describe your situation in medical terms. You might hear you are "2cm, 50% and a -2 station." This means the cervix is open 2cm (about 1 inch), it is halfway thinned out (50% effaced) and the presenting part (baby's head, feet or buttocks) is higher inside the birth canal.

Write down this information and have it at hand when you go to the hospital and are checked there. You can tell the medical personnel what your dilatation and effacement were at your last checkup so they can determine if your situation has changed.

How Your Actions Affect Your Baby's Development

Cesarean Delivery

Most women plan on a vaginal birth, but a Cesarean delivery is always a possibility. With a Cesarean, the baby is delivered through an incision made in the mother's abdominal wall and uterus. An *emergency Cesarean delivery* is one that is unplanned. An *elective Cesarean delivery* is planned.

The illustration on page 366 shows a Cesarean delivery. Other names for this type of surgery include *C-section* and *Cesarean section*.

The main advantage to having a Cesarean delivery is delivery of a healthy infant. A Cesarean may be the safest way for your baby to be born. The disadvantage is Cesarean delivery is a major operation and carries with it all the risks of surgery.

It would be nice to know you're going to need a Cesarean so you wouldn't have to go through labor. Unfortunately, we don't know beforehand whether you will have problems.

. . . .

It's possible for you to dilate during labor without the baby moving down through the pelvis. When baby's head is too large to fit through the birth canal, it results in failure to progress. This situation is one of the most common reasons for a Cesarean delivery.

. . . .

Some women believe if they have a Cesarean, "it won't be like having a baby." They falsely believe they won't experience the birth process. That's not true. If you have a Cesarean delivery and deliver a healthy baby, you haven't failed in any way!

Remember, having a baby has taken 9 long months. Even with a Cesarean delivery, you have accomplished an amazing feat.

Reasons for Cesareans. Cesareans are often performed when there's a problem during labor. The most common reason for having one is a previous Cesarean delivery. Nine out of 10 women who had a Cesarean delivery choose a repeat Cesarean for the next birth. Other reasons for having a Cesarean include maternal choice, more conservative practice guidelines and legal pressures. A Cesarean delivery may be performed if:

- you're exhausted when you begin labor
- you have pre-eclampsia or an active herpes sore
- baby is too big to fit through the birth canal, called *cephalo-pelvic disproportion (CPD)*
- an ultrasound shows your baby is 9½ pounds or larger
- baby shows signs of fetal stress
- the umbilical cord is compressed
- you're older
- baby is in a breech presentation
- you have placental abruption or placenta previa

Some women who have had Cesareans may be able to have a vaginal delivery with later pregnancies; this is called *vaginal birth after Cesarean (VBAC)*. See the discussion that begins on page 367.

Rising Rate of Cesarean Deliveries. In 1965, only 4% of all deliveries were by C-section. Today in the United States, Cesarean deliveries account for over 30% of all deliveries. In some areas, this percentage is even higher.

The rising rate is related in part to closer monitoring during labor and safer procedures for Cesarean deliveries. Part of the increase can also be attributed to the increase in multiple births, but the Cesarean rate actually increased more for singletons than for multiples.

Elective Cesarean Deliveries. Part of the increase in Cesarean deliveries in the United States is due to Cesarean delivery on maternal request (CDMR). It is also called *patient-requested Cesarean*. There are many reasons a woman may think she wants a Cesarean delivery, including fear of labor, concern over vaginal tearing and worry about incontinence. Some women believe a Cesarean will help them retain their prepregnancy figure; others believe a Cesarean is safer for baby.

In many Latin American countries, the rate of elective Cesareans is 40 to 50%. One survey conducted in Brazil showed private hospitals, where the wealthiest patients go, had an 80 to 90% rate of elective Cesareans.

U.S. doctors are split on the question of elective Cesarean delivery. There's evidence supporting both sides. Some believe with improved anesthesia, infection control and pain management, a Cesarean is no riskier than vaginal delivery. However, many believe we

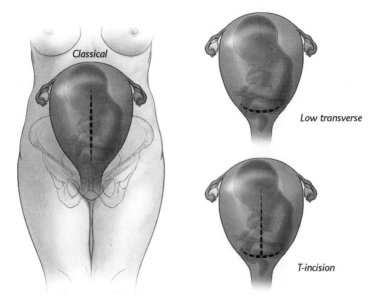

Classical

Low transverse

T-incision

Three common Cesarean incisions; the low-transverse incision is the one most commonly used.

should look more closely at the present Cesarean-delivery rate.

The point in pregnancy when a Cesarean is scheduled is important. ACOG recommends a Cesarean delivery not be scheduled any earlier than 39 weeks unless tests show the baby's lungs are mature. Research shows a baby will do better if he or she is born within 7 days of its due date.

. . . .

Babies delivered by a scheduled Cesarean delivery between 37 and 39 weeks have more respiratory problems than babies born vaginally or by emergency Cesarean at the same point in pregnancy. It's believed hormones released during labor help baby deal with fluid in the lungs. The compressions of baby's chest from labor are also believed to help clear amniotic fluid from baby's lungs.

. . . .

How Is a Cesarean Delivery Performed?
In most areas, an obstetrician performs a Cesarean. In small communities, a general surgeon or a family practitioner may perform Cesarean deliveries.

If you're scheduled to have a Cesarean, follow directions for eating before surgery. You are often awake when a Cesarean is done. If you are awake, you may be able to see your baby immediately after delivery!

You're first visited by the anesthesiologist to discuss pain-relief methods. Up to 90% of all elective Cesarean deliveries are done with spinal anesthesia.

Today, most Cesarean deliveries are *low-cervical Cesareans* or *low-transverse Cesareans*. This means the incision is made low in the uterus. Or a *T-incision* may be used. It goes across and up the uterus in the shape of an inverted T to

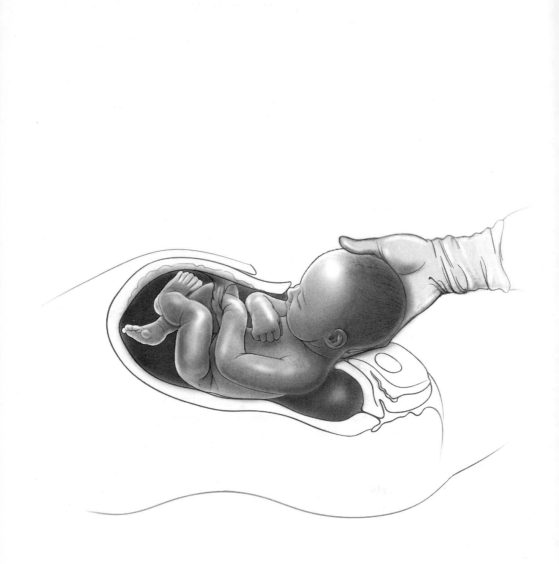

Delivery of a baby by Cesarean section.

provide more room to get baby out. If you have a T-incision, you may need a Cesarean delivery with all subsequent pregnancies.

After you receive anesthesia, your doctor makes a 5- to 6-inch incision in the area above your pubic bone, through tissue down to the uterus. There a horizontal incision is made into the lower part of the uterus. After all incisions are made, the doctor reaches into the uterus and removes the baby, then the placenta. Each layer is sewn together with absorbable sutures; the entire procedure takes 30 minutes to an hour.

In the past, a Cesarean was often done with a *classical incision*, in which the uterus was cut down the midline. This incision doesn't heal as well and is more likely to pull apart with contractions. If a woman had a classical Cesarean section, she must have a Cesarean delivery every time she has a baby.

After Your Cesarean Delivery. If you're awake for baby's birth, you may be able to hold him or her immediately. You may also have a chance to begin nursing.

You may need pain relief for the incision. *ON-Q* is a device to help deal with pain after a Cesarean. A small catheter is inserted underneath the skin to send a local painkiller to the incision area so very little, if any, medication gets to baby through breast milk. Studies show moms who use ON-Q are able to get out of bed and walk around sooner, and hospital stays are shorter. Ask your healthcare provider about it at a prenatal visit.

You'll probably stay in the hospital 2 to 4 days. Recovery at home from a Cesarean delivery takes longer than recovery from a vaginal delivery; usually full recovery takes 4 to 6 weeks.

. . . .

For a discussion of depression after pregnancy—postpartum distress syndrome—see Appendix B, page 423.

. . . .

Vaginal Birth after Cesarean (VBAC)
Should you attempt a vaginal delivery after having had a Cesarean delivery? In some cases, you may not have any choice in the matter. In other cases, you and your healthcare provider may decide to let you labor for a while to see whether you can deliver vaginally. Medically speaking, the method of delivery isn't as important as the well-being of you and your baby.

Research indicates up to 65% of women who have had a Cesarean delivery with their first baby may be successful if they choose to have a vaginal delivery with their second baby. However, one study shows nearly 90% of women who delivered their first baby by Cesarean delivery also had a Cesarean with their second child. Studies show women younger than 25 are most likely to try to deliver their second baby by VBAC.

The reason a Cesarean delivery was done with the first baby impacts on the success of a vaginal birth with the next baby. If a woman failed with induced labor with the first baby, and that was the reason for a Cesarean delivery, she is twice as likely to fail with VBAC with her second child.

ACOG states if a woman has had only one or two Cesarean deliveries, she can try to deliver her next baby vaginally if the incision for her previous C-section was low and horizontal. They also state that 24-hour availability of emergency care is necessary for VBAC to be attempted.

Some women like having a repeat Cesarean delivery because they don't want to go through labor only to end up with a Cesarean delivery. Discuss it with your healthcare provider.

Reasons Not to Choose VBAC. If you are small and the baby is large, you may need another Cesarean. Multiple fetuses may also make vaginal delivery difficult or impossible without danger to the babies.

Inducing labor with VBAC may be necessary; however, there's an increased risk of the uterine scar from the earlier Cesarean stretching and pulling apart with induction. This is especially true if hormones are used to ripen the cervix and/or induce labor. Contractions may be too strong for a uterus scarred by previous surgery. A repeat Cesarean may be advised to avoid rupturing the uterus.

Risk also increases for a woman who gets pregnant within 9 months of having a previous Cesarean. In this case, the uterus is more likely to rupture during a vaginal delivery because it can take from 6 to 9 months for the uterine scar to heal (this is the scar on the uterus—not your abdomen). The uterus may not be strong enough to stand up to the stress of a vaginal delivery. VBACs are safest when at least 18 months have passed between the previous Cesarean and the attempted vaginal delivery.

VBAC Advantages. Advantages of VBAC include a decreased risk of problems associated with Cesarean surgery. Recovery after a vaginal delivery is shorter. You can be up and about in the hospital and at home in a much shorter amount of time.

If you want to try VBAC, discuss it with your healthcare provider in advance so plans can be made. Consider the benefits and risks, and discuss them with your partner before making a final decision. Don't be afraid to ask your healthcare provider his or her opinion of your chances for a successful vaginal delivery. He or she knows your health and pregnancy history.

If you decide to try VBAC, you may have to deliver at a different hospital; not all hospitals are equipped for VBAC. During labor, you will probably be monitored more closely. You may be attached to I.V.s in case a Cesarean delivery becomes necessary.

Your Nutrition

You and your partner have been invited to a big party. You've been careful about your nutrition, and your pregnancy is almost over. Should you let yourself go

> ## *Dad Tip*
> . . . .
> You may not understand how nervous your partner may be about getting in touch with you when she needs you. Be sure to let her know how she can reach you at work or when you're out. Keep your cell phone with you all the time. This can comfort her and provide her with peace of mind.

and eat and drink whatever you want? Probably not. Maintain your good eating habits, and party healthfully. Before you go, eat or drink something to take the edge off your appetite. It may be easier to avoid high-fat, high-calorie foods if you're not ravenous.

At the party, eat food when it's fresh or hot. As the party goes on, food may not be chilled or heated enough to prevent bacteria from growing. Eat early or when dishes are refilled.

Avoid alcohol. Drink fruit juice "spiked" with ginger ale or lemon-lime soda. If it's the holiday season and they're serving eggnog, have a glass if it's pasteurized and alcohol-free.

Raw fruits and vegetables can be satisfying. Avoid raw seafood, raw meat and soft cheeses, such as Brie, Camembert and feta; they may contain listeriosis.

Stay away from the refreshment table if you can't resist the goodies. It may feel better to sit down (away from food), relax and talk with friends.

. . . .

If a woman experiences gestational diabetes during pregnancy, she should undergo a glucose-tolerance test within 12 weeks of delivery to make sure she does not have prediabetes or diabetes.

. . . .

You Should Also Know

Will You Have an Enema?

Will you be required to have an enema when you arrive at labor and delivery? An *enema* is a procedure in which fluid is injected into the rectum to clear out the bowel. An enema before labor can make the birth of your baby more pleasant for you. When the baby's head comes out through the birth canal, anything in the rectum also comes out. An enema decreases the amount of contamination from feces during labor and at the time of delivery, which may also help prevent infection.

Most hospitals offer an enema at the beginning of labor, but it's not always mandatory. There are certain advantages to having one early in labor. You may not want to have a bowel movement soon after your baby's birth because of discomfort. Having an enema before labor can prevent this discomfort.

Ask your healthcare provider if an enema is routine or considered helpful. Tell him or her you'd like to know about the benefits of an enema and the reasons for giving one. It isn't required by all doctors or all hospitals.

What Is Back Labor?

Some women experience back labor. *Back labor* refers to a baby coming through the birth canal looking straight up. With this type of labor, you will probably experience lower-back pain, which can last a long time.

The mechanics of labor work better if baby is looking down at the ground so it can extend its head as it comes through the birth canal. If the baby can't extend its head, its chin points toward its chest, which may cause pain in your lower back. Your doctor may need to rotate baby so it comes out looking down at the ground rather than up at the sky.

Will Your Doctor Use a Vacuum Extractor or Forceps?

The goal with every birth is to deliver a baby as safely as possible. Sometimes baby needs a little help. Your doctor may use a vacuum extractor or forceps to help safely deliver baby. Vacuum and forceps delivery methods each have about the same risks. Use of either is associated with a more frequent need for mechanical ventilation in infants and with more 3rd- and 4th-degree perineal tears.

Vacuum extractors are used more than forceps. There are several types of vacuum extractors. Some have a plastic cup that fits on baby's head by suction. Another type has a metal cup that fits on baby's head so the doctor can gently pull on it to deliver baby's head and body.

Forceps is a metal instrument that looks like two large metal hands. Use of forceps has decreased in recent years. If a lot of traction with forceps is needed to deliver baby, a Cesarean may be a better choice. Cesarean deliveries are also used more often to deliver a baby that is high up in the pelvis.

If the possible use of a vacuum extractor or forceps causes you concern, discuss it with your healthcare provider. It's important to discuss issues that may come up during labor and delivery so you can communicate your concerns.

Exercise for Week 37

• • • • • • •

Sit on a chair or on the floor in a crossed-leg position. Inhale, and slowly tilt your head to the right until you feel a stretch in your neck. Breathe deeply 3 times while holding the stretch. Slowly bring your head to the center, then tilt your head to the left. Hold while you breathe deeply 3 times. Do 4 times on each side. *Helps stretch the neck, and relieves neck and shoulder tension.*

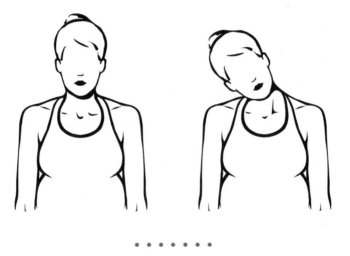

• • • • • • •

Week 38

Age of Fetus—36 Weeks

How Big Is Your Baby?

At this time, your baby weighs about 6¾ pounds (3.1kg). Crown-to-rump length is still about 14 inches (35cm). Total length is around 19⅔ inches (49.5cm).

How Big Are You?

You may feel uncomfortable during the last weeks of pregnancy because your uterus is so large. It's about 14½ to 15¼ inches (36 to 38cm) between your uterus and the pubic symphysis. From your bellybutton to the top of your uterus is about 6½ to 7¼ inches (16 to 18cm).

How Your Baby Is Growing and Developing

Specific cells in the lungs produce chemicals needed for breathing immediately after birth; an important one is *surfactant*. A baby born before its lungs are mature may not have surfactant in its lungs. But it can be introduced directly into a newborn's lungs and baby can use it immediately. Many premature babies who receive surfactant do not have to be put on respirators—they can breathe on their own!

Changes in You

Tests You May Have during Labor

If you think you may be in labor and go to the hospital, you will have a *labor check* to find out if you're in labor and if your pregnancy is doing OK. Vital signs are taken, a monitor will be placed on your abdomen and a pelvic exam will be done. If you're not in labor, you'll be sent home. No one wants to be sent home, but don't fret—you'll be back soon.

If you are not sent home, other tests may be done. *Fetal blood sampling* measures how well a baby can stand the stress of labor. Before the test can be done, your water must have broken, and the cervix must be dilated at least 2cm (about an inch). An instrument is placed into the vagina, through the cervix, to the top of the baby's head to make a small nick in baby's scalp. Baby's blood is collected, and acidity is checked to help your healthcare team decide whether

Tip for Week 38

• • • • • • • • • • •

If baby may be in a breech presentation, your healthcare provider may order an ultrasound to determine how baby is lying in your uterus.

labor can continue or if a Cesarean is needed.

In many hospitals, a baby's heartbeat is monitored. *External fetal monitoring* can be done before your water breaks. A pair of belts is strapped to your tummy. One strap holds a device that monitors baby's heart rate, the other holds a device to measure the length of contractions and how often they occur.

Internal fetal monitoring monitors the baby more precisely. An electrode, called a *scalp electrode*, is placed through the vagina and attached to baby's scalp to measure its heart rate. A thin tube is used inside the uterus to monitor the strength of contractions. This is done only after membranes have ruptured. It may be a little uncomfortable, but it's not painful. Results can usually be seen in your room, at the nurses' station and maybe on your healthcare provider's computer.

How Your Actions Affect Your Baby's Development

Breech and Other Abnormal Presentations

It's common for a baby to be in the *breech presentation* (baby's bottom comes first into the birth canal) early in pregnancy. However, when labor starts, only 3 to 5% of babies, not including multiple pregnancies, are a breech or other abnormal presentation.

Although we don't always know why a baby is in the breech presentation, we know breech births occur more often when you have had more than one pregnancy, you're carrying multiple fetuses, there is too much or too little amniotic fluid, you have an abnormally shaped uterus, you have abnormal uterine growths, you have placenta previa or baby has hydrocephalus. Certain factors can make a breech presentation more likely; one main cause is baby's prematurity.

There are different kinds of breech presentations. A *frank breech* occurs when the legs are flexed at the hips and extended at the knees. This is the most common type of breech found at the end of pregnancy; feet are up by the face or head. With a *complete breech* presentation, knees are flexed. See the illustration on page 375.

Other unusual presentations include a *face presentation*, in which baby's head is hyperextended so the face comes into the birth canal first. In a *shoulder presentation*, the shoulder presents first. In a *transverse lie*, the baby is lying as if in a cradle in the pelvis. The baby's head is on one side of your abdomen, and its bottom is on the other side.

Delivering a Breech Baby. For many years, breech deliveries were done vaginally. Then it was believed the safest

Grandma's Remedy
. . . .

If you want to avoid using medication, try a folk remedy. If you have a stomach-ache, drink a 4-ounce glass of warm water to which you've added 1 teaspoon of baking soda.

method was by Cesarean. Today, experts believe a baby in the breech position can probably be delivered more safely by Cesarean delivery before labor begins or during early labor.

Some experts believe a woman can deliver a breech presentation vaginally if the situation is right. This usually includes a frank breech in a mature baby if the woman has had previous normal deliveries.

. . . .

Studies show 30% of all abnormal presentations aren't detected before labor begins; your risk increases if you're overweight. Your healthcare provider may order a fetal ultrasound to check baby's position toward the end of pregnancy if you're overweight.

. . . .

Most agree a *footling breech* presentation (one leg extended, one knee flexed) should be delivered by Cesarean delivery. Cesarean delivery may be the only a way to deliver a face presentation and a transverse lie.

If you know baby is breech, tell them when you get to the hospital. If you call with a question about labor and have a breech presentation, tell the person you talk with.

Turning a Breech Baby. Attempts may be made to turn the baby from a breech to a head-down (vertex) position before your water breaks, before labor begins or in early labor. Using his or her hands, the healthcare provider turns baby into the head-down birth position. This is called *external cephalic version (ECV)* or just *version*. More than 50% of the time, turning baby is successful. However, some stubborn babies shift again into a breech presentation. ECV may be tried again, but version is harder to perform as your delivery date draws closer.

Problems can occur with ECV. Possible risks include the rupture of membranes, placental abruption, effect on baby's heart rate and/or onset of labor.

. . . .

If your baby is in an abnormal presentation, your healthcare provider may suggest you get on your hands and knees during labor, with your hips above your heart, then lower yourself onto your forearms. This position may help baby turn into a head-down position.

. . . .

Your Nutrition

You may not feel much like eating now, but it's important to eat healthfully. Snacks might be the answer—eat small snacks throughout the day to keep your energy levels up and to help avoid heartburn. You may also be tired of the foods you've been eating. The list below offers

Dad Tip
. . . .

Ask your partner if there are things she'd like you to bring to the hospital for her, such as an iPod or special CDs and a CD player. If you take a tour of the hospital or birthing center, you might get other ideas. Discuss your role in labor and delivery with her; learn what you can do. You may be able to help maintain privacy. Let your partner rest and recover; be her knight in shining armor.

some smart snacks for your healthy nutrition:

- bananas, raisins, dried fruit and mangoes to provide you with iron, potassium and magnesium
- string cheese; it's high in calcium and protein
- fruit shakes made with skim milk and yogurt, ice milk or ice cream for calcium, vitamins and minerals
- high-fiber crackers, spread with a little peanut butter for protein
- cottage cheese and fruit, flavored with a little sugar and some cinnamon, for milk and fruit servings
- salt-free chips or tortillas with salsa or bean dip for fiber
- humus and pita slices for fiber
- fresh tomatoes, flavored with some olive oil and fresh basil; eat with a few thin slices of Parmesan cheese for a vegetable serving and dairy serving
- chicken or tuna salad and crackers or tortilla pieces for protein and fiber

You Should Also Know

What Is a Retained Placenta?
The placenta is usually delivered within 30 minutes after baby's birth; it's a routine part of delivery. In some rare cases, a piece of placenta remains inside the uterus and doesn't deliver on its own. This is called a *retained placenta*. When it occurs, the uterus can't contract enough, resulting in vaginal bleeding that can be heavy.

A retained placenta can occur for many reasons. The placenta may attach over scars on the uterus. The placenta may also attach over an area that was scraped or once infected. The placenta may also grow through the uterine wall, resulting in a retained placenta.

When the placenta doesn't separate from the uterine wall, bleeding is usually severe after delivery, and surgery may be necessary to stop it. An attempt may be made to remove the placenta by D&C.

Your healthcare provider will pay attention to the delivery of your placenta while you pay attention to baby. Some people ask to see the placenta after delivery; you may wish to have your healthcare provider show it to you.

. . . .

Experts now believe it's better to wait 18 to 24 months before trying to get pregnant with your next child. If you get pregnant within 6 months, your chances of having a low-birthweight baby or a premature baby increases significantly.

. . . .

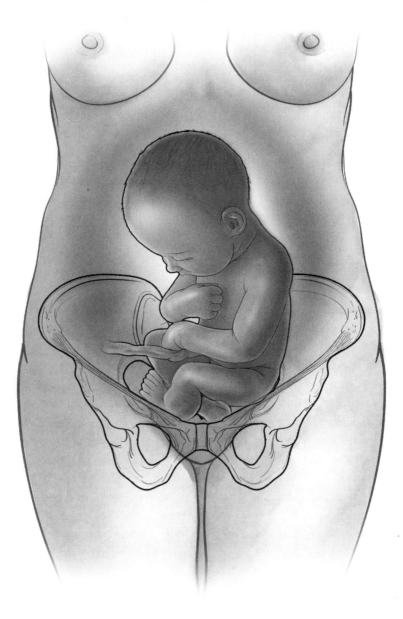

Baby aligned in the pelvis bottom first, with knees flexed,
is called a *complete breech presentation*.

Will You Need to Be Shaved?

Many women want to know if they have to have their pubic hair shaved before birth. It's not a requirement; many women are not shaved today. However, some women who chose not to have pubic hair shaved later told us it hurt a lot when their hair became tangled in their underwear due to the normal vaginal discharge after birth. You might want to think about this and discuss it with your healthcare provider.

Exercise for Week 38

· · · · · · ·

Stand with your feet shoulder-width apart and your knees soft, with your arms by your side. Hold your tummy in. Using light weights (2 to 3 pounds each to start; if you don't have weights, use a 16-ounce can), keep your hands by your hips, your head up and back straight. Inhale as you squat about 6 inches; hold for 5 seconds. Exhale as you squeeze your buttocks muscles and return to the standing position. Repeat 8 times. *Strengthens quadriceps.*

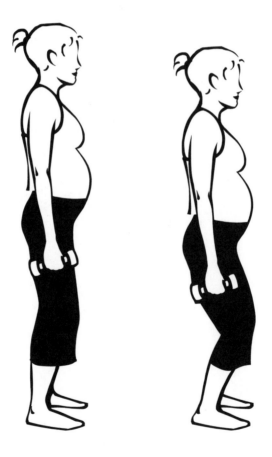

· · · · · · ·

Week 39

Age of Fetus—37 Weeks

How Big Is Your Baby?

Your baby weighs about 7¼ pounds (3.3kg). Crown-to-rump length is about 14½ inches (36cm). The baby's total length is close to 20 inches (50.5cm).

How Big Are You?

The illustration on page 380 shows a side view of a woman's uterus with baby inside it. She's about as big as she can get. You probably are too! Your weight gain should remain between 25 and 35 pounds (11.4 and 15.9kg) until delivery.

If you measure from the pubic symphysis to the top of the uterus, the distance is 14½ to 16 inches (36 to 40cm). Measuring from the bellybutton, the distance is about 6½ to 8 inches (16 to 20cm).

How Your Baby Is Growing and Developing

Your baby continues to gain weight. It doesn't have much room to move. All the organ systems are developed. The last organ to mature is the lungs.

Can Baby Get Tangled in the Cord?

You may have been told by friends not to raise your arms over your head or to reach high because it may cause the cord to wrap around the baby's neck. There doesn't seem to be much truth to this old wives' tale.

The term *nuchal cord* refers to an umbilical cord wrapped around a baby's neck. It occurs in nearly 25% of all births. Nothing you do during pregnancy causes or prevents this. A tangled umbilical cord isn't necessarily a problem during labor. It only becomes a problem if the cord is stretched tight around the baby's neck or is in a knot. The good news is this situation is not always dangerous for baby.

Changes in You

It would be unusual for you not to be uncomfortable and feel huge at this time. Your uterus fills your pelvis and most of your abdomen. It has pushed everything else out of the way. You may want baby to be born soon because you're so uncomfortable.

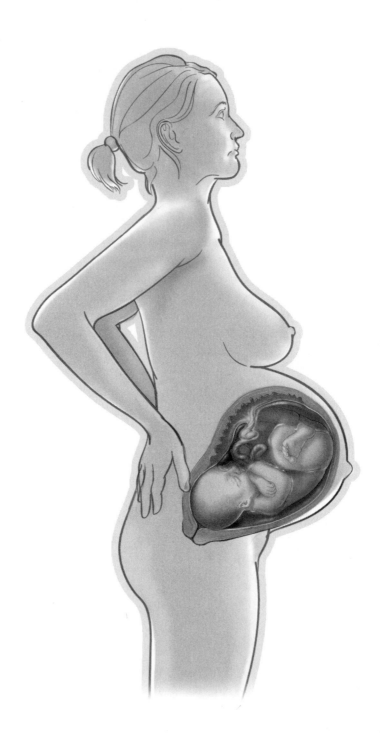

Comparative size of the uterus at 39 weeks of pregnancy
(fetal age—37 weeks) with a baby that is close to full term.

How Your Actions Affect Your Baby's Development

Feeding Your Baby

Feeding your baby is one of the most important tasks you will perform. The nutrition you provide after birth will have an effect on the rest of his life. If you have any questions, discuss them with your healthcare provider.

You may decide to breastfeed baby; it may be the best nutrition you can give him. Baby receives more than just breast milk from you. He will also receive important nutrients, antibodies to help prevent infections and other important substances for growth and development. However, you may choose not to breastfeed—if you bottlefeed, you can still provide good nutrition for your baby.

In Appendix C, page 426, we discuss breastfeeding and bottlefeeding. Read each section, make a list of questions about both types of feeding and talk them over with your healthcare provider at a prenatal visit.

ACOG discourages elective delivery of a baby before the 39th week of pregnancy. The best time to deliver is between 39 weeks and one day before you reach 42 weeks.

Your Nutrition

If you're going to breastfeed, you need to think about your nutrition because it can affect the quality of your milk. You may have to avoid some foods because they can pass into breast milk and cause baby stomach distress. You'll need to continue to drink lots of fluids and keep up your calcium intake. Ask your healthcare provider about any vitamins you should take.

If you choose to bottlefeed, you have a few more options. However, it's still important to follow a nutritious eating plan. You may need fewer calories, but don't drastically cut your calories in hopes of losing weight quickly. You need good energy levels. Keep up your fluid intake.

If a woman has type-1 or type-2 diabetes, after pregnancy she should be tested for diabetic retinopathy. If there is damage to the retina, it should be treated before another pregnancy is attempted.

You Should Also Know

Pain Relief during Labor

Your uterus contracts a lot so your baby can be born. Labor can be painful. You won't have any idea what your labor is going to be like until it begins. If you're afraid of the pain of labor and delivery, you may tense up, which can make it worse. If you choose anesthesia, studies show it can speed up labor because you're more relaxed. Anesthesia in early labor does not seem to increase the Cesarean-delivery rate.

Focusing on your breathing can help you stay relaxed during labor.

Labor-pain relief is approached in many ways. When you use medication, there are two patients to consider—you and baby. Find out in advance what options are available for pain control, then see how your labor goes before making a final decision.

An *analgesic* is full or partial pain relief. Narcotic analgesics pass to baby through the placenta and may decrease respiratory function in a newborn and affect baby's Apgar scores. These medications should not be given close to the time of delivery.

Anesthesia is a complete block of all pain sensations and muscle movement. When it is given to affect a particular area of the body, it is called a *block*, such as a pudendal block, an epidural block or a cervical block. Medication is similar to the type used to block pain when you have a tooth filled.

Occasionally, it's necessary to use general anesthesia for delivery, usually for an emergency Cesarean delivery. A pediatrician attends the birth because baby may be asleep following delivery.

What Is an Epidural Block? An epidural block provides relief by blocking painful sensations between the uterus and cervix and your brain. Medication in the epidural prevents pain messages from traveling up your spinal cord to your brain.

An epidural is very popular and provides relief from the pain of uterine contractions and delivery. It should be administered only by someone trained and experienced in this type of anesthesia. Some obstetricians have this experience, but in most areas an anesthesiologist or nurse anesthetist administers it.

While you are sitting up or lying on your side, a needle is placed through numbed skin; anesthetic flows through the needle and around the spinal cord but not into the spinal canal. A catheter is left in place to deliver anesthesia, and pain medication may be delivered by a pump at regular intervals or as needed. Many hospitals use patient-controlled epidurals (PCEA)—you press a button for more medication when you need it.

. . . .

On the average, epidurals slow labor by 45 minutes.

. . . .

Most experts believe an epidural block should be given based on your level of pain. They agree a woman can have an epidural anytime after she begins active labor; you may not be required to be dilated to a specific point before getting an epidural.

Some medical conditions may keep you from having an epidural, such as a serious infection when you begin labor, scoliosis, previous back surgery or some blood-clotting problems. If you have one of these problems, discuss it at a prenatal visit.

You may have problems pushing if you have an epidural, but you should be able to feel enough pressure to push. An epidural may increase the chances forceps or a vacuum extractor may be needed during delivery.

An epidural block can make your blood pressure drop. Low blood pressure may affect blood flow to the baby. Fortunately, I.V. fluids given with the epidural help reduce the risk.

Epidural anesthesia does not increase the risk of Cesarean delivery. And no link between use of epidurals during labor and back pain after delivery has been established.

An epidural can cause shaking as well as itching and headache. If you have trembling (nearly 50% of all women do), ask for blankets or a hot-water bottle. If you itch, wait a bit. Itching is usually mild

Nitrous Oxide

· · · · · · · · · · ·

Have you heard nitrous oxide is making a comeback here in the United States as a pain-relief method during labor? Nitrous oxide has been used for this purpose in European countries and Canada for many years.

Once popular in this country, it fell out of favor when the epidural was introduced in the 1930s. Since then, it has been little used in American delivery rooms. However, in 2011 the FDA (Food and Drug Administration) approved new nitrous-oxide equipment for use in delivery rooms. Today, it is believed several hundred hospitals in this country are using it or investigating its use. The gas has a very good safety record in delivery rooms in other countries. More studies need to be done to ensure its safety.

and goes away on its own. Put pressure on the area with a towel, or apply lots of lotion. If itching doesn't go away, your healthcare provider may recommend medication, such as naloxone (Narcan).

Very occasionally, you'll get a headache. Drink a caffeinated beverage, such as coffee, tea or a caffeinated soda. Try resting on your back. If the headache persists for more than 24 hours, talk to your healthcare provider. If you become nauseous, breathe deeply; inhale through your nose, and exhale through your mouth.

Combined Spinal-Epidural Analgesia (CSE). Combined spinal-epidural analgesia (CSE) uses epidural and spinal techniques to relieve pain and is a popular epidural option. The combination provides the quick relief of a spinal block with the option of an epidural if your labor is longer. It is sometimes called a *walking epidural.*

A walking epidural doesn't have much to do with walking. It refers to regional labor-pain relief in which a woman maintains some strength in her legs. Few women actually walk after receiving pain relief.

With CSE, there is a lower incidence of spinal headache. There may be less numbness with a CSE, and you may be able to control the amount of anesthesia you receive.

Other Pain Blocks. When contractions are regular and the cervix begins to dilate, uterine contractions can be uncomfortable. For the early stage of labor, medication may be given through an I.V. or by injection into a muscle. A mixture of a narcotic analgesic drug, such as meperidine (Demerol), and a tranquilizer, such as promethazine (Phenergan), may be used. It reduces pain and may cause sleepiness or sedation. These medications also enter baby's bloodstream and can make baby groggy.

Spinal anesthesia is often used for a Cesarean delivery. It works within seconds and is effective for up to 45 minutes. Pain relief lasts long enough for the Cesarean delivery to be done.

Other types of blocks may be used. A *pudendal block* is given through the vaginal canal and decreases pain in the birth canal. You still feel contractions and pain in the uterus. A *paracervical*

> ### *Dad Tip*
> ....
> Having a baby is a personal experience. Some couples choose the intimacy and privacy of being alone during the birth. Other couples want family members and friends to share the experience with them. If you talk about it ahead of time, you can decide together what you both want. After all, it's your baby's birth.

block provides pain relief for the dilating cervix but doesn't relieve contraction pain. *Intrathecal anesthesia* is delivered into the area surrounding the spinal cord. It isn't a total block; the woman feels contractions so she can push.

There is no perfect method for pain relief during labor and delivery. Discuss all possibilities with your healthcare provider, and mention any concerns. Find out what types of anesthesia are available and the risks and benefits of each. Most complications with anesthesia affect the baby; with general anesthesia, increased sedation, slower respiration and a slower heartbeat may be observed in baby. The mother is usually "out" for more than an hour and is unable to see her newborn infant until later.

Before labor, it may be impossible to determine which anesthesia will be best for you. But it's helpful to know what's available. If you're interested in nonmedical pain-relief methods, see the discussion in Week 40.

Umbilical-Cord-Blood Banking
You may have heard about storing blood from your baby's umbilical cord after birth. *Umbilical-cord blood* (UCB) is blood in the umbilical cord and placenta; it contains stem cells. Stem cells have proved useful in treating some diseases. In cord blood, stem cells are undeveloped and can become many different kinds of blood cells. Cord blood doesn't need to be matched as closely for a transplant. This feature can be important for people who have difficulty finding acceptable donor matches.

How Cord Blood Is Used. Cord-blood transfers have been in use since about 1990. UCB has been used to treat over 75 life-threatening diseases, especially those that affect the blood and immune systems.

If you or your partner have a family history of some specific diseases, consider saving and banking your child's umbilical-cord blood in case it's needed for treatment in the future. Siblings or parents can also use the blood. In fact, the most common use for stem cells from cord blood is between siblings. However, stored blood can't be used to treat a genetic disease in the child from whom the blood was collected. Those stem cells have the same genetic problems. If you're interested, discuss it at a prenatal appointment. You only have one chance to collect and to save baby's umbilical-cord blood.

Before making a decision, ask about how and where blood is stored and the cost of storing it. Blood storage is expensive and may not be covered by insurance.

Tip for Week 39
• • • • • • • • • • •

Don't take tags off shower gifts and other gifts until after baby is born. You may need to exchange the gift if its size, color or "sex" isn't correct.

In many hospitals, expecting mothers learn about cord-blood donation when they are admitted to the hospital. Donating cord blood is free.

Collecting and Storing Blood for Your Family's Use. The cord-blood storage bank you choose sends you a collection kit. Blood is collected within minutes after birth, before you deliver the placenta. It's taken directly from the umbilical cord; there's no risk or pain to mom or baby. You can also bank the blood if you have a Cesarean delivery.

After cord blood is collected, it's taken to a banking facility where it is frozen and stored. At this time, we don't know how long frozen cells will last. Cord blood has been banked only since 1990.

It's expensive to collect and to store umbilical-cord blood. Collection and storage can run between $1000 and $2000. A single year's storage can cost around $100.

There are two types of banks—private blood banking and public blood banking. You may be advised to use private blood banking if you have a history of some illnesses. With private banking, access is guaranteed to your own or a relative's stored blood. Cord blood is available for you or a family member if you need it in the future.

Most banks, whether private or public, require the mother to be tested for various infections before blood is accepted.

This can add to the cost of saving cord blood. Your insurance company may pay for this testing if you have a family history of a disease that might be treated with umbilical-cord blood. Some insurance companies pay collection and storage fees for families at high risk of cancer or genetically based diseases. Cord-blood banking services may waive fees for at-risk families who are unable to afford them.

The blood bank you choose should be accredited by the American Association of Blood Banks. They have established procedures for collecting and storing umbilical-cord blood.

Donating Cord Blood. If you don't think you'll need cord blood, you may want to donate it. If cord blood isn't used for patients, it may be used for research. Public UCB banks provide those who need it with cord blood. Needs-based help may be available. If you donate your child's cord blood to a public bank, his or her name is added to the national registry. If the child ever needs cord blood, he or she is guaranteed it.

There are over 40 public cord-blood banks in the United States at this time. They work with hospitals that ask women to donate their baby's cord blood. Collection is an expensive procedure, so not all hospitals participate in the program. If you're interested, ask your healthcare provider for information.

Exercise for Week 39

· · · · · · ·

Stand with your feet slightly apart and your knees soft. Hold onto a counter or a chair with your left hand for stability, if you need it. Holding in your tummy muscles, lift your right leg up behind you until you can touch your bottom with your foot. Return your foot to the floor, then turn around. Hold onto the support with your right hand, and lift your left foot. Repeat 8 times for each leg. *Tones quadriceps.*

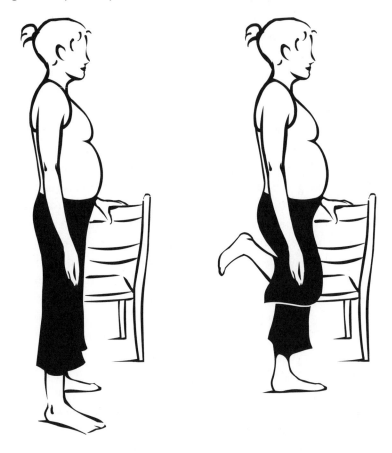

· · · · · · ·

Week 40

Age of Fetus—38 Weeks

How Big Is Your Baby?

Your baby weighs about 7⅔ pounds (3.5kg). Its crown-to-rump length is about 14¾ to 15¼ inches (37 to 38cm). Total length is 20⅔ inches (51cm). Baby fills your uterus and has little room to move. See the illustration on page 388.

How Big Are You?

You probably don't care an awful lot about how much you measure. You feel you're as big as you could ever be, and you're ready to have your baby. From the pubic symphysis to the top of the uterus, you probably measure between 14½ and 16 inches (36 to 40cm). From your bellybutton to the top of your uterus is 6½ to 8 inches (16 to 20cm).

How Your Baby Is Growing and Developing

Your baby is fully grown at this point. If you were correct about the date of your last period and your due date is this week, baby may be born very soon. However, it's helpful to realize only 5% of all babies are born on their due date. Don't get frustrated if you see your due date come and go. Baby will be here soon!

Changes in You

While You Wait to Go to the Hospital

If you're waiting to go to the hospital and are in pain, there are a few things you can do at home to help you manage your pain. At the beginning of each contraction, take a deep breath. Exhale slowly. At the end of the contraction, again breathe deeply. When a contraction begins, try to distract yourself with soothing mental pictures.

Get up and move! Walk around. It may relieve back pain. Ask your partner to give you a massage to help ease tension. Hot and/or cold compresses can help reduce cramping and aches and pains. A warm shower or bath can feel very good.

Your chances of having your baby on the way to the hospital are pretty small. Labor with a first baby often lasts between 12 and 14 hours.

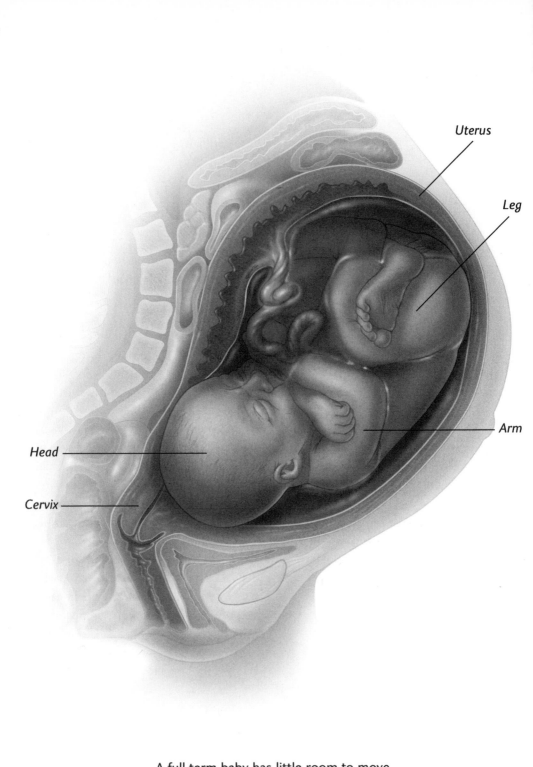

Uterus

Leg

Arm

Head

Cervix

A full-term baby has little room to move.
This is one reason fetal movements may slow down in
the last few weeks of pregnancy.

How Your Actions Affect Your Baby's Development

Going to the Hospital

If you preregistered at the hospital before your due date, it'll save time checking in. If you didn't, fill out forms early. Have your insurance card or insurance information at hand. It's helpful to know your blood type and Rh factor, your healthcare provider's name, the pediatrician's name and your due date.

Ask your healthcare provider how you should prepare to go to the hospital; he or she may have specific instructions for you. Many couples are advised to go to the hospital after an hour of contractions that are 5 to 10 minutes apart. However, leave sooner if the hospital is far away or hard to get to or if the weather is bad. When you get there, you'll be checked for signs of labor.

In the Hospital. A copy of your office chart is usually kept in labor and delivery. When you're admitted, you may also be asked many questions, such as when your membranes ruptured, whether you're bleeding, when you last ate and what you ate. Personnel will also want to know if you're having contractions, how often and how long they last.

A brief pregnancy history is taken. Vital signs are noted. Tell them about any medical problems you have and any medications you take or have taken during pregnancy. If you've had complications, tell them. This is the time to tell them any information your healthcare provider gave you about your last pelvic exam.

A pelvic exam is done to see what stage of labor you're in and to use as a reference point for future labor exams. This exam and vital signs are done by a labor-and-delivery nurse (the nurse can be male or female). Only in unusual situations, such as an emergency, will your healthcare provider do this initial exam. In fact, it may be quite a while before you see him or her. He or she may not arrive until close to delivery.

. . . .

Some couples choose to bring young children to see the birth of a new brother or sister. Ask your healthcare provider's opinion ahead of time. The delivery of the baby might be frightening to a young child. Many places offer special classes for older siblings to help prepare them for the new baby. This may be a better way to help your older children feel they're part of the birth experience.

. . . .

Once You're Admitted. If you're in labor, you'll be admitted to the hospital. You'll be informed about the procedures that may be done for you and any risks involved. You may be asked to sign forms from the hospital, your healthcare provider and/or the anesthesiologist acknowledging you received this information.

After you're admitted, you may receive an enema. Blood may be drawn. Your healthcare provider may want to discuss pain relief, or you may have an epidural put in place if you requested one. If you have decided to have an epidural or if it looks as if labor will last quite awhile, an I.V. will be started. You may still be able to walk around.

Tip for Week 40
· · · · · · · · · · ·

If you want to use a different labor position, massage, relaxation techniques and/ or hypnotherapy to relieve labor pain, don't wait until you're in labor to ask about it. Discuss it with your healthcare provider at one of your prenatal visits.

During this time, you and your partner may be alone, with nurses coming in and out of the room. A monitoring belt may be used to record your contractions and baby's heartbeat. The monitoring record can be seen in the room and at the nursing station.

Blood pressure is regularly checked, and pelvic exams are done to follow labor's progress. The healthcare provider is usually notified upon your admission to labor and delivery; he or she is called at regular intervals as labor progresses or if problems arise.

In some cases, when you get to the hospital, you may learn someone else will deliver baby. If your healthcare provider believes he or she might be out of town when your baby is born, ask to meet those who "cover" when he or she is unavailable. It's not always possible for your healthcare provider to be there for the birth of your baby.

Keep Your Options Open

An important consideration in planning for your labor and delivery is the method(s) you may use to get through the process. Every woman is different, and every labor is different. You don't know what will happen and what you will need for pain relief. It's impossible to know how long labor will last—3 hours or 20 hours. It's best to be flexible.

Understand what's available and what options you can choose during labor.

Pain Relief without Medication

Some women do not want medication during labor to relieve pain. Nondrug techniques to manage labor pain include continuous labor support, water therapy, hypnosis and acupuncture/acupressure.

Continuous labor support is provided by a nurse, midwife or doula, and includes touch, massage, application of cold or heat, and other methods to provide physical comfort. It also includes emotional support.

For some women, *water therapy (hydrotherapy)* has been shown to reduce stress hormones in the body and may also decrease the frequency of contractions. Some women experience less pain in the water. The water also softens the perineal area, so it may stretch more easily. A warm shower can relax and massage you. Water immersion involves a warm bath during early labor and is most often used then. Birth pools may be available in some hospitals. You may have to get out of the pool to give birth.

Hypnosis to relieve labor pain is sometimes called *hypnobirthing*; it may not be available everywhere. Visualization, relaxation and deep breathing help you relax so you can deal with your fear of pain. If you choose hypnotherapy to help you deal with pain, you must prepare and practice for months before baby's birth.

Acupuncture uses needles at specific points to relieve pain. It must usually be started at the beginning of labor. *Acupressure* uses pressure on specific parts of the body to help relieve pain and to relax you.

Other Techniques. Swaying from side to side, changing positions and rolling on a birthing ball (like a big exercise ball) can help ease discomfort. Because you're upright, the force of gravity may help your labor progress. Walking also keeps you upright, which helps dilate the cervix naturally.

Aromatherapy—massage with certain aromatic oils—can be helpful for relaxation. Listening to instrumental music for at least 3 hours during early active labor may also help you deal with pain by helping you relax.

Massage for Pain Relief

The touching and caressing of massage can help you relax and helps reduce pain. One study showed women who were massaged 20 minutes every hour during active labor felt less anxiety and pain. Many parts of the body of a laboring woman can be massaged. The person doing the massage should pay close attention to the woman's responses to determine correct pressure.

. . . .

You may not realize it, but having a baby is hard work!

. . . .

Different types of massage affect a woman in various ways. You and your partner may want to practice the two types of massage described below before labor.

Effleurage is light, gentle fingertip massage over the abdomen and upper thighs used during early labor. Stroking is light but doesn't tickle; fingertips never leave the skin. Place hands on either side of the navel. Move them upward and outward, and come back down to the pubic area. Then move hands back up to the navel. Massage may extend down the thighs. It can also be done as a crosswise motion, around fetal-monitor belts. Move fingers across the abdomen from one side to the other between the belts.

Counterpressure massage can relieve back-labor pain. Ask your labor coach to place the heel of his or her hand or the flat part of the fist (you can also use a tennis ball) against your tailbone. Firm pressure is applied in a small, circular motion.

Laboring Positions

Different laboring positions may allow you and your partner (or labor coach) to work together during labor to find relief. This interaction can help you feel closer, and it lets you share the experience. Some women say using these methods brought them closer to their partner and made the birth experience a more joyful one.

Most women in North America and Europe give birth in bed on their backs. However, some women are trying different positions to find relief from pain and to make birth easier. In the past,

> ### Dad Tip
> . . . .
>
> Baby can come at any time. When your little one decides to make his or her appearance, take care of some things your partner might forget about. If she works outside the home, call her workplace and let them know she's at the hospital. Find out if she has any appointments or plans you may need to change for her. Ask her what might need to be done at home to finish preparing for baby's arrival.

women often labored and gave birth in an upright position that kept the pelvis vertical. Kneeling, squatting, sitting or standing up lets the abdominal wall relax and the baby descend more rapidly. Because contractions are stronger and more regular, labor is often shorter.

. . . .

If your labor slows down, your healthcare provider may give you oxytocin.

. . . .

Today, many women are asking to choose the birth position that is most comfortable for them. Freedom to do so can make you feel more confident about managing labor and birth and help you feel more satisfied with the entire experience.

If it's important to you, discuss it with your healthcare provider. Ask about the facilities at the hospital you will use; some have special equipment, such as birthing chairs, squatting bars or birthing beds.

Walking and standing are good positions to use during early labor. Walking may help you breathe more easily and relax more. Be sure someone is with you to offer support. Standing in a warm shower may provide relief.

There has been some debate about walking during labor. Some believe walking helps move the baby into position more quickly, dilates the cervix faster and makes labor more pain free. Others believe walking puts the woman at risk of falling and doesn't allow for fetal monitoring. We believe the bottom line is that it's a personal decision, and together with your healthcare provider, you should be allowed to decide what feels best for you.

Sitting can slow labor. Sitting to rest after walking or standing is OK, but sitting can be uncomfortable during a contraction.

Kneeling on hands and knees is a good way to relieve the pain of back labor. Kneel against a support, such as a chair or your partner, to stretch back muscles. The effects of kneeling are similar to those of walking and standing.

When you can't stand, walk or kneel, lie on your side. If you receive pain medication, you'll need to lie down. Lie on your left side, then turn onto your right side.

Although lying on your back is the most common position used, it can slow labor. It can also make your blood pressure drop and cause baby's heart rate to drop. If you lie on your back, elevate the head of the bed and put a pillow under one hip so you're not flat on your back.

If you were diagnosed with gestational diabetes, you should be tested regularly for diabetes. This is especially important before you become pregnant again.

Your Nutrition

In the past, women were not allowed to eat or drink during labor. One of the major concerns was if a woman needed general anesthesia at any time, any food or liquid in the stomach could be aspirated into her lungs. However, general anesthesia is used less frequently today; when it is necessary, administration has improved greatly, which has reduced risks. In addition, many women choose epidural for anesthesia—with an epidural, aspiration isn't a concern.

ACOG has issued new guidelines and states women in labor do not have to forego *all* nutrition. If a woman has a normal, uncomplicated labor, she may drink modest amounts of clear liquids, such as water, fruit juice without pulp, carbonated beverages, clear tea, black coffee, sports drinks, even a protein shake. Labor is hard work, similar to strenuous exercise. Letting a mom-to-be have a protein shake during labor gives her some energy to do this hard work and makes her feel less hungry.

The common belief today is if a woman is healthy and has a low-risk pregnancy, giving her clear liquids or a protein shake during labor is OK. If you have any risk factors, such as morbid obesity or diabetes, or if you may be at risk for a Cesarean delivery or one involving forceps or a vacuum extractor, your fluid intake may be limited or curtailed.

If you're scheduled for a Cesarean delivery, you may drink clear liquids up to 2 hours before anesthesia is given. Don't eat solid food for 6 to 8 hours before surgery.

If your labor is long, your body may be hydrated with an I.V. After your baby's birth, if everything is OK, you may be able to eat and drink without much restriction.

You Should Also Know

Your Labor Coach

Your labor coach may be one of your most valuable assets during labor and delivery. He (or she) can help you prepare. He can support you as you go through the experience of labor together. He can share with you the joy of the birth of your baby.

An important role of the labor coach is to make sure you get to the hospital! Work out a plan during the last weeks of pregnancy so you know how to reach your coach. It's helpful to have an alternate driver who's available in case you can't reach your labor coach immediately and need to be taken to the hospital.

In most instances, your partner is your labor coach. However, this isn't an absolute requirement. A close friend or relative, such as your mother or sister, may act as your labor coach. Or you may choose the services of a doula. Ask someone ahead of time; don't wait until the last minute. Give the person time to prepare for the experience and to make sure he or she will be able to be there with you.

Not everyone feels comfortable watching the entire labor and delivery. This may include your partner. Don't force your partner or labor coach to watch the delivery if he or she doesn't want to. It's not unusual for a labor coach to get lightheaded, dizzy or pass out during labor and delivery. On more than one occasion, coaches or partners have fainted or become extremely lightheaded just from talking about plans for labor and delivery or a Cesarean delivery!

Before going to the hospital, your labor coach can time your contractions. Once you're at the hospital, your coach can talk to you while you're in labor to distract you and to help you relax, encourage and reassure you during labor and when it comes time for you to push, keep a watch on the door and protect your privacy.

If you don't want to be touched during labor, tell your coach. But do ask him to reassure you it's OK for you to deal vocally with your pain. He can also wipe your face or your mouth with a washcloth, rub your abdomen or back, and support your back while you're pushing. Your labor coach can do other things, such as help create a mood in the labor room and take pictures. Many couples find photographs taken of baby after the delivery help them best remember these wonderful moments of joy.

It's all right for your labor coach to rest or to take a break during labor, especially if it lasts a long time. It's better if your coach eats in the lounge or hospital cafeteria. A labor coach should not bring work into the labor room.

Many couples do different things to distract themselves and to help pass time during labor. These include picking names for the baby, playing games, watching TV or listening to music.

Talk to your healthcare provider about your coach's participation in the delivery, such as cutting the umbilical cord or bathing baby after birth. These things vary from one place to another. The responsibility of your healthcare provider is the well-being of you and your baby—don't make requests or demands that could cause complications.

Decide ahead of time about who needs to be called after baby's birth. Bring a list of names and phone numbers with you. There are some people you may want to call yourself. In most places, a telephone is available in the labor and delivery area, or you may be able to use your cell phones.

If you want to be with your partner when friends or relatives first see the baby, make it clear. In most instances, you need some cleaning up. Take some time for yourselves with your new baby. After that, you can show baby to friends and relatives, and share the joy with them.

Vaginal Delivery of Your Baby

We have already covered Cesarean delivery in Week 37. Most women don't have a Cesarean delivery—they have a vaginal birth.

There are three distinct stages of labor, as previously discussed. In the first stage, your uterus contracts with enough intensity, duration and frequency to cause effacement and dilatation of the cervix. This stage ends when the cervix is fully dilated and sufficiently open to allow the baby's head to come through it.

The second stage of labor begins when the cervix is completely dilated at 10cm. Once full dilatation is reached, pushing begins. Pushing can take 1 to 2 hours (first or second baby) to a few minutes (an experienced mom). This stage ends with baby's delivery.

* *

Studies show if you wait about 3 or 4 minutes before cutting the umbilical cord, the extra blood flowing to your baby increases his or her iron levels for the first 6 months of life.

* *

The third stage of labor begins after baby's delivery and ends with delivery of the placenta and membranes that have surrounded the fetus. Delivery of the baby and placenta and repair of the episiotomy (if you have one) usually takes 20 to 30 minutes.

Following delivery, you and the baby are evaluated. During this time, you get to see and to hold your baby; you may even be able to feed him or her.

Depending on whether you deliver in a hospital or birthing center, you may deliver in the same room you've labored in. Or you may be moved to a delivery room nearby. After birth, you will go to recovery for a short time, then move to a hospital room until you're ready to go home.

You will probably stay in the hospital 24 to 48 hours after delivery if you have no complications. If you do have any complications, you and your healthcare provider will decide what is best for you.

Exercise for Week 40

· · · · · · ·

Stand with your feet slightly apart and your knees soft. Cross your chest with your right arm. With your left hand, gently push your right elbow toward you. Pat yourself on the back for a pregnancy job well done! Hold stretch for 10 seconds; repeat 4 times for each arm. *Provides a good stretch for the upper back.*

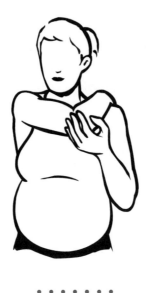

· · · · · · ·

When You're Overdue

Your due date has come and gone. You haven't delivered, and you're getting tired of being pregnant. You keep hearing, "I'm sure it'll be soon. Just sit tight." You feel ready to scream. But hang in there. It will be over soon—the wait just seems never-ending right now.

What Happens When You Pass Your Due Date?

If you pass your due date, you're not alone—nearly 10% of all babies are born more than 2 weeks late. A pregnancy is considered *overdue (postterm)* only when it exceeds 42 weeks or 294 days from the first day of the last menstrual period. (A baby born at 41 weeks, 6 days is not overdue, even if it feels like it to you!)

Your healthcare provider can determine whether baby is moving around and that the amount of amniotic fluid is healthy and normal. If baby is healthy and active, you're usually monitored until labor begins on its own. Tests may be done as reassurance an overdue baby is OK and can remain in the womb. If signs of fetal stress are found, labor may be induced.

Take Good Care of Yourself

It may be hard to keep a positive attitude when you're overdue, but don't give up yet! Eat healthfully, and keep up your fluid intake. If you can do so without problems, get some mild exercise, like walking or swimming. You may feel better.

One of the best exercises you can do at this point is water exercises. You can swim or exercise in the water without fear of falling or losing your balance. Even just walking back and forth in the pool can feel good!

Rest and relax now because your baby will be here soon, and you'll be very busy. Use the time to get things ready so you'll be all set when you and baby come home from the hospital.

Postterm Pregnancies

Most babies born 2 weeks or more past their due date are delivered safely. However, carrying a baby longer than 42 weeks can cause some problems, so tests may be done and labor may be induced if necessary.

When a pregnancy is overdue, the placenta may not provide the respiratory function and essential nutrients baby needs. A baby may begin to suffer nutritional loss. The baby is called *postmature*. At birth, a postmature baby may have dry, cracked, peeling, wrinkled skin, long fingernails and lots of hair. It also has less vernix covering its body. The baby may have less fat and appear almost malnourished.

Because a postmature infant is in danger of losing nutritional support from the placenta, it's important to know the true dating of your pregnancy. This is yet another reason why it's important to go to all of your prenatal visits.

Tests You May Have

Various tests may be done to reassure you and your healthcare provider baby is doing OK and can remain in the womb. To evaluate baby, tests are done on you to determine the health of your baby.

One of the first tests is a vaginal exam. This test will probably be done every week to see if your cervix has begun to dilate. You may also be asked to record kick counts. A weekly ultrasound may be done to determine how big baby is and how much amniotic fluid is present and to identify any problems with the placenta.

Three other tests may be done when a baby is overdue to check baby's well-being inside the womb. They are the *nonstress test*, the *contraction stress test* and the *biophysical profile*. Each is discussed below.

The Nonstress Test (NST)

When baby moves, its heart rate usually goes up. The findings from a nonstress test help measure how well baby is tolerating life inside the uterus. Your healthcare provider can decide if further action is necessary.

The NST is performed in your healthcare provider's office or in the labor-and-delivery department of a hospital. While you're lying down, a fetal monitor is attached to your tummy. Every time you feel your baby move, you push a button that makes a mark on monitor paper. At the same time, the monitor records baby's heartbeat.

The Contraction Stress Test (CST)

The contraction stress test (CST), also called a *stress test*, gives an indication of how well baby will tolerate contractions and labor. If baby doesn't respond well to contractions, it can be a sign of fetal stress. Some believe this test is more accurate than the nonstress test in assessing baby's well-being.

To perform a CST, a monitor is placed on your abdomen. You are attached to an I.V. that dispenses small amounts of oxytocin to make your uterus contract. If nipple stimulation is used, an I.V. isn't necessary. Baby's heartbeat is monitored for its response to contractions. If baby doesn't respond well to contractions, it can be a sign of fetal stress.

The Biophysical Profile (BPP)

A biophysical profile uses a scoring system. Four tests are done with ultrasound; the fifth is done with external fetal monitors. A score is given to each area. The five areas evaluated include fetal breathing movements, fetal body movements, fetal tone, the amount of amniotic fluid and reactive fetal heart rate (nonstress test [NST]).

An abnormal score is 0 for any of these tests; a normal score is 2. A score of 1 is a middle score. A total score is obtained by adding all the values together. Evaluation may vary depending on the sophistication of the equipment used and the expertise of the person doing the test. The higher the score, the better the baby's condition. A lower score may cause concern about the well-being of the fetus.

If the score is low, a recommendation may be made to deliver the baby. If the score is reassuring, the test may be repeated at a later date. If results fall between these two values, the test may be repeated the following day. Your healthcare provider will evaluate all the information before making any decision.

Research from the Centers for Disease Control and Prevention (CDC) indicates about 25% of all inductions are elective or medically unnecessary. If labor is induced at 37 or 38 weeks for nonmedical reasons, baby's chances of having complications greatly increase. Or you may end up having a Cesarean delivery.

Inducing Labor

There may come a point in your pregnancy when your healthcare provider decides to induce labor, which means labor is started to deliver your baby. It's a fairly common practice; each year, healthcare providers induce labor for about 450,000 births. In addition to inducing labor for overdue babies, it is also used when a woman has other problems or when baby is at risk.

When your healthcare provider does a pelvic exam at this point in your pregnancy, it probably also includes an evaluation of how ready you are for induction. Indications for induction of labor include a pregnancy 2 weeks past the due date, baby isn't thriving in the uterus (determined from tests), you have pre-eclampsia or there are signs the placenta is no longer functioning as well as it should. Other reasons for inducing labor include illness that threatens your well-being or baby's well-being, pregnancy-induced high blood pressure or premature rupture of membranes. If your water breaks but contractions don't begin in a reasonable amount of time or there is concern about infection, labor may be induced.

The Bishop score may be used to predict the success of inducing labor. Scoring includes dilatation, effacement, station, consistency and position of the cervix. A score is given for each point, then they are added together to give a total score to help the healthcare provider decide whether to induce labor.

Sometimes labor should *not* be induced. Your healthcare provider will take into account any contraindications to inducing labor.

Ripening the Cervix for Induction
The cervix may be ripened before labor is induced. Medicine is used to help the cervix soften, thin and dilate. Various preparations are used for this purpose. The two most common are Prepidil Gel and Cervidil. In most cases, Prepidil

You may want to try some "natural" labor inducers that have been known to work for some women. They include:
- walking
- eating fresh pineapple (it contains bromelain, which may help soften cervical tissues)
- nipple stimulation
- sexual intercourse (semen contains prostaglandins, which help soften cervical tissues)

Gel and Cervidil are used to prepare the cervix the day before induction. Both preparations are placed in the top of the vagina, behind the cervix. Medication is released directly onto the cervix to help ripen it. This is done in the labor-and-delivery area of the hospital so baby can be monitored.

Labor Induction

If labor is induced, you may first have your cervix ripened, as described above, then you will receive oxytocin (Pitocin) through an I.V. The oxytocin starts contractions to help you go into labor.

The length of the entire process—ripening your cervix until the birth of your baby—varies from woman to woman.

Oxytocin is gradually increased until contractions begin. The amount you receive is controlled by a pump so you can't receive too much. While you receive oxytocin, you're also monitored for the baby's reaction to labor.

It's important to realize being induced does not guarantee a vaginal delivery. In many instances, induction doesn't work. Inducing labor may increase your chances of having an emergency Cesarean delivery.

Your New Life Begins

After Your Pregnancy Ends

The birth of your baby is a wonderful new beginning. You and your partner are probably filled with wonder and happiness at the incredible miracle that has occurred. You're enjoying your new baby and are probably anxious to begin your new life together.

The first 6 weeks immediately after baby's birth is called the *postpartum period*. During this time, you and your partner will go through periods of great adjustment. You may want to read the information as we present it, or you may want to check out the sections that are of most interest to you right now.

What Happens to Your Baby after Birth?

When your baby is delivered, the umbilical cord is cut and clamped, and the baby's mouth and throat are suctioned out. Then baby is usually passed to a nurse or pediatrician for initial evaluation and attention. Apgar scores (see below) are recorded at 1 and 5 minutes after birth. An identification band is placed on the baby. The nurse will dry baby and wrap her in warm blankets.

If your labor is complicated, baby may need to be evaluated more thoroughly in the nursery. You probably want to hold and to nurse her, but if she's having trouble breathing or needs special attention, immediate evaluation is the most appropriate procedure at this time.

Your baby will be weighed, measured and footprinted. Drops to prevent infection are placed in her eyes. A vitamin-K shot is given to help with her blood-clotting factors. Your baby may receive the hepatitis vaccine if you request it. Then she may be put in a heated bassinet for 30 minutes to 2 hours.

Your pediatrician is notified immediately if there are problems or concerns. Otherwise, he or she will be notified soon after birth, and a physical exam will be performed within 24 hours.

Tests for Your Baby

A baby is examined and evaluated at 1 minute, 5 minutes and, sometimes, 10 minutes after birth with the *Apgar score*.

It is a method of evaluating the overall well-being of a newborn infant. The higher the score, the better the infant's condition. Areas scored include the baby's heart rate, respiratory effort, muscle tone, reflex irritability and color.

A baby with a low 1-minute Apgar may need to be stimulated to breathe and to recover from delivery. In most cases, the 5-minute Apgar is higher than the 1-minute score as baby becomes more active and more accustomed to being outside the uterus.

Blood is taken from baby's heel for a *blood screen*. Results often indicate whether baby needs further evaluation. The *Coombs test* is administered if the mother's blood is Rh-negative, type O or if the mother has not been tested for antibodies. Test results indicate whether Rh-antibodies have been formed in the mother.

The *reflex assessment* tests for several reflexes in baby. If a particular reflex is not observed, further evaluation will be done. In the *neonatal maturity assessment*, baby's neuromuscular and physical maturity are evaluated. Each characteristic is assigned a score, and the sum indicates baby's maturity.

The *Brazelton neonatal behavioral assessment scale* covers a broad range of newborn behavior. It provides information about how a newborn responds to his or her environment. It is usually used when a problem is suspected, but some hospitals test all babies.

All 50 states and the District of Columbia require every newborn be screened for many life-threatening disorders. State laws and rules vary, but all states require screening for 21 or more of the 29 serious genetic or functional disorders. New York requires hospitals to check every newborn for HIV. Results are reported to the mother or guardian.

In the Hospital after Baby's Birth

You may be disappointed if you're expecting to lose 30 or 40 pounds immediately after baby's birth. It takes awhile for things to get back to normal, so be patient. In the first 10 days after birth, many women lose about 18 to 20 pounds. You may be very tired physically after labor and delivery. Your muscles may feel sore. It's the result of the hard physical work you did.

The time you spend in the hospital after delivery can be very helpful. Take advantage of educational channels, DVDs or videotapes on various subjects. The nursing staff is available to answer questions about your care, breastfeeding or the care of your baby. They can also show you how to bathe or diaper baby. They will advise you how to deal with your episiotomy and care for your breasts. They also allow you to get some rest—something you probably need very much!

Immediately Following Birth

Whether you had a vaginal birth or a Cesarean delivery, you are checked closely for the first few hours after birth for bleeding, pain and fever. If you had a Cesarean delivery, your abdomen may be sore, and you may not be able to move very quickly. If you had a vaginal birth, you may be able to get out of bed and walk around or go to the bathroom within a few hours.

When you feel able, get out of bed and go for a walk. Most healthcare providers want you to get up and get moving. It's also a good time to begin nursing baby. Many women breastfeed their babies as soon as they are able to—on the delivery table or in the recovery room.

During this time, food and fluids may be restricted for your safety. If you have a problem, such as heavy bleeding, it may be necessary to perform minor surgery, such as a D&C. It's safer for you to have an empty stomach if a procedure is necessary.

You will be offered medication to relieve any pain you experience after delivery. Your urine output may be checked to ensure your kidneys and bladder are working. Nurses check your incision if you had an episiotomy or a Cesarean.

You may have thought once you delivered, contractions would disappear, but your uterus contracts to control bleeding. Nursing your baby helps make contractions stronger and helps control bleeding. Contractions continue for several days after birth and signal the uterus is shrinking to its prepregnancy size (or as close as it will come to it). You may notice the same discomfort when you breastfeed.

You will experience a discharge of blood, called *lochia*. This occurs with a vaginal delivery *and* a Cesarean delivery, although it may not be quite as heavy with a C-section.

Your breasts may feel sore or tender. You can't stop the natural process of breast milk coming in, even if you do not plan to nurse your baby.

You may be surprised how hungry you are. When you get the OK, order something you really want. Or ask your partner to bring special food into the hospital.

Constipation, uncomfortable bowel movements and hemorrhoids may be leftover effects of pregnancy. In addition, delivery can slow the movement of food through the intestines, which may cause you to feel bloated or make you constipated. Taking pain medicine, changes in your diet and spending more time in bed may also keep your bowel from functioning normally. Drink plenty of fluids, eat bran and prunes, and take stool softeners.

Following a normal pregnancy, your body retains about 3 liters of water. It can take several weeks to get rid of this extra fluid. You may experience incontinence for a short time. As your uterus contracts and gets smaller, it'll improve.

Exercise may help you feel better faster. Walking is also good exercise. Ask your healthcare provider or the nurses taking care of you if it's OK to do these activities. If you get their OK, do light exercises, such as gently stretch your legs and arms. You can do some neck and shoulder rolls, shoulder shrugs, and foot and ankle circles. If you have done yoga exercises in the past, some of the gentler stretches may be good to do. Let your body and your healthcare provider be your guides as to how much you can do.

You may find you're emotional at times after baby's birth. Mood swings are usually mild, but some women experience more-severe feelings. These feelings are normal.

Friends and family will probably want to visit you in the hospital, which can be enjoyable, but don't be afraid to limit visiting time—either in person or on the telephone. Put a hold on your phone calls or hang a "Do not disturb" sign on your door when you want to rest.

Relax in the hospital before you go home with baby. Take advantage of the "built-in" room service and babysitting provided. Most women are discharged within a day or two after their baby's birth if labor and delivery were normal and the baby is doing well. With a Cesarean delivery, that time could be 3 to 4 days.

Physical Changes after Birth

Changes in the Uterus

Immediately after delivery, you should feel your uterus around your navel; it should be very hard. You are checked frequently to make sure it remains hard. If it feels soft, you or a nurse can massage it so it becomes firm—this is called *Credé*. The uterus shrinks about a finger's width every day, called *involution*. You will be checked daily while you're in the hospital to ensure your uterus is shrinking normally. This exam can be a little uncomfortable, but it is necessary.

Afterpains

Afterpains are just what they sound like—pains you experience after the birth of your baby. They are normal; expect to feel them for several days as your uterus contracts. Contractions occur to prevent heavy bleeding and to enable the uterus to return to its normal size.

If you breastfeed, afterpains may intensify when you nurse. Contractions help control bleeding, but they can be uncomfortable. Mild pain medication, such as acetaminophen or ibuprofen, can offer relief.

Perineum Pain

Stretching, cutting or tearing the area between the vagina and anus during labor and delivery can cause pain in the perineum. An episiotomy can add to this discomfort.

Pain doesn't last too long; most soreness should improve daily and be gone in about 3 weeks or by the time you see your healthcare provider for your 6-week checkup. If you have severe discomfort, use ice packs to numb the area and help reduce swelling. After 24 hours, a hot bath or soaking in a sitz tub several times a day can help.

Urinating may be painful because urine can sting the cut area. You may find it less painful to urinate standing or in the shower with running water washing over the area.

Bleeding after Delivery

It's common to lose some blood during labor and delivery. However, heavy bleeding after the baby is born can be a concern. A loss of more than 17 ounces in the first 24 hours after baby's birth is called *postpartum hemorrhage*. The most common causes of heavy bleeding include a uterus that doesn't contract, a large or bleeding episiotomy, clotting or coagulation problems, retained

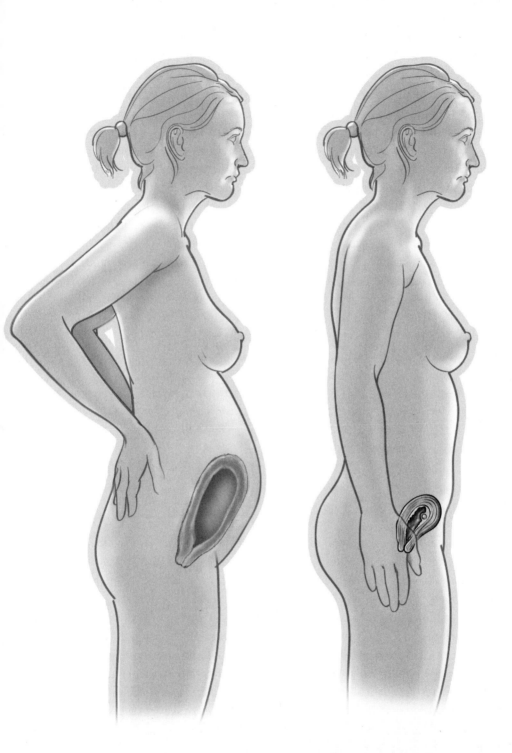

The illustration on the left shows the uterus is still enlarged
immediately after birth. It will take weeks before it is as small as it was
at 4 weeks of pregnancy (see the illustration on the right).

placental tissue, retained blood clots in the uterus, rips or tears in the vagina or cervix during birth or a tear, rupture or hole in the uterus (rare). Bleeding is controlled by massaging the uterus (Credé) and use of certain medications, such as Pitocin or methergine.

Normal bleeding after delivery gradually decreases each day until it stops. It may become a little heavier when you increase your activities. Do not use tampons; they have been associated with an increase in toxic-shock syndrome.

If you experience an *increase* in bleeding, call your healthcare provider immediately! In addition, if bleeding suddenly becomes heavy or you pass large blood clots, contact your healthcare provider. He or she may want to see you or to prescribe medication.

Headaches

Headaches can be a problem for some women after delivery. A headache can be caused or influenced by a long labor, having to push for a while or not sleeping in 24 to 36 hours. If you had pre-eclampsia or pregnancy-induced hypertension, either could cause a headache after delivery. An epidural or spinal anesthetic for labor or a Cesarean delivery can result in a headache called a *spinal headache.*

Tell your healthcare provider if you have a headache that doesn't go away or doesn't get better, especially if it is severe or is accompanied by blurred vision or nausea. He or she can recommend a course of treatment for you. Usually rest, fluids and mild pain medicine offer relief.

Hyperemesis after Pregnancy?

It has been commonly believed that symptoms associated with hyperemesis gravidarum (severe morning sickness; see Week 5) disappear after pregnancy. This is the case for most women, but studies show some women experience symptoms well beyond delivery that can take months to overcome. Women who received I.V. feedings during pregnancy because they couldn't eat had the highest rate of symptoms.

Recovery can take a few months to as long as 2 years. Some believe it takes 1 to 2 months of recovery for *every month* you were ill. Talk to your healthcare provider if your hyperemesis gravidarum persists after baby's birth. You may need to see a nutritionist. It is especially important to seek help before you plan another pregnancy.

Tubal Ligation

Some women choose to have a form of surgical sterilization performed, called *tubal ligation, postpartum tubal ligation* or *PTL*, while they are in the hospital after baby's birth. Tubal ligation is the number-one birth control method in the United States.

Surgery involves blocking a woman's Fallopian tubes to prevent further pregnancies. If you have decided before baby's birth to have a tubal ligation, doing it after delivery while you're still in the hospital can make sense. If you received an epidural for your labor and delivery, you're already anesthetized.

If you have a postpartum tubal ligation, your healthcare provider may want to examine you 10 to 14 days after you leave the hospital. He or she will check the incision to see if it is healing properly and to look for signs of infection.

Bonding with Your Baby

Have you heard how important it is to "bond with your baby"? What is bonding? Is it really important in your life with baby? When does it happen? How does it happen? *Bonding* is a process that usually takes longer than one instance to occur. It's the *process* of becoming emotionally attached to your child, and it deepens over time.

We once believed bonding was a purely emotional response, but today we believe there is also a physical aspect to bonding. Some researchers theorize that bonding stimulates production of prolactin and oxytocin in you, which causes you to feel more motherly toward your baby.

You can bond with your baby in the delivery room, your hospital room or at home. Don't be afraid the bond will be weaker if you and baby cannot "meet in the delivery room." A mother and her infant are programmed to connect after baby's birth. Both need each other.

Bonding often begins in the delivery room and can continue in your hospital room. Breastfeeding is one of the best ways for a mom to bond with her baby, especially if baby is fed on demand. If you don't breastfeed, you can still bond when you bottlefeed.

As your infant begins to mature, the bonding process will be strengthened. Dad also needs to bond with baby.

Encourage your partner to hold the baby close and make eye contact and skin contact. He can feed baby when you begin expressing your breast milk.

The key to bonding is to focus on the baby and the experiences you share. Include baby in your daily activities. Holding, cuddling and cooing are great ways to bond. Your baby will connect with you both when she feels the love and security you offer.

Recovery from a Vaginal Birth

A source of discomfort after you deliver vaginally will be in the vagina and the perineum. Pain or discomfort should lessen every day. You will be given a prescription for mild pain medications if necessary.

It's normal to bleed after delivery; bleeding continues for several days up to a couple of weeks. In the hospital, nurses will check bleeding to be sure it isn't excessive. When you go home, you'll still be bleeding, but the amount of bloody discharge should be decreasing. Sometimes when you become more active, bleeding may get a little heavier, but it should slow down again.

When you go home, gradually increase activities. Walk around, eat more normally and become more active each day. You may need to rest frequently—that's normal. Most healthcare providers recommend you wait until after your 6-week postpartum checkup before you begin any strenuous activity, exercise or become sexually active again. If you take pain medicines or have problems, don't drive. It's OK to use stairs, but plan ahead so you're not running up and down stairs all day.

Full recovery is different for every woman. If you had problems, it may take longer. From 2 to 6 weeks, you should be feeling a little better every day. You probably won't need pain medicine, and bleeding will decrease or stop. After 6 weeks, it's usually OK to resume routine activities.

Recovery from a Cesarean Delivery

The length of time a woman stays in the hospital after a Cesarean delivery varies from 2 to 4 days after delivery. With a Cesarean, pain control is accomplished in different ways. If you had an epidural or spinal anesthetic for the surgery, pain medicine may be injected through the epidural or spinal catheter; this is called *Duramorph* or *epidural morphine*. Medication usually offers pain relief for the first 24 hours.

Other pain-relief methods include injections of pain medications (Demerol or morphine) into an I.V. or a muscle during the first 24 hours after delivery. Once you can eat, you may be offered oral pain medications, such as acetaminophen with codeine or Lortab, or anti-inflammatory pain medications, such as ibuprofen.

. . . .

Research shows if a woman has a Cesarean delivery, she is less likely to breastfeed.

. . . .

With most Cesarean deliveries, a catheter is placed in your bladder through the urethra (the small tube from the bladder to the outside) to keep the bladder empty and out of the way during surgery. The catheter is usually left in place for 12 to 24 hours after the surgery.

Problems with gas or bowel movements are more common following a C-section than with a vaginal delivery. Although it may seem unpleasant, passing gas is a good sign your bowels are working. Get up and walk around as soon as possible. Drink plenty of liquids. Laxatives and stool softeners are available if necessary.

Light activity is important. In the hospital, you'll probably have to practice coughing or deep breathing to keep lungs clear. Wiggle toes to aid circulation. Move arms in circles. Walking may not be easy, but try—it helps minimize the chances of developing a blood clot.

Nurses will check your incision daily for infection or bleeding. Staples are usually removed before you leave the hospital. This may seem a little soon, but don't worry; the layers of tissue that really hold you together are deeper. Deeper sutures dissolve on their own, which can take weeks or months. If sutures were used to close abdominal skin, they may be removed or they may dissolve on their own. Most healthcare providers place steri-strips (small pieces of tape) on the incision; they stay on for 3 or 4 days. Before you leave the hospital, the nurses can show you how to take care of the incision and advise you of warning signs to watch for when you go home.

When you go home, you'll still be bleeding, but the amount of bloody discharge should be decreasing. Sometimes when you become more active, bleeding may get a little heavier, but this shouldn't last more than a few hours before it slows down again. Many healthcare providers will encourage you to take stool softeners or laxatives.

Your incision will probably be sore. Most women need mild pain medication; you will be offered prescriptions for pain medicine before you leave the hospital.

You should be able to get in and out of bed on your own. Certain activities, such as bending or lifting, may be uncomfortable, so during the first few weeks, don't lift anything heavier than your baby. Take things slowly, rest when necessary and increase activities gradually. Your healthcare provider may recommend you not drive if you're taking pain medicine. You may not want to drive for a while if you're uncomfortable or have trouble getting in or out of your car.

Most healthcare providers want you to come in for an exam following a Cesarean 10 to 14 days after you leave the hospital. Your incision will be checked to see whether it's healing properly and to look for signs of infection. A pelvic exam is usually *not* done at this visit.

From week 2 to week 6, you should notice gradual improvements in your energy every day. By 6 weeks, you can usually do anything you want. In the months to come you may not see big changes, but you will experience subtle improvements. Be aware—if you feel something isn't right, call your healthcare provider's office.

If you want to start exercising again, discuss it with your healthcare provider at your first postpartum visit, about 2 weeks after baby's birth. Before seeing the healthcare provider, you can do some nonstrenuous walking, Kegel exercises and breathing exercises. At your 6-week checkup, talk to your healthcare provider about more strenuous exercising, such as brisk walking, stretching and lifting light weights. Swimming can be very beneficial.

Life at Home

You probably have many questions about your postpartum recovery period. Your "problems" are probably normal, whether they are physical or emotional. If you have questions about any of this information or if you're concerned about your situation, call your healthcare provider. He or she is there to answer your questions and to reassure you.

Things should go well for you after your baby's birth—you shouldn't feel ill. However, women do occasionally experience problems. Below is a list of symptoms and warnings signs to be alert for:

- temperature of 101°F or more, except in the first 24 hours after birth
- painful or red breasts
- chills
- loss of appetite for an extended period
- pain in the lower abdomen or in the back
- pain, tenderness, redness and/or swelling in your legs
- painful urination or feeling an intense need to urinate

- failure to pass gas or severe constipation (no bowel movements for a few days)
- severe pain in the vagina or perineum area
- unusually heavy bleeding or a sudden increase in bleeding (more than your normal menstrual flow or soaking more than two sanitary pads in 30 minutes)
- vaginal discharge with strong, unpleasant odor

If you experience any of the above symptoms, call your healthcare provider. He or she may want to see you and prescribe a course of treatment.

If you have a chronic illness, such as diabetes or asthma, it may impact your recovery. You may need to watch for specific problems or to make particular adjustments. You may need to take medications or to adjust your activities. Discuss your situation with your healthcare provider at your 6-week checkup.

If pregnancy and birth have affected you in some particular way, you may be referred to a healthcare provider who specializes in treating the problem. He or she will work with your pregnancy healthcare provider if necessary.

Your Changing Bowel Habits
Your bowel habits will probably change for a few days after baby's birth. Your digestive system slows down during labor and after delivery because of medications, changes in your activity level or because you sit or lie in bed.

Many women don't want to have to deal with having a bowel movement for the first 4 or 5 days after delivery because it hurts. If you had vaginal tearing, an episiotomy or if you have hemorrhoids, your bowel movements may be difficult or painful. If you don't have a bowel movement within a week or if you become uncomfortable, contact your healthcare provider.

To help avoid constipation, eat a high-fiber diet, and drink lots of fluid to keep your system working efficiently. Prunes, prune juice, apple juice and bran are all natural laxatives; include them in your diet. Over-the-counter stool softeners may also be beneficial. Many stool softeners and laxatives are safe to use if you breastfeed.

Changes in Your Breasts
Whether you breastfeed or bottlefeed, sore breasts are fairly common after delivery. In the natural course of pregnancy and delivery, your body has prepared you to breastfeed, so your breasts will fill with milk. Fullness in your breasts is called *engorgement* and usually lasts a few days; it may be uncomfortable. If you breastfeed, empty your breasts when baby nurses, and the situation will resolve itself in a few days.

It's a little more difficult if you choose *not* to breastfeed because milk still comes in. Medication is not given to stop production of breast milk. Ease discomfort by wearing a support bra or binding your breasts with an Ace bandage or a towel. Ice packs also help milk dry up.

Try *not* to empty your breasts. This may be difficult; emptying your breasts may be the only way to get relief.

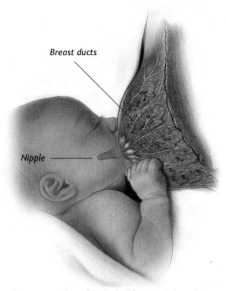

Breast ducts

Nipple

Nursing the first 4 weeks of baby's life provides the most protection
for baby and the best hormone release for you.

However, when you empty your breasts, your body replaces the expressed breast milk with more milk! Avoid nipple stimulation and warm water on the breasts because these practices also stimulate breasts to produce milk. Hearing a baby cry—yours or someone else's—may also make you lose milk.

Urinary Incontinence

Bladder function and/or urination may be different after delivery. After a baby is born, some women experience *urinary incontinence*. It may last briefly, or it can last a few weeks or longer. Most women report the more pregnancies and deliveries they have, the greater their problem with incontinence.

Help yourself regain bladder and urine control by practicing Kegel exercises. See Week 14. Do not hold your urine; empty your bladder fairly often.

It takes time for things to get better. Even after you're fully recovered, bladder control may not be the same as before pregnancy. Let your healthcare provider know if a urinary problem continues or worsens. Improvement may not come until you begin to get back in shape.

Swelling and Water Retention

After baby's birth, it takes some time to get rid of extra fluid your body has retained. To help lessen swelling, do the same things you were advised to do during pregnancy. Lie on your side several times during the day and at night when you sleep. Get up and get moving; if you just sit in bed, it'll take longer to get rid of extra fluid. Exercise regularly. Contact your healthcare provider if these measures don't help or if problems continue after your recovery.

Getting Enough Sleep and Rest

Fatigue and exhaustion may become more of a problem after baby's birth. As many parents can tell you, it's no easy task to adjust to night after night of interrupted sleep. A baby usually wakes up every 2 to 4 hours to feed, which can be disruptive to parents.

Don't be afraid to ask for help; most people enjoy it. It's fun to take care of a new baby! Your partner will want to help, but he may not know what to do. He may appreciate suggestions from you, such as getting up to feed the baby (this works best if you're not nursing), changing baby at night or bringing baby to you in the middle of the night.

Get sleep whenever and wherever you can. Until baby is about 2 months old, you probably won't be able to put a long-term sleep plan into action.

The Postpartum Checkup

Your body changes a lot during the 4 to 6 weeks following delivery. By the time you visit your healthcare provider for your 6-week postpartum checkup, your uterus will be about the size of a grapefruit. That's an incredible feat, considering it was the size of a small watermelon only a few weeks ago!

At your visit, your healthcare provider checks your weight and blood pressure. Any incision you have will be checked. Breasts are examined, and your uterus, ovaries and cervix are checked—yes, that means another pelvic exam. Your healthcare provider may discuss postpartum depression with you; you may undergo screening for the condition.

If you had a vaginal birth, your healthcare provider will examine any tears or incisions. If you had a C-section, your incision will be examined. If you

developed hemorrhoids or varicose veins during pregnancy, your healthcare provider will also check those.

If you took any medication before or during pregnancy, ask about continuing it or resuming it now. If you have any questions about your recovery, address them at this time. It's a good time to discuss birth-control options if you don't want to get pregnant again immediately.

Your 6-week postpartum checkup is also a good time to ask questions about future pregnancies. Discuss concerns about, and complications from, your recent delivery. This information can be helpful if you move or deliver with a different healthcare provider or hospital in the future.

Birth Control after Pregnancy

Contraception after the birth of your baby is something you probably need to think about. If you don't want to have another baby very soon, it's important to discuss birth-control options with your partner and your healthcare provider in the hospital or at your postpartum checkup.

If You Breastfeed

Breastfeeding usually inhibits the production of gonadotropin for an average of 17 weeks. However, be aware research shows that 80% of all breastfeeding women ovulate *before* their first period! About 40% of women who use breastfeeding for birth control get pregnant. Don't rely on breastfeeding alone if you don't want another pregnancy right away. *Take precautions.*

Breastfeeding may help you lose baby weight, but studies show you need to do it for at least 3 months to get any benefit.

In the past, oral contraceptives were not prescribed for a breastfeeding woman. However, today we have progesterone-only pills that do not decrease milk production, and there are no known harmful effects on the baby. Most healthcare providers do not prescribe these oral contraceptives until a woman's milk supply is fully established, usually 1 to 2 weeks after birth or at your 6-week postpartum checkup.

Or you may choose an IUD; it has been proved safe for nursing. An IUD has no effect on milk production and can be inserted 6 weeks after delivery. You may also choose Norplant or Depo-Provera. Either method can be started immediately after delivery; both are safe to use during breastfeeding.

If You Bottlefeed

If you bottlefeed, you have many birth-control options. If you want to use an oral contraceptive that contains estrogen and progestin (the regular birth-control pill), wait at least 2 weeks after delivery to begin. Oral contraceptives are easy to use and pose few health risks. A hormone-releasing patch is also a good choice. It is very effective and releases the same hormones as the pill. One patch is good for 1 week.

Implanon is a flexible plastic implant placed under the skin, like Norplant. It releases hormones to prevent pregnancy and has proved 99.9% effective for up to 3 years. A flexible ring, called *NuvaRing*, can provide you with protection for 3 weeks. It is inserted into the vagina like a diaphragm, then removed for 1 week, during which you have periodlike bleeding. A new ring is then inserted for the next 3 weeks.

Methods for Any Woman to Use

Some birth-control methods can be used by any woman whether she breastfeeds or bottlefeeds. Barrier methods may be considered; they include condoms, a diaphragm or a cervical cap. The size of a woman's cervix can change after she has a baby, so if you used a diaphragm or cervical cap before pregnancy, you need to be refitted after the birth.

Talk to your healthcare provider if you practice any of the "rhythm" methods of contraception. This refers to three different methods of avoiding pregnancy, including periodic (rhythmic) abstinence, calendar-rhythm method and temperature-rhythm method.

Will We Ever Have Sex Again?

In the past, we advised a woman to wait at least 6 weeks before having intercourse. Today, we tell a woman to let her body be her guide, but 6 weeks is still a good suggestion. You probably won't feel like it anyway until then. If you feel no pain or discomfort, and your episiotomy is healed, you can resume sexual relations when you feel up to it if bleeding has stopped. For most women, this is often 4 to 6 weeks after delivery.

Belly Bands after Pregnancy?
. . . .

You've probably heard about belly bands during pregnancy. What about after pregnancy—will a belly band help you recover your figure? Some new mothers swear by them.

Belly bands and wraps, also called *abdominal binders*, have been around for quite a while. They've been used to help support the back and to help ease pain in people who suffer from back pain. They are also used after some surgeries, such as tummy tucks or liposuction.

Belly bands can be used after a vaginal or Cesarean delivery to provide abdominal support and to help with posture. Women often ask for them while they are still in the hospital—many hospitals now supply them on request. A belly band gently compresses abdominal muscles and may help the uterus return to its normal, after-pregnancy size more quickly. This may help a new mom reduce the size of her after-baby tummy. And it may help you get moving more quickly and easily after delivery.

Some healthcare providers recommend a belly band as part of postbaby recovery. But you must realize you won't have your prepregnancy figure back in a week. Most experts recommend you don your belly band after delivery and wear it off and on for 4 to 6 weeks after birth for the best results.

A belly band can cost from $20 to $100. You may need to buy more than one to fit you as you get smaller. Or if you bought various sizes to fit you as you grew during pregnancy, you may be able to wear the larger ones after delivery, gradually fitting into the smaller ones as your body recovers from your pregnancy.

Be aware—belly bands are not a substitute for exercise and healthy eating after pregnancy. You'll still have to exercise and eat a well-balanced diet after baby's birth. If you're interested, talk to your doctor about belly bands after pregnancy.

Maybe the last thing on your mind right now is resuming sexual relations. However, many couples look forward to resuming intimacy after baby's birth. In fact, studies show over 80% of couples enjoy sex again at 12 weeks postpartum.

Resuming sexual relations can be a little difficult. Your sex drive, and that of your partner, can be affected by stress, emotions and fatigue. Share your feelings and concerns. There are physical reasons you may not feel like having sex. You may still be bleeding. If you had an episiotomy, that may add to your discomfort. And with all the changes your body has gone through, you just may not feel sexy right now. That's OK. Take it easy and go slowly.

Talk to your partner to make sure he isn't expecting to resume relations with you 1 or 2 weeks after delivery when you're thinking it will be 4 to 6 weeks. When you do decide to have intercourse, take precautions if you don't want to get pregnant again immediately.

Getting Back in Shape

After a woman gives birth, often one of her first concerns may be regaining her prepregnancy figure. Your body needs some time to recover from the grueling 9-month experience that has just ended. Don't obsess about weight loss after baby's birth.

Some experts suggest a woman wait until her baby is at least 2 months old before she tries to shed extra pregnancy pounds. If you begin dieting too early, your body may release environmental toxins stored in your body fat. These can pass into your breast milk and, thus, to your baby if you breastfeed.

. . . .

Wait a couple of weeks to get on the scale after delivery. It takes some time for your body to get rid of excess fluid you added during pregnancy.

. . . .

What you eat after pregnancy has an effect on your weight, energy level and emotional state. Be sure to get enough protein—if you don't, your body will break down muscle to get it. Do *not* crash diet—even if you're bottlefeeding. Your body needs a balanced diet for energy. Drink plenty of fluids, especially water. Avoid junk food and empty-calorie foods. Eat protein, complex carbohydrates and dairy products. For most women, it takes about a year to lose all their pregnancy weight.

One of the most frequently asked questions after a baby is born is, "How soon can I start exercising?" After months of watching their bodies change so dramatically, many women want to get their prepregancy figures back and are eager to begin exercising soon after baby is born.

If you exercised regularly during pregnancy, you may be able to continue with many of the same exercises. Your body is probably still in good condition, so after delivery you can begin exercising and increase your activity levels a little more quickly.

Do an activity you enjoy and will stick with. Begin with light exercise; gradually work into a more-strenuous program. Let your body be your guide as to how much you can do and the level of intensity you put into your workout. Changes in your cardiovascular system from pregnancy can last for a while, which can affect your ability to exercise.

After about 6 weeks, strenuous exercise shouldn't impact your milk supply. If you breastfeed and do weightbearing exercises during that time, it will benefit your health because you lower your risk of developing osteoporosis later in life.

Talk to your healthcare provider *before* you start an exercise program. **If you had a Cesarean delivery or birth complications, it's necessary to check with your healthcare provider before starting an exercise routine or exercise program of any kind.**

Planning and Preparing for Your Next Pregnancy

It may seem strange to discuss your next pregnancy when you've just had a baby, but it's an important consideration. Most women want to wait for a while after they have a baby before even thinking about pregnancy again. They're busy with baby and recovering from pregnancy, labor and delivery.

Getting pregnant right away can affect your ability to breastfeed. Most experts recommend stopping breast-feeding if you're pregnant, which can shorten the time you can provide the benefits of breastfeeding to your baby.

Most recommend you not get pregnant for at least 18 months after delivery. A short interval between pregnancies increases your chances of many problems. If you conceive too soon, your body may not have time to replenish vitamins or blood lost after your last pregnancy. Having your children 2½ to 3 years apart may be an ideal length of time. Consider waiting 18 to 28 months after giving birth to get pregnant again.

. . . .

Recent research indicates a baby born within 2 years of an older sibling may be at higher risk of autism. The incidence of siblings being born closely together has risen as many older mothers complete their families more quickly. It was once believed older parents were a major element in the increased autism rate. However, experts now theorize biological factors, such as depleted maternal nutrients due to the short amount of time between pregnancies, could be more important in the increased autism rate. More research needs to be done.

. . . .

If you had any problems or complications during or after your pregnancy, take care of them now. Talk to your healthcare provider about receiving any vaccinations you had to put off during pregnancy.

Many women are able to lose most, but not all, of the weight gained during a previous pregnancy. With each pregnancy they start out 5 to 10 pounds heavier. It's a good idea to lose all your pregnancy weight *before* getting pregnant again. If you don't, you double your risk of having a large baby with your next pregnancy and may increase your risks of high blood pressure and gestational diabetes.

Whenever you decide to have another baby, it's important to be prepared. Take good care of yourself so if you decide to become pregnant again, you'll have already gone a long way in ensuring the good health of yourself and your next baby.

. . . .

For further information about baby after birth, read our book Your Baby's First Year Week by Week. *It contains a lot of information you may find useful.*

. . . .

Appendix A

Getting Pregnant

At any one time, over 7 million couples in the United States are having difficulty conceiving. Many couples struggle with infertility—the inability or decreased ability to achieve pregnancy. Problems that affect fertility can be present in either partner. When evaluating fertility, both parents-to-be should be examined. This discussion explores some of the reasons a couple may have trouble conceiving.

Age can be a factor in infertility—fertility decreases as a couple gets older. If you're healthy and in your 20s, don't get concerned unless a year has passed and you aren't pregnant. If you're over 30, talk to your doctor if you aren't pregnant in 6 months.

If you have health issues, you may want to talk to your doctor after trying to get pregnant for 6 months. Some things may impact your ability to conceive, including endometriosis, pelvic inflammatory disease (PID), painful or irregular periods, recurrent miscarriages or sexually transmitted diseases. Endometriosis is most common in women in their 30s and 40s, especially those who have not had children. It also runs in families, so if a sister or your mother had the problem, you may also experience it.

We know maternal age and lifestyle choices, such as smoking and obesity, can impact fertility. But stress does *not* seem to reduce fertility. Studies show no difference in the rates of pregnancy between women who were stressed and those who were not.

Check your diet; what you eat and drink is important. Eating at least two servings a day of full-fat dairy products has been shown to help increase fertility by as much as 25%! If you eat low-fat dairy foods every day, you may be reducing your chances of conceiving. If you eat a lot of protein, it may interfere with embryonic development. Studies show taking in more than 300mg/day of caffeine can also impact fertility. In addition, eating disorders can cause infertility.

Taking specific vitamins and minerals may help increase your chances of pregnancy. Decreased levels of iron, protein, vitamin C and zinc have been tied to less-frequent ovulation. A daily multivitamin can help you increase your levels of these important vitamins and nutrients.

. . . .

Men play an important role in prenatal health. However, the study of male reproductive health falls far behind that of women.

. . . .

Ovulation Monitors and Other Tests

Many tests are available to predict when ovulation occurs. Tests detect a surge in luteinizing hormone (LH). Most tests can be done at home and are easy to use. The tests work well if you have a fairly regular menstrual cycle. But you need to be consistent in your testing.

If your menstrual cycle is not regular, consider using a daily ovulation test. It provides testing for 20 days every month to help ensure you don't miss a surge in luteinizing hormone. Your best chance of getting pregnant is actually the *day before* a surge in LH. The second best day is the day of the surge, and the third best day is the day after the surge.

Types of Tests

Today we're lucky to have many tests available to predict when ovulation occurs. Below is a discussion of some ovulation-predictor tests available.

The *First Response Easy-Read Ovulation Test* may help you learn the most fertile time during your cycle. You use it for 7 days, during the time you believe you're ovulating, and it shows the day you are most fertile.

The *Clear-Plan Easy Fertility Monitor* helps you track where you are in your menstrual cycle. All you have to do is press a button at the start of a new menstrual period to begin tracking your cycle. For 10 days during the cycle, you use a urine sample to test hormone levels. The monitor judges where you are in your fertility cycle.

The *Donna Saliva Ovulation Tester* uses saliva to predict ovulation. The salt content of a woman's saliva is the same as the woman's cervical fluid when she ovulates. Saliva is placed on the microscope lens, and the pattern is examined after it dries. When a woman is not ovulating, random dots appear; however, 1 to 3 days before ovulation, short hairlike structures can be seen. On the day of ovulation, a fernlike pattern appears that makes it easy to distinguish from other patterns.

The *OV-Watch* is a device you wear on your wrist to help you determine when you're most fertile. The device measures the concentration of chloride on your skin, which can be an indicator of increased fertility. When you read the OV-Watch, it tells you whether you are fertile (preovulation), ovulating, less fertile (after ovulation) or not fertile. It is worn at night; in the morning, you read the results.

The *TCI Ovulation Tester* measures the level of estrogen throughout your cycle using your saliva. Some saliva is placed on a slide, and when it's dry, you examine it with a small lens or eye piece. When your saliva has a fernlike appearance, you're fertile.

The *Ovulite* microscope is similar to the TCI test; however, it allows for unlimited testing of saliva. You sample your saliva daily, and when you see a change, you know you're ovulating.

Other Fertility Tests

Home tests for men measure whether sperm is moving and provide an approximate sperm count. Sperm concentration is one of the factors doctors use to help determine male fertility.

One test for men is a home screening test called *Baby Start*. It's a quick test that looks at sperm concentration in semen. It measures sperm as above or below the cutoff of 20 million sperm cells per milliliter (ml). Two test results of less than 20 million cells/ml may indicate male infertility. If a man uses this test and results indicate a low sperm count, he should see a urologist for further testing.

Should a Man Prepare for Pregnancy?
. . . .

Is a father-to-be's health important in getting pregnant? Research over the years has proved a man's health before pregnancy is just as important as a woman's! We know about 40% of all infertility problems are caused by a father-to-be. And because it takes 74 days for sperm to mature, anything a man ingests or is exposed to during that time can impact sperm, which can affect pregnancy.

A man's eating habits, exercise routine and vitamin/supplement intake are very important in preparing for pregnancy. So are lifestyle issues, such as the use of tobacco and/or marijuana products, alcohol intake and use of some over-the-counter and prescription medications.

So when should a man starting preparing for pregnancy? He should start at least 3 months before conception—that's the same amount of time as a woman needs to prepare. A dad-to-be should be as healthy as possible before pregnancy, and he should continue these habits until pregnancy is achieved. By doing so, he will help give baby the best start in life.

One fertility test is for couples to use at home; it is called *Fertell* and contains tests for each partner. The tests measure the number of sperm that can swim through mucus in the man and the level of follicle-stimulating hormone (FSH) in a woman at a particular point in her cycle.

A Man's Health and Fertility

A man can affect a woman's ability to get pregnant. We know about 40% of all infertility problems can be placed directly on the shoulders of the male partner.

Men have a biological clock. After age 30, a man's level of testosterone decreases about 1% each year. Men over 40 are at increased risk for infertility. In addition, if a man fathers a child after he reaches 40, the child has a greater chance of problems. Risks are even higher for men 55 and older.

Women who have a partner over age 40 have an increased risk of miscarriage, no matter what the woman's age. The miscarriage rate for partners of men under 30 is about 14%. For men over 45, that rate more than doubles to over 30%!

If a man's parents underwent fertility treatments to conceive him, he may have fertility issues. Some problems in men born after fertility treatments include lower sperm count, smaller testicles and fewer motile sperm.

Many things can impact a man's fertility. Below is a discussion of some of the elements that can affect a man.

Foods and Supplements

The foods a man eats can affect a woman's chances of getting pregnant. Studies show men who eat and/or avoid certain foods for at least 3 months may increase fertility. Beneficial foods to eat and foods to avoid include those listed in the box on page 420.

. . . .

Alcohol and caffeine can cause sperm deformities that result in problems in child development.

. . . .

Supplements can also affect fertility. Men should take a multivitamin every day, especially one with zinc. Zinc supplements should not contain cadmium, which can damage testes. A man also needs an

Fertility Food Facts

Foods Beneficial to Fertility
- Grains and seeds
- Nuts, such as cashews and almonds
- Chocolate
- Vitamin-C-rich organic fruits and vegetables, grown without pesticides
- Dark, green, leafy vegetables
- Total of 6 to 8 ounces a day of chicken, meat or fish, including red meat and cooked oysters (but keep total weekly fish intake to 12 ounces or less)
- Calcium-rich foods, such as yogurt, cheese and milk
- Fortified breakfast cereals

Foods that May Contribute to Infertility
- Chips, cookies and crackers made with partially hydrogenated oils
- Fruits and vegetables commercially grown with pesticides
- Fried foods
- High-meat diet

adequate intake of selenium, either in the foods he eats or as a 60mcg supplement every day. Selenium-rich foods include garlic, fish and eggs.

It's important for a man to consume folate (the folic acid found in food) before conception. One study showed men who took in more than 700mcg each day from food sources passed on 20% fewer chromosomal abnormalities. Good sources of folate include asparagus, bananas, tuna and spinach. In addition, walnuts improve sperm quality in men under age 35. Eating 2½ ounces of walnuts a day for 3 months improves sperm motility. In older men, intake of antioxidants helps sperm quality. To produce sperm with less DNA damage, increase your intake of foods containing vitamins C and E and zinc.

Be careful with manganese—higher blood levels have been found to lower sperm quality. Calcium supplements made from seashells may be contaminated with metals.

Lifestyle Issues

Lifestyle choices and changes by a man may increase a woman's chances of getting pregnant. These choices may provide a growing baby a healthy start in life. There are many issues in a man's life to examine.

Use of tobacco products can affect sperm production. Smoking one or two packs of cigarettes a day may cause sperm to move slowly and/or be misshapen. Second-hand and third-hand smoke can also affect fertility.

Men who smoke have a higher occurrence of sperm containing the wrong number of chromosomes. In addition, smoking by a dad-to-be has been linked to childhood cancers in their offspring.

Smoking marijuana can damage sperm and lower the number of sperm produced. It takes up to several months to rid the body of THC (tetrahydrocannabinol), even after a person quits smoking marijuana.

Alcohol use can lower testosterone levels, contribute to erectile dysfunction and cause chromosome abnormalities in sperm cells. One study showed men who drank heavily around the time of conception increased their partner's risk of miscarriage.

Men who are too thin may be malnourished. Men who are too heavy may have lower testosterone levels.

. . . .

There are many ways men can increase the health of their sperm. Being physically active is a good start. Studies show men who are active have better-formed, faster-swimming sperm than men who are inactive. For most men, exercise does not impact the quality or quantity of sperm. The exception is cycling, which can negatively affect sperm. Men who are sedentary for more than 20 hours a week have a lower sperm count than men who are active.

. . . .

Women whose partners were exposed to heavy metals, such as lead and mercury, had a higher number of miscarriages. Men who worked in industries involving solvents, dyes, paints and cleaning solutions fathered a higher number of children with birth defects. Long-term exposure to solvents affects a man's sperm.

Use of anabolic steroids and nonsteroidal anti-inflammatory medications may slow or reduce sperm production. Even antibiotics can affect sperm production.

Limit time in the hot tub. The scrotum is a few degrees cooler than the rest of the body, so soaking a long time in hot spa water may affect sperm.

Medical Problems

About 10% of American men who are trying to achieve a pregnancy with their partner experience some sort of fertility problem. However, many men don't know they have a problem. For example, a low sperm count

may be caused by infection, hormone problems, certain medications or undescended testicles. A man's doctor can explore these conditions with him.

One of the most common medical problems is a *varicocele*, a collection of enlarged veins in the scrotum that leads to lower sperm production. Another problem is an obstruction in the ducts that carry sperm from the testes. Often, both of these can be taken care of with microsurgical techniques to improve a man's sperm count and increase the chances of a couple achieving pregnancy.

Treatments for Infertility

If a doctor suggests a couple have a fertility workup, it helps to understand what's involved. For a man, a physical and semen analysis may be done and a detailed medical history may be taken.

Testing is more involved for a woman. A detailed medical history is taken, and a pelvic exam is done. Hormone levels may be checked. A vaginal ultrasound to examine ovaries and the uterus may also be done. If the doctor wants to check Fallopian tubes, a hysterosalpingogram (HSG) may be performed.

After test results are back for the couple, they will meet with the doctor to discuss results. Then together, options will be examined for care and/or treatment, if necessary.

Cinnamon to Help Infertility?

Polycystic ovary syndrome affects up to 5 million American women in the United States of childbearing age. Believed to be caused by an insensitivity to insulin, the syndrome often contributes to a woman's infertility.

Treatment frequently involves weight loss, ovulation-inducing medications and some diabetes drugs. However, research has demonstrated the spice cinnamon (in approved quantities) may improve a woman's ability to process glucose and insulin. This could help relieve the problem of irregular menstrual cycles that many women with polycystic ovary syndrome experience. If you have questions about this treatment, discuss them with your healthcare provider.

Assisted-Reproductive Technologies (ART)

Assisted-reproductive technologies (ART) can often help a couple achieve pregnancy. ART account for more births today and include ovarian stimulation, superovulation and in-vitro fertilization.

. . . .

Implanting only one embryo during in-vitro fertilization is now recommended. With one embryo, a woman is 5 times more likely to give birth to a healthy baby than a woman who chooses to have two embryos implanted. In addition, implantation of only one embryo improves the live-birth rate and decreases costs.

. . . .

Ovarian stimulation is used to stimulate ovaries to produce an egg. Several different medications are used for this purpose; a common one is clomiphene (Clomid). It is used most often in women who don't ovulate and may result in controlled ovarian hyperstimulation. The chance of twin fetuses is somewhat less with clomiphene than with other fertility medicine, but an increased chance exists. A complication that may occur is ovarian hyperstimulation syndrome—ovaries become enlarged and the abdomen becomes distended.

The use of fertility drugs can result in *superovulation*, which results in multiple eggs and increases the chance of multiple fetuses. A large percentage of births resulting from assisted-reproductive techniques are multiples.

In-vitro fertilization (IVF) is the process in which eggs are placed in a medium and sperm are added for fertilization. The zygote produced is then placed inside the uterus in an attempt to result in pregnancy. Since 1989, over 5 million babies have been conceived via in-vitro fertilization. Nearly 2½ million were conceived since 2008!

Assisted-reproductive technologies account for nearly 65% of all multiple births today. Fertility treatments are expensive and can cost up to $15,000 for each attempt at conception. Often, health insurance does not cover fertility treatments.

Appendix B

Postpartum Distress Syndrome (PPDS)

You may experience many emotional changes after baby is born. Mood swings, mild distress or bouts of crying are not uncommon and are often a result of hormonal changes you experience after birth, just as they were when you were pregnant.

Many women are surprised by how tired they are emotionally and physically in the first few months after baby's birth. Sleep and rest can help you deal with mood shifts, which seem to occur more often when a woman is exhausted.

After pregnancy, many women experience some degree of depression. This is called *postpartum distress syndrome (PPDS)*. Some experts believe PPDS may begin during pregnancy, but symptoms may not appear until after delivery. They may occur when a woman starts getting her period again and experiences hormonal changes.

Postpartum distress syndrome can resolve on its own, but it can often take as long as a year. With more severe problems, treatment may relieve symptoms in a matter of weeks, and improvement should be significant within 6 to 8 months. Often medication is necessary for complete recovery.

If your baby blues don't get better in a few weeks or if you feel depressed, call your healthcare provider. You may need medication to help deal with the problem.

Different Degrees of Depression

There are different degrees of depression. The mildest form is *baby blues*. Up to 80% of all women have "baby blues." They usually appear between 2 days and 2 weeks after birth. They are temporary and usually leave as quickly as they come. This situation lasts only a couple of weeks, and symptoms do not worsen.

A more serious version of postpartum distress is called *postpartum depression (PPD)*. It affects about 10% of all new mothers. The difference between baby blues and postpartum depression lies in the frequency, intensity and duration of symptoms.

PPD can occur from 2 weeks to 1 year after birth. A mother may have feelings of anger, confusion, panic and hopelessness. She may experience changes in her eating and sleeping patterns. She may fear she will hurt her baby or feel as if she is going crazy. Anxiety is one of the major symptoms of PPD.

The most serious form of postpartum distress is *postpartum psychosis (PPP)*. The woman may have hallucinations, think about suicide or try to harm the baby. Many women who develop postpartum psychosis also exhibit signs of bipolar disorder, which is unrelated to childbirth. Discuss this situation with your physician if you are concerned.

After you give birth, if you believe you are suffering from some form of postpartum distress syndrome, contact your healthcare provider. Every postpartum reaction, whether mild or severe, is usually temporary and treatable.

It's normal to feel extremely tired, especially after the hard work of labor and delivery and adjusting to the demands of being a new mom. However, if after 2 weeks of motherhood you're just as exhausted as you were shortly after you delivered, you may be at risk of developing postpartum depression.

. . . .

The Family and Medical Leave Act provides for up to 12 weeks of maternity leave, but research indicates this amount of time may not be enough time for a new mom. She may need more time than this to recover fully and to help reduce the risk of PPDS. In the year following the birth of their babies, many women experience some degree of postpartum distress, so a longer time away from work may be beneficial. A minimum of 6 months may help reduce the risk of PPDS.

. . . .

Causes of Postpartum Distress Syndrome

We aren't sure what causes postpartum distress; not all women experience it. A woman's individual sensitivity to hormonal changes may be part of the cause. The drop in estrogen and progesterone after delivery may contribute to the problem.

A new mother must make many adjustments, and many demands are placed on her. Either or both of these situations may cause distress. If you had a Cesarean delivery, you may also be at greater risk for postpartum depression.

Other possible factors include a family history of depression, lack of familial support after the birth, isolation and chronic fatigue. You may also be at higher risk of suffering from PPDS if your mother or sister suffered from the problem; it seems to run in families. If you suffered from PPDS with a previous pregnancy, chances are you'll have the problem again. Fertility treatments to achieve this pregnancy may contribute to PPDS—hormone fluctuations may be more severe. Suffering from extreme PMS before the pregnancy can cause hormonal imbalances after birth, adding to the problem.

If you have a personal history of depression or you suffered from untreated depression before pregnancy, you may experience PPDS. Anxiety, low self-esteem, a struggling relationship with baby's father or limited access to finances and health care can all contribute to postpartum distress syndrome. If you don't have enough social support, if you had more than one baby or if you have a colicky or high-maintenance baby, this can add to the problem. Lack of sleep, sleeping less than 6 hours in a 24-hour period or waking 3 or more times in a night can also be a cause.

In addition, if you answer "most of the time" or "some of the time" to any of the following questions, you may be at increased risk.

- I blame myself when things go wrong (even if you have nothing to do with them).
- I often feel scared or panicked without good reason.
- I am anxious or worried without good reason.

Handling the Baby Blues

One of the most important ways you can help yourself handle baby blues is to have a good support system. Ask family members and friends to help. Ask your mother or mother-in-law to stay for a while. Ask your husband to take some work leave, or hire someone to come in and help each day.

Rest when your baby sleeps. Find other mothers who are in the same situation; it helps to share your feelings and experiences. Don't try to be perfect. Pamper yourself.

Do some form of moderate exercise every day, even if it's just going for a walk. Eat nutritiously, and drink plenty of fluids. Get out of the house every day. Eating more complex carbohydrates may help raise your mood. And giving baby a massage may help you because it helps you connect with your baby.

Talk to your healthcare provider about temporarily using antidepressants if the above steps don't work for you. Some women who suffer from postpartum depression require medication.

Dealing with More Serious Forms of PPDS

Beyond the relatively minor symptoms of baby blues, postpartum distress syndrome can appear in two ways. Some women experience acute depression that can last for weeks or months; they cannot sleep or eat, they feel worthless and isolated, and they are sad and cry a great deal. For other women, they are extremely anxious, restless and agitated. Their heart rate increases. Some unfortunate women experience both sets of symptoms at the same time.

If you experience symptoms, call your healthcare provider immediately. He or she will probably see you, then prescribe a course of treatment. Do it for yourself and your family.

Your Distress Can Affect Your Partner

If you experience baby blues or PPD, it can also affect your partner. Prepare him for this situation before baby is born. Explain to him that if it happens to you, it's only temporary.

There are some things you might suggest to your partner that he can do for himself. Tell him not to take the situation personally. Suggest he talk to friends, family members, other fathers or a professional. He should eat well, and get enough rest and exercise. Ask him to be patient with you, and ask him to provide his love and support to you during this difficult time.

Appendix C

Feeding Your Baby

Feeding your baby is one of the most important things you will do as a mother. Will you breastfeed or bottlefeed? Until the 1940s, babies were breastfed almost exclusively. Today, about 70% of all new moms start out breastfeeding their babies, but by 3 months, over 65% of all babies are bottlefed exclusively. Some women choose not to breastfeed. The decision is yours. You won't be considered a "bad mother" if you choose to bottlefeed.

Some experts believe you can start feeding baby a bottle almost as soon as you get home from the hospital. If you do, give baby expressed breast milk because its taste is familiar. Feed a bottle an hour or two after breastfeeding. It's easier to get baby to try a bottle when she's not starving.

Breastfeeding Baby

Breastfeeding is the healthiest way to feed baby because breast milk provides the best nutrition. For many women, it completes the birth experience. Breast milk provides many benefits for baby that can't be duplicated by formula feeding.

You can usually begin breastfeeding within an hour (or sooner) after birth. This helps establish your milk supply and provides baby with colostrum, the first milk your breasts produce. Breast milk comes in 12 to 48 hours after birth.

If you have problems breastfeeding, people are available to help you. Your local La Leche League can put you in contact with a breastfeeding counselor who can offer support and share experiences. If she believes your situation is beyond her scope, she can refer you to a lactation consultant.

Benefits of Breastfeeding

All babies receive some protection from mom against disease before birth. Breast-fed babies receive continued protection in breast milk. Nursing the first 4 weeks of baby's life provides the most protection for baby and the best hormone release for you. Breastfeeding for as short as 3 months may reduce baby's risk of developing allergies and infections. Breastfeeding for the first 6 months may help reduce the risks of many other problems, and it may lower your child's risk of SIDS by 50%!

The American Academy of Pediatrics (AAP) recommends breastfeeding exclusively for the first 6 months. Breast milk contains many substances to help prevent infection. However, microwaving breast

Lactation Consultants
• • • • • • • • • • •

A *lactation consultant* is a qualified professional who can help with basic breastfeeding issues, assess and observe you and your baby, develop a care plan, inform healthcare providers of the situation and follow up with you as needed. You can contact a lactation consultant before baby's birth. Contact the International Lactation Consultant Association for further information. They can be reached at 919–861–5577 or through their website at www.ilca.org.

milk can kill antibodies that help protect baby from illness and disease, so *never* microwave breast milk.

DHA (docosahexaenoic acid) and ARA (arachidonic acid) in breast milk are important for baby. Studies show a baby who has them in his diet may have a higher IQ and greater visual development.

Breastfeeding and You
Breastfeeding baby affects you as well. It may help you lose weight, but studies show you need to breastfeed baby for at least 3 months to get any benefit. After your milk supply is well established (about 6 weeks), strenuous exercise shouldn't impact it. However, sleep loss can affect your milk supply.

Breastfeeding may reduce your risks of diabetes, high blood pressure and heart disease in later life. It may cut your breast-cancer risk by nearly 60%! If there's a history of breast cancer in your family, breastfeeding may help protect you against developing breast cancer.

Caffeine may affect baby. Drinking one to two cups of coffee a day should be OK, but if you notice baby becoming agitated, cut down your intake. Be careful with alcohol consumption. Drinking beer will *not* increase your milk supply. If you have an alcoholic drink, drink it immediately after breastfeeding and only have one. Wine and beer have a lower percentage of alcohol than hard liquor and pass from your body in about 3 hours. Studies show it can take up to 13 hours for hard liquor to leave the body.

Disadvantages of Breastfeeding
Let's be honest—there are disadvantages to breastfeeding. Breastfeeding ties you completely to baby. Breast milk empties rapidly from baby's stomach, so most newborns need to feed every couple of hours. You may spend more time feeding baby than you anticipated. Pay careful attention to your diet. Most substances you eat or drink (or take orally, such as medicine) can pass to baby in your breast milk.

• •
Breastfeeding won't make your breasts sag.
• •

Problems You May Have during Breastfeeding
A common breastfeeding problem is *breast engorgement*. Breasts become swollen, tender and filled with breast milk. The best cure is to drain the breasts, as you do when breastfeeding. Some women take a hot shower and empty their breasts in the warm water. Ice packs may also help.

To help prevent the problem, feed baby from both breasts each time you feed. When you're away from baby, express some breast milk to keep milk flowing and breast ducts open. You'll also feel more comfortable.

Over-the-counter pain relievers are often helpful. You might need to use stronger medications, such as acetaminophen with codeine, if pain is more severe. Call your healthcare provider; he or she will decide on treatment.

It is possible to get a *breast infection*; it can cause red, swollen breasts and pain. You may notice red streaks on the breast; you may also feel as though you have the flu. If you think you have an infection, call your healthcare provider. He or she can devise a treatment plan and/or prescribe medication for you.

Most nursing mothers have *sore nipples* at some point, particularly when they begin breastfeeding. To lessen soreness, keep your breasts dry and clean. Don't air dry them; it encourages scab formation and can take longer for a sore breast to heal. Moist healing is best, such as applying lanolin. Use it after every feeding. Or express a little breast milk after breastfeeding, and rub it over your nipples. Research shows it contains antibiotic qualities that can help prevent and/or heal sore, cracked nipples.

Good news! Before too long—a few days to a few weeks—your breasts will become accustomed to breastfeeding, and problems will lessen.

. . . .

For a more complete discussion of breast-feeding baby, read our books Your Baby's First Year Week by Week *and* Your Pregnancy Quick Guide to Feeding Your Baby.

. . . .

Your Nutrition If You Breastfeed

Your nutrition is important in making breast milk. You will probably be advised to eat about 500 extra calories each day to help maintain good health. They should be nutritious, like the ones you ate during pregnancy.

Choose 9 servings from the bread/cereal/pasta/rice group and 3 servings from the dairy group. Fruit servings should number 4, and vegetable servings should number 5. The amount of protein in your diet should be 8 ounces a day during breastfeeding. Be careful with fats, oils and sugars; limit intake to 4 teaspoons.

Some foods can pass into breast milk and cause baby stomach distress. Avoid chocolate, foods that produce gas in you, highly spiced foods and any other foods you have problems with.

Continue to drink lots of fluids. Keeping hydrated can help increase energy levels and milk production. Drink at least 2 quarts of fluid every day. You'll need more fluid in hot weather. Avoid caffeine-containing foods and drinks; they can act as diuretics.

Ask about the kind of vitamin supplement you should take. Some mothers take a prenatal vitamin as long as they breastfeed. Some new moms take lactation supplements that contain higher doses of some vitamins and minerals than prenatal vitamins and lower doses of iron. Breastfeeding depletes your supply of choline; you need 550mg a day to replace it.

. . . .

If you nurse your baby for at least 3 months, you may have a smaller waistline for many years to come.

. . . .

Breastfeed with Confidence— Tips to Get Started

You may have some problems when you begin breastfeeding, so don't get discouraged. It takes time to discover what works for you and baby. Although breastfeeding is a natural way to feed baby, it takes time and practice to get the hang of it.

Feed baby on demand—this could be as many as 8 to 10 times a day or more! A baby usually cuts back to eating 4 to 6 times a day by 4 months. A breastfed baby will take in only as much breast milk as he needs, so your milk production usually adjusts to his needs.

Hold baby across your chest, or lie in bed so he can easily reach your breast. His tummy should touch you; tuck his lower arm between your arm and your side. Help him latch onto your breast. Brush your nipple across his lips. When he opens his mouth, place your nipple and as much of the areola as possible in his mouth. You should feel him pull the breast while sucking, but it shouldn't hurt.

Nurse baby 5 to 10 minutes on each breast; he gets most of his milk at the beginning of the feeding. Don't rush him—it can take as long as 30 minutes to finish. Baby may not need burping. As you begin, burp between feedings at each breast and when baby finishes. If he doesn't burp, he may not need to.

Breastfeeding More than One Baby
Feeding more than one baby can be a challenge. Breastfeeding for one or two feedings a day gives them the protection from infection your breast milk provides. Research has shown even the smallest dose of breast milk gives baby an advantage over babies only fed formula.

If babies are early and you can't nurse them, begin pumping! Pump from day one, and store your breast milk for the time babies are able to receive it. In addition, pumping tells the body to produce breast milk—pump and the milk will come. It just takes some time.

You may find your babies do well with breast and bottlefeeding. You can bottlefeed expressed breast milk. Supplementing with formula allows your partner and others to help you feed the babies.

Medications You May Take while Breastfeeding
Be careful with any medicine you take if you breastfeed, even in the hospital. Take a medication only when you need it, and take it only as prescribed. Ask for the smallest dose possible. Ask about possible effects on baby so you can be alert for them. Consider taking medication immediately after nursing to have less of an effect on baby.

If a medicine could have serious effects on your baby, you may decide to bottlefeed while you take the medication. Maintain your milk supply by pumping (then throwing away) expressed milk.

There are many safe antibiotics to take if you breastfeed. Talk to your healthcare provider if you have concerns.

Is Baby Getting Enough Milk?
You may be concerned about how much breast milk baby gets at a feeding. There are clues to look for. Watch his jaws and ears while he eats—is he actively sucking? At the end of a feeding, does he fall asleep or settle down easily? Can he go 1½ hours between feedings? You'll know your baby is getting enough to eat if he nurses every 2 to 3 hours or 8 to 12 times in 24 hours, has 6 to 8 wet diapers and/or 2 to 5 bowel movements a day, gains 4 to 7 ounces a week or at least 1 pound a month and appears healthy, has good muscle tone and is alert and active.

If your breasts show little or no change during pregnancy, there's no engorgement after birth or no breast milk by the fifth day, you may have a problem. If you can't hear baby gulping while he feeds or he loses more than 10% of his birth weight, it's cause for concern. If baby never seems satisfied, discuss it with your pediatrician.

Bottlefeeding Your Baby

Bottlefeeding is the other way to feed baby. Your baby will receive good nutrition if you bottlefeed her iron-fortified formula. And a baby can still get all the love, attention and nutrition she needs with bottlefeeding.

Choosing to Bottlefeed

Some women try to breastfeed, but it doesn't work out. Sometimes a woman can't breastfeed because she's very underweight or has a medical condition and breastfeeding isn't possible. Some babies have problems breastfeeding or can't breastfeed due to a physical problem. Lactose intolerance can also cause breastfeeding problems.

There may be many reasons you may choose to bottlefeed. A woman may choose not to breastfeed because of other demands on her time. You don't have to be concerned about feeding baby in front of other people. It may be easier to bottlefeed if you plan to return to work soon after baby's birth.

Some women enjoy the freedom bottlefeeding provides. It can make it easier for someone else to help care for baby. When you bottlefeed, dad can feed baby, and mom can get a bit of rest. You can determine exactly how much formula your baby takes at each feeding. Bottlefeeding is easy to learn; it never hurts if done incorrectly. Bottlefed babies may go longer between feedings because formula is usually digested more slowly than breast milk.

If you feed iron-fortified formula, baby won't need iron supplements. If you use fluoridated tap water to mix formula, you may not have to give baby fluoride supplements.

Bonding with Baby

Some parents fear bottlefeeding won't encourage closeness with their child. They fear bonding won't happen. It's not true that a woman must breastfeed her baby to bond with her. Skin-to-skin contact while bottlefeeding helps bring mom (or anyone else feeding baby) and baby closer.

Your Nutrition If You Bottlefeed

Even if you bottlefeed, it's important to follow a nutritious eating plan, such as the one you followed during pregnancy. Continue to eat foods high in complex carbohydrates, such as grain products, fruits and vegetables. Lean meats, chicken and fish are good sources of protein. For your dairy products, choose the low-fat or skim types.

. . . .

It takes about 10 to 15 days for your milk production to decline and stop if you don't breastfeed. The greatest discomfort is usually experienced between the third and fifth day after delivery. To help ease soreness, wear a sports bra day and night, take acetaminophen or ibuprofen, and use cold packs.

. . . .

You need fewer calories than you would if you were breastfeeding. But don't drastically cut your calories in the hopes of losing weight quickly. You still need to maintain good energy levels.

Here is a list of the types and quantities of foods you should try to eat each day. Choose 6 servings from the bread/cereal/pasta/rice group and 3 servings of fruit. Eat 3 servings of vegetables. From the dairy group, choose 2 servings. Eat about 6 ounces of protein each day. We still advise caution with fats, oils and sugars; limit intake to 3 teaspoons. And keep up your fluid intake. You can also use the pregnancy nutrition plan as a reference; see Week 6.

Formulas to Consider

Commercial formula first became available in the 1930s. Today, we have many types and brands of formula available to feed baby. Ask your pediatrician about the type of formula you should feed your baby.

When choosing formula, there isn't much difference among the brands of regular formula available. Most babies do well on milk-based formula, which comes from cow's milk and is modified to make it more like human breast milk. It's easier to digest than regular cow's milk. Most formulas are iron fortified; a baby needs iron for normal growth.

Formulas are packaged in powder form, concentrated liquid and ready-to-feed—the end product is the same. Powdered formula is the least expensive. When choosing formula, choose the powdered type in cans. Cans containing liquid formula often are lined with plastic containing BPA. To avoid BPA exposure, many companies sell products in glass or BPA-free containers.

All formulas sold in the United States must meet the same minimum standards set by the FDA, so they are all nutritionally complete. Many formulas on the market include two nutrients found in breast milk—DHA and ARA. DHA (docosahexaenoic acid) contributes to baby's eye development. ARA (arachidonic acid) is important in baby's brain development.

The American Academy of Pediatrics recommends baby be fed iron-fortified formula for the first year of her life. Feeding for this length of time helps maintain adequate iron intake.

If you make formula from tap water, use cold water. Many pipes contain lead; heated tap water releases lead from pipes. If you want to warm up the formula, use hot water on the outside of the bottle.

Bottlefeeding is not cheap—you'll spend $1500 to $2000 to feed your baby formula for the first year.

Feeding Equipment to Use

Don't buy plastic bottles or containers with the number 7 on the label or bottom to avoid exposing baby to BPA. Use a slanted bottle; this design keeps the nipple full so baby takes in less air. And a slanted bottle also helps ensure baby is sitting up to drink, so milk doesn't pool in the eustachian tube, leading to ear infections.

A wide, round, soft flexible nipple helps baby latch on, similar to nursing. Another type of nipple allows formula or pumped breast milk to be released at the same rate as breast milk flows during nursing. A twist adjusts the nipple flow to slow, medium or fast. You can find the flow that works best for your baby. The nipple fits on most bottles. Check local stores if you're interested.

Bottlefeeding Pointers

Bottlefed babies take from 2 to 5 ounces of formula at a feeding. They feed about every 3 to 4 hours for the first month (6 to 8 times a day). If baby fusses when her bottle is empty, it's OK to give her a little more. When baby is older, the number of feedings decreases, but the amount of formula you feed at each feeding increases.

If baby pulls away from the bottle, it's usually a sign she's finished. However, you may want to try burping her before ending the feeding.

You know baby's getting enough formula if she has 6 to 8 wet diapers a day. She may also have 1 or 2 bowel movements. Stools of a bottlefed baby are more solid and greener in color than a breastfed baby's.

If your baby poops after a feeding, it's caused by the *gastrocolic reflex*. This reflex causes squeezing of the intestines when the stomach is stretched, as with feeding. It's very pronounced in newborns and usually decreases after 2 or 3 months of age.

After baby drinks 2 ounces, burp her. Burp after every feeding to help her get rid of excess air. If baby doesn't want a feeding, don't force it. Try again in a few hours. But if she refuses two feedings in a row, contact your pediatrician. Baby may be sick.

Glossary

Abdominal measurement— Measurement at prenatal visits of baby's growth inside the uterus. Made from pubic symphysis to top of fundus; also called *fundal measurement.*

Abnormal placentation—Placenta that grows into or through uterine wall; possible complication of multiple Cesarean deliveries.

Abruptio placenta—See *placental abruption.*

Acquired immunodeficiency syndrome (AIDS)—Illness that affects the body's ability to respond to infection; caused by the human immune deficiency virus (HIV).

Active labor—Woman's cervix is dilated between 4 and 8cm. Contractions are usually 3 to 5 minutes apart.

Advance-practice nurse—Nurse who has received postgraduate education in a medical specialty; must be nationally certified, such as in women's health. Licensed through a state nursing board. Also called a *nurse practitioner (NP).*

Aerobic exercise—Exercise that increases heart rate and causes person to consume oxygen.

Afterbirth—Placenta and membranes expelled after baby is delivered. See *placenta.*

Alpha-fetoprotein (AFP)—Substance produced by unborn baby inside the uterus. Large amounts of AFP are found in amniotic fluid. Part of triple- or quad-screen test.

Alveolar gland—Grapelike cluster of cells in the breast where milk is produced.

Amino acids—Substances that act as building blocks in developing baby.

Amniocentesis—Procedure in which amniotic fluid is removed from amniotic sac for testing for some genetic defects and for fetal lung maturity.

Amniotic fluid—Fluid surrounding baby inside the amniotic sac.

Amniotic sac—Membrane that surrounds the baby inside the uterus; contains baby, placenta and amniotic fluid. Also called *amnion.*

Anatomy scan—Ultrasound that measures baby's length and head size, and checks for organ development. Also called a *level-2 ultrasound.*

Anemia—Condition in which the number of red blood cells is less than normal.

Anencephaly—Defective development of baby's brain, combined with absence of bones normally surrounding the brain.

Aneuploidy—Abnormal number of chromosomes.

Angioma—Tumor or swelling composed of lymph and blood vessels; usually benign.

Anovulatory—Woman doesn't ovulate.

Anti-inflammatory medications—Drugs to relieve pain and/or inflammation.

Apgar scores—Measurement of baby's response to birth and life on its own. Taken 1 minute and 5 minutes after birth.

Areola—Colored ring surrounding the nipple of the breast.

Arrhythmia—Irregular or missed heartbeat.

Aspiration—Swallowing or sucking foreign body or fluid into an airway.

Asthma—Disease marked by recurrent attacks of shortness of breath and difficulty breathing.

Atonic uterus—Uterus that lacks tone.

Augmented labor—When progress is not being made during labor, medication is given.

Autoantibodies—Antibodies that attack parts of the body or tissues.

Baby blues—Mild depression in a woman after delivery.

Back labor—Labor pain felt in the lower back.

Bilirubin—Product formed in the liver when red blood cells are destroyed.

Biophysical profile (BPP)—Method of evaluating baby before birth.

Biopsy—Removal of a small piece of tissue for microscopic study.

Birthing center—Facility specializing in delivering babies; may be part of hospital or a free-standing unit.

Bishop score—Method used to predict success of inducing labor.

Blood pressure—Push of blood against artery walls; blood-pressure changes may indicate problems.

Blood-sugar tests—See *glucose-tolerance test.*

Blood typing—Test to determine whether a woman's blood type is A, B, AB or O.

Bloody show—Small amount of vaginal bleeding late in pregnancy; often precedes labor.

Board certification (of physician)—Doctor has received additional training and testing in a particular specialty.

Braxton-Hicks contractions—Irregular, painless tightening of the uterus during pregnancy.

Breech presentation—Buttocks or legs come into the birth canal before the head.

Carrier—Person with recessive disease-causing gene, which can be passed to his or her children.

Cataract, congenital—Cloudiness of the eye lens; present at birth.

Cell antibodies—See *autoantibodies.*

Cell-free DNA (cfDNA)–Screening test performed on fetal placental DNA found in mother-to-be's blood; performed after 10 weeks of pregnancy to detect chromosomal abnormalities 21, 18 and 13. Placental DNA is the same as fetal DNA.

Cephalo-pelvic disproportion—Baby is too big to fit through the birth canal.

Certified nurse-midwife (CNM)—Registered nurse who has received additional training for delivering babies and providing prenatal and postpartum care to women.

Cervical cultures—Test for STDs.

Cervix—Opening of the uterus.

Cesarean section or delivery—Delivery of baby through an abdominal incision rather than through the vagina. Also called *C-section.*

Chadwick's sign—Dark-blue or purple discoloration of vagina and cervix during pregnancy.

Chemotherapy—Treatment of a disease with chemical substances or medication.

Chlamydia—Sexually transmitted venereal infection.

Chloasma—Colored patches of irregular shape and size on the face or other body parts. Also called *mask of pregnancy.*

Chorion—Outermost fetal membrane around amniotic sac.

Chorionic villus sampling (CVS)— Diagnostic test done to determine some pregnancy problems. Tissue is taken from the placenta through the abdomen or cervix.

Chromosomal abnormality—Abnormal number or abnormal makeup of chromosomes.

Chromosomes—Structures within cells that carry genetic information via DNA. Humans have 22 pairs of chromosomes and 2 sex chromosomes. One chromosome of each pair is inherited from the mother; the other is inherited from the father.

Cleft lip—Birth defect of the lip.

Cleft palate—Birth defect in part of the roof of the mouth.

Clubfoot—Birth defect in which a foot is misshaped and twisted.

Colostrum—Thin yellow fluid; first milk to come from the breast.

Complete blood count (CBC)—Blood test to check cellular elements of the blood and iron stores, and to check for infections.

Condyloma acuminatum—Sexually transmitted skin tags or warts; caused by human papilloma virus (HPV). Also called *venereal warts.*

Congenital deafness screening—Blood test to help identify problem in a baby if a couple has a family history of inherited deafness.

Congenital problem—Problem present at birth.

Conjoined twins—Twins connected at a point on their bodies; may share vital organs. Previously called *Siamese twins.*

Constipation—Infrequent or incomplete bowel movements.

Contraction stress test (CST)—Test to evaluate baby's well-being during pregnancy.

Contractions—Uterus squeezes or tightens to push baby out during birth.

Crown-to-rump length—Measurement from top of baby's head (crown) to baby's buttocks (rump).

Cystic fibrosis—Inherited disorder that causes breathing and digestion problems.

Cystitis—Bladder inflammation.

Cytomegalovirus (CMV) infection— Common virus passed from mom to baby during pregnancy.

Cytotoxic—Substance that can terminate a pregnancy.

D&C (dilatation and curettage)— Surgical procedure in which the cervix is dilated and the lining of the uterus scraped.

Developmental delay—Condition in which child's development is slower than normal.

Diagnostic test—Test done to determine if a problem is present; often done after a screening test indicates a problem may be present. See *screening test.*

Diastasis recti—Separation of abdominal muscles.

Diethylstilbestrol (DES)—Synthetic estrogen; used in the past to try to prevent miscarriage.

Dilatation—Amount, in centimeters, cervix has opened before birth. When woman is fully dilated, she is at 10cm.

Dizygotic twins—Twins born from two different eggs. Also called *fraternal twins.*

Dominant gene—Trait will be evident even if only one gene is present (from one parent); an example is dimples.

Doppler—Device that amplifies a fetal heartbeat so it can be heard.

Down syndrome—Chromosomal disorder in which baby has three copies of chromosome 21; results in mental retardation, distinct physical traits and other problems.

Due date—Date baby is expected to be born. Most babies are born near this date, but only 1 of 20 are born on the actual date.

Dysuria—Difficulty or pain when urinating.

Early labor—Woman experiences regular contractions for longer than 2 hours. Cervix usually dilates to 3 or 4cm.

Eclampsia—Convulsions and coma in a woman with pre-eclampsia. Not related to epilepsy. See *pre-eclampsia*.

Ectodermal germ layer—Layer in developing baby that produces skin, teeth and glands of the mouth, nervous system and pituitary gland.

Ectopic pregnancy—Pregnancy that occurs outside the uterus, most often in the Fallopian tube. Also called *tubal pregnancy*.

ECV (external cephalic version)—Procedure in which doctor manually attempts to move a baby in the breech presentation into normal head-down birth presentation.

EDC (estimated date of confinement)—Estimated due date for delivery of a baby.

Effacement—Thinning of the cervix.

Electroencephalogram—Recording of electrical activity in brain.

Embryo—Organism in early stages of development; from conception to 10 weeks.

Embryonic period—First 10 weeks of gestation.

Endodermal germ layer—Area of tissue that produces digestive tract, respiratory organs, vagina, bladder and urethra in a baby.

Endometrial cycle—Regular development of mucous membranes that line inside of uterus. Begins with preparation for acceptance of pregnancy and ends with shedding of the lining during menstrual period.

Endometrium—Mucous membrane that lines inside of uterine wall.

Enema—Fluid injected into the rectum for the purpose of clearing out the bowel.

Engorgement—Filled with fluid; usually refers to breast filled with milk.

Enzyme—Protein that improves or causes chemical changes in other substances.

Epidural block—Anesthesia medication is injected around the spinal cord during labor or other types of surgery.

Episiotomy—Surgical incision used during delivery to avoid tearing the vaginal opening and rectum.

Essential nutrient—Nutrient that can't be made by the body; must be provided in the diet.

Expressing breast milk—Manually forcing milk out of the breast.

Face presentation—Baby comes into the birth canal face first.

Fallopian tube—Tube that leads from the uterine cavity to the area of the ovary. Also called *uterine tube*.

False labor—Tightening of uterus without dilatation of the cervix.

Fasting blood sugar—Blood test to evaluate the amount of sugar in blood following a period of fasting.

Fertilization—Joining of the sperm and egg.

Fertilization age—Dating a pregnancy from the time of fertilization; 2 weeks shorter than gestational age. Also see *gestational age*.

Fetal anomaly—Birth defect.

Fetal fibronectin (fFN)—Test done to evaluate premature labor.

Fetal goiter—Enlargement of baby's thyroid gland.

Fetal monitor—Device used before or during labor to record fetal heartbeat.

Fetal period—Time period from after the first 10 weeks of gestation until birth.

Fetal stress—Problems with baby that occur before birth or during labor; often requires immediate delivery.

Fetoscopy—Test that enables doctor to look through a fiberoptic scope to detect problems in a fetus.

Fetus—Refers to an unborn baby after 10 weeks of gestation until birth.

Fibrin—Elastic protein important in blood coagulation.

Fistula—Abnormal opening from one part of the body to another, such as from the vagina to the rectum.

Forceps—Instrument sometimes used to deliver a baby.

Fortification—Addition of one or more essential nutrients to a food.

Frank breech—Baby presenting buttocks first; legs and knees are straight.

Fraternal twins—See *dizygotic twins*.

Fundus—Top part of the uterus; often measured during pregnancy.

Genes—Basic units of heredity; each gene carries specific information and is passed from parent to child.

Genetic counseling—Consultation between a couple and specialists about the possibility of genetic problems in a pregnancy.

Genetic screening—Performing one or more genetic tests.

Genetic tests—Various screening and diagnostic tests done to determine whether a couple may have a child with a genetic defect.

Genital herpes simplex—Herpes simplex infection involving the genital area.

Genitourinary problems—Problems involving genital organs and bladder or kidneys.

Germ layers—Layers or areas of tissue important in fetal development.

Gestational age—Dating pregnancy from the first day of the last menstrual period; 2 weeks longer than fertilization age. Also see *fertilization age*.

Gestational diabetes—Occurrence of diabetes only during pregnancy.

Gestational trophoblastic disease (GTN)—Abnormal pregnancy in which embryo does not develop. Also called *molar pregnancy* or *hydatidiform mole*.

Globulin—Family of proteins from plasma or serum of blood.

Glucose-tolerance test (GTT)—Blood test done to evaluate body's response to sugar.

Glucosuria—Glucose (sugar) in urine.

Gonorrhea—Contagious venereal infection, transmitted primarily by intercourse.

Grand mal seizure—Loss of body control and functions during major seizure.

Group-B streptococcal (GBS) infection—Serious infection occurring in mother's vagina, throat or rectum.

Group-B streptococcus (GBS) test—Samples may be taken from woman's vagina, perineum and rectum to check for GBS. Urine tests may also be done.

Habitual miscarriage—Occurrence of three or more miscarriages.

Health Information Portability and Accountability Act (HIPAA)—Legislation creating national standards protecting personal health information.

Heartburn—Discomfort or pain that occurs in the chest, often after eating.

Height of fundus—Top of the uterus.

Hematocrit—Determines proportion of blood cells to plasma.

Hemoglobin—Pigment in red blood cells that carries oxygen to body tissues.

Hemolytic disease—Destruction of red blood cells. See *anemia*.

Hemopoietic system—System that controls the formation of blood cells.

Hemorrhoids—Dilated blood vessels, most often found in rectum or rectal canal.

Heparin—Medication used to prevent blood clotting and to treat or to prevent thrombosis.

Hepatitis-B antibodies test—Test to determine if a pregnant woman has hepatitis B.

High-risk pregnancy—Pregnancy with complications that require special medical attention, often from a specialist. Also see *perinatologist*.

Homan's sign—Pain caused by flexing toes toward knees when a person has a blood clot in the lower leg.

Home uterine monitoring—Pregnant woman's contractions are recorded at home, then transmitted to healthcare provider.

Human chorionic gonadotropin (HCG)—Hormone produced in early pregnancy; measured in a pregnancy test.

Human placental lactogen—Hormone of pregnancy produced by the placenta, found in the bloodstream.

Hyaline membrane disease—Respiratory disease of a newborn.

Hydatidiform mole—See *gestational trophoblastic disease*.

Hydramnios—Increased amount of amniotic fluid.

Hydrocephalus—Excessive accumulation of fluid around baby's brain. Also called *water on the brain*.

Hyperbilirubinemia—Extremely high level of bilirubin in the blood.

Hyperemesis gravidarum—Severe nausea, dehydration and vomiting during pregnancy.

Hyperglycemia—Increased blood sugar.

Hypertension, pregnancy-induced (PIH)—High blood pressure that occurs during pregnancy.

Hyperthyroidism—Higher-than-normal levels of thyroid hormone in the bloodstream.

Hypoplasia—Defective or incomplete development or formation of tissue.

Hypotension—Low blood pressure.

Hypothyroidism—Low or inadequate levels of thyroid hormone in the bloodstream.

Identical twins—See *monozygotic twins*.

Imaging tests—Tests that look inside body; includes X-rays, CT scans (or CAT scans) and magnetic resonance imaging (MRI).

Immune globulin preparation—Substance used to protect against infection with certain diseases, such as hepatitis or measles.

In utero—Within the uterus.

Incompetent cervix—Cervix dilates painlessly, without contractions.

Incomplete miscarriage—Miscarriage in which part, but not all, of uterine contents are expelled.

Inducing labor—Medication is used to start labor.

Inevitable miscarriage—Pregnancy complicated with bleeding and cramping. Usually results in miscarriage.

Infertility—Inability or decreased ability to get pregnant.

Insulin—Hormone made by the pancreas; promotes use of sugar and glucose.

Intrauterine-growth restriction (IUGR)—Inadequate fetal growth during pregnancy.

In-vitro fertilization—Process in which eggs are fertilized outside the body; fertilized egg is placed inside the uterus in attempt to result in pregnancy.

Iron-deficiency anemia—Anemia produced by a lack of iron in the diet; often seen in pregnancy.

Isoimmunization—Development of a specific antibody directed at the red blood cells of another individual, such as baby inside the uterus.

Jaundice—Yellow staining of skin, eyes and body tissues. Caused by excessive amounts of bilirubin.

Ketones—Breakdown product of metabolism found in blood, particularly from starvation or uncontrolled diabetes.

Kick count—Record of how often a pregnant woman feels her baby move.

Kidney stone—Small mass or lesion found in the kidney or urinary tract.

Labor—Process of expelling fetus from the uterus.

Laparoscopy—Less-invasive surgical procedure performed for tubal ligation, diagnosis of pelvic pain or diagnosis of ectopic pregnancy.

Leukorrhea—Vaginal discharge characterized by white or yellowish color.

Lightening—Change in the shape of a pregnant uterus a few weeks before labor. Often described as the baby "dropping."

Linea nigra—Darker-than-normal line that runs down the abdomen from bellybutton to pubic area.

Lochia—Vaginal discharge that occurs after delivery of the baby and placenta.

Macrosomia—Abnormally large fetus.

Malignant GTN—Cancerous change of gestational trophoblastic disease. See *gestational trophoblastic disease.*

Mammogram—X-ray study of breasts.

Mask of pregnancy—Increased pigment over the area of face under each eye.

Maternal serum screen—Blood test done between 15 and 20 weeks of pregnancy on mother-to-be to screen for Down syndrome, trisomy 18 and neural-tube defects.

McDonald cerclage—Surgical procedure performed on an incompetent cervix; drawstring-type suture holds cervical opening closed during pregnancy.

Meconium—First intestinal discharge of a newborn; green or yellow in color.

Melanoma—Cancerous pigmented mole or tumor.

Meningomyelocele—Birth defect in which membranes and spinal cord protrude through an opening in the vertebral column.

Menstrual age—See *gestational age.*

Menstruation—Regular or periodic discharge of endometrial lining and blood from the uterus.

Mesodermal germ layer—Embryonic tissue that forms connective tissue, muscles, kidneys, ureters and other organs.

Microcephaly—Abnormally small head development.

Microphthalmia—Abnormally small eyeballs.

Miscarriage—Premature end of pregnancy; usually defined as before 20 weeks of pregnancy.

Missed miscarriage—Failed pregnancy without bleeding or cramping; often diagnosed by ultrasound weeks or months after a pregnancy fails.

Mittelschmerz—Pain that coincides with release of an egg from the ovary.

Molar pregnancy—See *gestational trophoblastic disease.*

Monilial vulvovaginitis—Yeast infection affecting the vagina and vulva.

Monozygotic twins—Twins conceived from one egg. Often called *identical twins.*

Morning sickness—Nausea and vomiting usually occurring during the first trimester of pregnancy. Also see *hyperemesis gravidarum.*

Morula—Cells resulting from early division of a fertilized egg at the beginning of pregnancy.

Mucus plug—Secretions in the cervix often released just before labor.

Multiple-markers test—See *quad-screen test* and *triple-screen test.*

Mutations—Change in the character of a gene; passed from one cell division to another.

Natural childbirth—Labor and delivery in which a woman has as few interventions as possible.

Neural-tube defects—Abnormalities in the development of the spinal cord and brain in a fetus.

Nonstress test (NST)—Test that records fetal movement felt by a woman or observed by a healthcare provider, along with changes in fetal heart rate.

NSAIDs—Nonsteroidal anti-inflammatory drugs, such as ibuprofen, Motrin, Aleve and Advil.

Nuchal translucency screening—Detailed ultrasound to measure space behind baby's neck; can help measure a woman's probability of having baby with Down syndrome.

Nurse-midwife—Registered nurse who has received extra training in the care of pregnant women and delivery of babies.

Obstetrician—Medical doctor or osteopathic physician who specializes in the care of pregnant women and delivery of babies.

Oligohydramnios—Lack or deficiency of amniotic fluid.

Omphalocele—Birth defect resulting in outpouching of the bellybutton containing internal organs.

Opioids—Synthetic compounds with effects similar to those of opium.

Organogenesis—Development of organ systems in an embryo.

Ossification—Bone formation.

Ovarian cycle—Regular production of hormones from the ovary in response to hormonal messages from the brain.

Ovarian hyperstimulation syndrome—Complication of infertility treatment involving ovarian enlargement and abdominal swelling, with changes in blood-fluid volumes.

Ovarian torsion—Twisting or rotation of the ovary.

Ovulation—Cyclic release of the egg from the ovary.

Ovulatory age—See *fertilization age.*

Oxytocin—Medicine that causes uterine contractions; used to induce or to help along labor. Brand name is *Pitocin.*

Palmar erythema—Redness of palms of the hands.

Pap smear—Test to evaluate presence of premalignant or cancerous conditions of the cervix.

Paracervical block—Local anesthesia to relieve pain of dilating cervix.

Pediatrician—Medical doctor or osteopathic physician who specializes in the care of babies and children.

Pelvic exam—Exam done inside pelvic area to assess various uterine conditions.

Percutaneous umbilical cord blood sampling (PUBS; cordocentesis)—Test done on fetus to diagnose Rh-incompatibility, blood disorders and infections.

Perinatologist—Physician who specializes in the care of high-risk pregnancies.

Perineum—Area between the rectum and vagina.

Phosphatidyl glycerol (PG)—Lipoprotein present when fetal lungs are mature.

Phospholipids—Fat-containing phosphorous; most important are lecithins and sphingomyelin, which are important in maturation of fetal lungs before birth.

Phototherapy—Treatment for jaundice in a newborn infant. Also see *jaundice.*

Physician assistant (PA)—Qualified healthcare professional who is licensed to practice medicine in association with a licensed doctor. Also called *physician associate.*

Physiologic anemia of pregnancy—Anemia during pregnancy caused by increase in the amount of fluid in blood compared to the number of cells in blood. Also see *anemia.*

Placenta—Organ inside the uterus attached to baby by the umbilical cord; essential for growth and development of an embryo and fetus. Also called *afterbirth.*

Placenta previa—Attachment of the placenta very close to, or covering, the cervix.

Placental abruption—Premature separation of the placenta from the uterus.

Pneumonitis—Inflammation of lungs.

Postmature baby—Baby born 2 weeks or more past its due date.

Postnatal—After baby's birth.

Postpartum—6-week period following baby's birth; refers to mother, not baby.

Postpartum blues—Mild depression after delivery.

Postpartum distress syndrome (PPDS)—Range of symptoms including baby blues, postpartum depression and postpartum psychosis.

Postpartum hemorrhage—Bleeding greater than 17 ounces (450ml) at the time of delivery.

Postterm pregnancy—Pregnancy of 42+ weeks gestation.

Pre-eclampsia—Group of important symptoms unique to pregnancy, including high blood pressure, edema, proteinuria and changes in reflexes.

Pregnancy diabetes—See *gestational diabetes.*

Premature birth or delivery—Birth before 37 weeks of pregnancy.

Premature infant—Infant who has immature lungs at the time of birth.

Premature rupture of membranes (PROM)—Rupture of fetal membranes (bag of waters) before onset of labor.

Prenatal care—Program of care for a pregnant woman before birth of baby.

Prepared childbirth—Situation in which woman has taken classes so she knows what will happen during labor and delivery.

Presentation—Describes which part of the baby comes into the birth canal first.

Preterm infant—Infant who is 32 weeks gestational age but has mature pulmonary or lung function at the time of birth.

Preterm premature rupture of membranes (PPROM)—Rupture of fetal membranes before 37 weeks of pregnancy.

Proteinuria—Protein in urine.

Pruritus gravidarum—Itching during pregnancy.

Pubic symphysis—Bony prominence in pelvic bone found in the middle of a woman's lower abdomen.

Pudendal block—Local anesthesia during labor.

Pulmonary embolism—Blood clot from another part of body that travels to the lungs.

Pyelonephritis—Serious kidney infection.

Quad-screen test—Measurement of four blood components—alpha-fetoprotein, human chorionic gonadotropin, unconjugated estriol and inhibin-A.

Quickening—Feeling baby move inside uterus.

Radiation therapy—Method of treating various cancers.

Radioactive scan—Diagnostic test in which radioactive material is injected into a particular part of the body then scanned to find the problem.

Recessive gene—Gene that shows its trait only if both parents had this gene (e.g., for cystic fibrosis).

Rh factor—Blood test to determine if a woman is Rh-negative.

Rh-negative—Absence of rhesus antigen in the blood.

Rh-sensitivity—See *isoimmunization*.

RhoGAM—Medication given to Rh-negative women during pregnancy and following delivery to prevent isoimmunization. Also see *isoimmunization*.

Ripening the cervix—Medicine is used to help the cervix soften, thin and dilate.

Round-ligament pain—Pain caused by stretching ligaments on the sides of the uterus.

Rubella titers—Blood test to check for immunity against rubella (German measles).

Rupture of membranes—Loss of fluid from the amniotic sac. Also called *breaking of waters* or *water breaking*.

Screening test—Test to determine if a problem may be present. If so, a diagnostic test may be done to determine if the problem actually is present. See *diagnostic test*.

Seizure—Sudden onset of a convulsion.

Sexually transmitted disease (STD)—Infection transmitted through sexual contact.

Sickle-cell disease—Anemia caused by abnormal red blood cells shaped like a sickle or cylinder.

Sickle-cell trait—Presence of the trait for sickle-cell anemia; not sickle-cell disease.

Sickle crisis—Painful episode caused by sickle-cell disease.

Silent labor—Painless dilatation of the cervix.

Skin tag—Flap or extra buildup of skin.

Sodium—Element found in many foods, particularly salt; may cause fluid retention and swelling.

Sonogram or sonography—See *ultrasound*.

Sperm motility—Spontaneous movement of sperm; ability of sperm to swim or move.

Spina bifida—Birth defect in which membranes of the spinal cord and the spinal cord itself protrude outside the body.

Spinal anesthesia—Anesthesia given in the spinal canal.

Spontaneous miscarriage—Loss of pregnancy during first 20 weeks of gestation.

Stasis—Decreased flow.

Station—Estimation of baby's descent into birth canal in preparation for birth.

Stillbirth—Death of a fetus before birth, usually defined as after 20 weeks gestation.

Stress test—Test in which mild uterine contractions are induced so fetal heart rate can be noted; same as contraction stress test.

Stretch marks—Stretched areas of skin; often found on abdomen, breasts, buttocks and legs.

Superovulation—Ovulation of a larger-than-normal number of eggs, usually from administration of fertility drugs.

Supplementation—Nutrients added to a normal diet.

Tay-Sachs disease—Inherited disease of the central nervous system.

Teratology—Study of abnormal fetal development.

Term—Baby is considered "term" when born after 38 weeks. Also called *full term*.

Thrombophilia—Disorder that causes blood to clot when and where it shouldn't.

Torsion—Twisting or rotation.

Trait—Refers to a characteristic of a person, such as blue eyes.

Transition—Phase after active labor during which the cervix fully dilates.

Trimester—Division of pregnancy into three equal periods of about 13 weeks each.

Triple-screen test—Measurement of three blood components—alpha-fetoprotein, human chorionic gonadotropin and unconjugated estriol.

Ultrasound—Noninvasive test that shows picture of a fetus inside womb.

Umbilical cord—Cord that connects placenta to developing baby. Brings oxygenated blood and nutrients from mother through placenta to baby, and removes waste products and carbon dioxide from baby.

Urinalysis and urine cultures—Tests for infections and to determine levels of sugar and protein in urine.

Uterine rupture—Splitting open of the uterus during labor or delivery; occurs most often in the area of a surgical scar, such as previous Cesarean delivery or uterine surgery.

Uterus—Organ the embryo/fetus grows in. Also called a *womb*.

Vacuum extractor—Device used to help deliver a baby.

Vagina—Birth canal.

Varicose veins—Dilated or enlarged blood vessels (veins).

Vasa previa—Condition in which blood vessels of the umbilical cord cross the interior opening of the cervix.

Vena cava—Major vein in the body that returns unoxygenated blood to the heart.

Venereal warts—See *condyloma acuminatum*.

Vernix—Fatty substance that covers fetal skin inside the uterus.

Vertex—Head first.

Villi—Projection from mucous membrane; important in exchange of nutrients from maternal blood to placenta and fetus.

Weight check—Measurement of mother's body weight done at every prenatal visit.

Womb—See *uterus*.

Yeast infection—See *monilial vulvovaginitis*.

Zygote—Cell that results from union of sperm and egg at fertilization.

Index

**When we use (B) following a page number,
it denotes the information can be found in a box on the designated page.**